FUNDAMENTALS OF

Obstetrics

and

Gynaecology

SIXTH EDITION

Derek Llewellyn-Jones

OBE, MD, MAO, FRCOG, FRACOG
Lately Professor of Obstetrics and Gynaecology
University of Sydney, New South Wales, Australia
Emeritus Obstetrician and Gynaecologist
St Margaret's Hospital, Sydney

Illustrations by Audrey Besterman

⋈ Mosby

London Baltimore Bogotá Boston Buenos Aires Caracas Carlsbad, CA Chicago Madrid Mexico City Milan Naples, FL
New York Philadelphia St. Louis Sydney Tokyo Toronto Wiesbaden

Copyright © 1994 D. Llewellyn-Jones

Figures 3.5, 3.6 and 3.10 are reproduced with permission from Buckley, C.H. and Fox, H., *Biopsy Pathology of the Endometrium*, Chapman and Hall, 1989, Figures 2.1, 2.8 and 2.15 respectively

Published in 1994 by Mosby, an imprint of Times Mirror International Publishers Limited

Reprinted 1995

1998 1997 1996

10 9 8 7 6 5 4 3 2

Printed by Grafos S.A. Arte sobre papel, Barcelona, Spain

ISBN 0 7234 2000 9

For full details of all Times Mirror International Publishers Limited titles, please write to Times Mirror International Publishers Limited, Lynton House, 7–12 Tavistock Square, London WC1H 9LB, England.

A CIP catalogue record for this book is available from the British Library.

Project Manager:	Penny Bourke
Developmental Editor:	Jennifer Prast
Cover Design:	Pete Wilder
Production:	Jane Tozer
Index:	Dr. Laurence Errington
Publisher:	Richard Furn

CONTENTS

Complications in elderly PRIMI >35 y.o.

Maternal

Pregnancy ind. HTN
Ess HTN.
Gestational diabetes.

Fetal

THE CONTENT OF OBSTETRICS AND GYNAECOLOGY

The expansion of medical knowledge over the past 20 years and its increasing complexity makes it difficult for medical students and interns to know what they need to know to be competent doctors and to pass the examinations set at the end of their assignments in various medical disciplines. This has led in the words of the General Medical Council to a situation in which 'it is distressing to see the progressive disenchantment [of many students] as they work their way through the course. Imagination and curiosity are soon dulled'. This opinion is echoed by the Dean of St. Bartholomew's Hospital Medical School who was horrified at the transformation of eager, bright school leavers into dull, demoralized doctors in the space of five years.

The question is: 'What has occurred to change the best and brightest into unhappy, disillusioned doctors, particularly in the intern year?'. In part, the change is due to the enormous collection of facts that students and interns appear to have to learn: in other words there is too much rote learning and too little encouragement of curiosity and of inquiry. In part it is because teachers in a discipline appear to believe that it is essential for students and interns to learn a great deal about that discipline and resent having to curtail the information they provide in the interests of the medical curriculum as a whole.

If teachers insist that students remember facts and gear their teaching sessions to encompass this, if teachers fail to inspire students to seek further, the situation will not change. If teachers 'put down' students in tutorials and fail to respect the patient's dignity during bedside teaching, the situation will not change.

Students are realists and if they know that they will be examined on matters they have memorized they will continue to rote learn facts and to forget most of the material as soon as they have passed the examinations. During the pre-registration year interns learn that to progress it is best to adopt the attitudes of their consultants towards patients, particularly when interns' working conditions often are appalling and not conducive to continued learning.

The difficulty in each of the medical disciplines is to determine what is the essential knowledge medical students and interns should acquire (and, equally importantly, what they do not need to know), and how to encourage them to retain their curiosity as well as to memorize facts.

This leads to the further question: 'Should women's health issues, that is, obstetrics and gynaecology (or, as I prefer, 'gyniatry') be a core subject or an optional subject?'. The General Medical Council considers that understanding of the human reproductive cycle and the understanding of human relationships are essential aspects of the undergraduate medical curriculum, which suggests that women's health issues should remain a core subject.

Fundamentals of Obstetrics and Gynaecology was first published over 25 years ago in two volumes. The contraction of the assignment in obstetrics and gynaecology in the undergraduate curriculum to 10 weeks or less means that the size of a text book should also be reduced. It is for this reason that the books, which have sold over 100,000 copies, have been completely rewritten as a single volume. In undertaking this task I have discussed the content with some of my colleagues and although we have not always agreed, there has been sufficient consensus for the book to be written. I am particularly grateful to Professor Malcolm Coppleson for reviewing Chapter 40; to Professor Ian Fraser for reviewing Chapter 30; to Professor David Henderson-Smart for reviewing the sections and chapters relating to the newborn infant; and to Dr Bernard Haylen for reviewing Chapter 41. However, the published opinions are mine and are based on the literature and on the discussions. If teachers do not agree with some of them I hope that students will be encouraged to find out why there is disagreement and to evaluate the information critically and creatively.

In the evolution of new medical curricula I believe that there will be a mix of teacher-centred information transfer and self-directed problem-based learning. I hope that this textbook will serve as a source book for both approaches, supplemented by literature searches and evaluation of chosen topics. This is the reason why I have limited the bibliography mainly to reference books.

Readers will note that some of the material may seem to be irrelevant for many students. Does a student need to know, for example, the steps required to perform a forceps delivery or a caesarean section?. These topics have been included, largely as illustrations with captions, as the book is used in several developing countries where this information has a practical value.

I have tried to describe the effect of a chosen procedure on the woman (and in many cases on her partner) as it appears that some teachers are brilliant diagnosticians and skilled surgeons, but are poor communicators. Modern medicine increasingly involves the patient in the treatment process, and the patient's fears, anxieties and psychosocial values need to be addressed.

It is my hope that *Fundamentals of Obstetrics and Gynaecology* will meet the needs of today's medical students and interns and will encourage self-learning skills whilst providing essential information in a readable manner.

Derek Llewellyn-Jones
Sydney, 1994

GYNIATRIC HISTORY AND EXAMINATION

EXAMINING A WOMAN WHO PRESENTS WITH GYNAECOLOGICAL PROBLEMS

It is generally accepted that most gynaecological problems are medical or psychological, rather than surgical. For this reason it is crucial that a careful history of the woman's complaints is obtained.

HISTORY

Doctors must be aware of the reluctance of many women to discuss gynaecological and sexual matters. The medical practitioner must be sensitive to this, tactful, communicative, courteous, gentle and unhurried. The history of the patient's complaints should be recorded sequentially.

The manner in which the woman answers questions may give a clue to the origin of the complaint. This is important as studies in Britain and Australia show that 10 per cent of women have psychiatric morbidity (measured by the Present State Examination). Other studies have noted a significant relationship between gynaecological symptoms, adverse life events and psychiatric morbidity. The doctor should exclude depression by inquiring about sadness, irritability, fatigue and so on.

The questions should seek information about the woman's:

- *Menstrual history.* Age at menarche; duration of the menstrual cycle; menstrual pain; and the duration and severity of menstruation. This may cause some confusion. For example, if the woman says that she bleeds for 5 days every 20 days, the doctor may believe that her periods are occurring too frequently. The doctor may need to explain that the menstrual cycle starts on day 1 of bleeding and includes the menstrual phase as well as the interval between menstrual bleeds. The woman in the example given in this designation, would bleed for 5 days every 25 days, which is normal. This designation is conveniently recorded as 5/25.
- *Obstetric history (if any).* The number of pregnancies and the outcome; that is, spontaneous miscarriages or induced abortions; children born and the year of the birth of each; complications occurring during pregnancy, labour or the puerperium.
- *Previous medical history* (family history, past illnesses and operations).
- *Psychological history.*
- *Sexual history.* This needs to obtained with great sensitivity, and should be left until late in the interview.
- *History of the main complaint.*

THE EXAMINATION

Unless the patient has been seen before, a general examination should be made, as the gynaecological complaint may only be a local manifestation of a general disorder. This examination, which can be performed quite quickly, should include inspection of the head and neck, palpation of the supraclavicular areas for enlarged lymph nodes, auscultation of the heart and determination of the pulse rate and blood pressure.

The gynaecological portion of the examination should include:
- A breast examination.
- An abdominal examination.
- An inspection of the external genitalia.
- A pelvic examination, by speculum and then digitally as a bimanual vagino-abdominal examination.
- A rectal examination in certain instances.

BREAST EXAMINATION *(SEE FIG. 2.1)*
With the patient sitting facing the examiner, the breasts are inspected, first with the patient's arms at her sides and then with her arms raised above her head. The shape, contour and size of the breasts, their height on the chest wall, and the position of the nipples are compared, any nipple retraction being noted. The supraclavicular regions and axillae are next palpated. The latter can only be palpated satisfactorily if the pectoral muscles are relaxed. This relaxation can be obtained if the physician supports the patient's arms whilst palpating the axillae. Palpation is then performed with the patient lying supine, her shoulders elevated on a small pillow. Palpation should be gentle and orderly, using the flat of the fingers of one hand. Each portion of the breast should be palpated systematically beginning at the upper, inner quadrant, followed by palpation of each portion sequentially until the upper, outer quadrant is finally examined.

ABDOMINAL EXAMINATION
The examination is conducted with the patient lying comfortably on her back, *having emptied her bladder immediately before.* Inspection of the abdomen will show its contour, the presence of striae and scars, or of dilated veins. If the patient raises her head and coughs, hernias and divarication of the recti abdominis muscles will be evident. Palpation of the viscera is performed systematically, the liver, the gall bladder, the spleen and the kidneys being palpated in turn. The caecum and colon are next palpated, the hand pressing down gently as the patient breathes out.

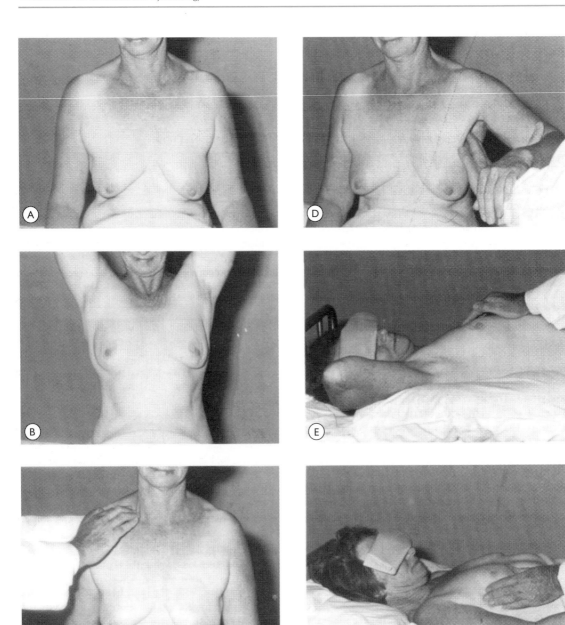

Fig 2.1 Sequence of examination of the breast.
(A) Inspection of the breasts – the patient's arms at her side.
(B) Inspection of the breasts – the patient's arms raised above her head. During the inspection, the contour of the breasts, the size and shape of the areolae and the condition of the nipples are examined. An indentation or a bulge in the contour may indicate a lesion.

(C) Supraclavicular palpation.
(D) Axillary palpation. Note that the patient's arm is supported on the gynaecologist's left forearm.
(E) Palpation of the inner half of the breast. Note the pillow under the patient's shoulder, and the position of her arms.
(F) Palpation of the outer half of the breast.

Percussion may be required if the presence of free fluid is suspected.

PELVIC EXAMINATION

The pelvic examination should follow the abdominal examination, and never be omitted unless the patient is a virgin. The external genitalia are first inspected under a good light with the patient in the dorsal position, the hips flexed and abducted, and knees flexed *(Fig. 2.2)*. If she or the doctor prefers, she may lie in the left lateral position *(Fig. 2.3)*. Some women are more comfortable and feel less exposed in the latter position. The patient must have voided just before the examination (unless stress inconti-

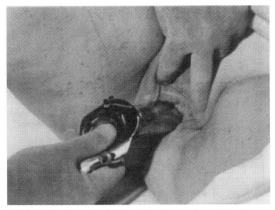

Fig 2.2 Introducing the bivalve (Cusco) speculum. Note the oblique position of the instrument; this avoids painful pressure on the urethra.

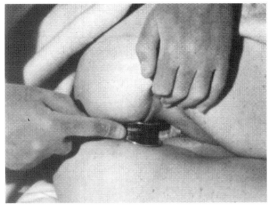

Fig 2.3 The patient in the left lateral position; a Sims speculum has been inserted into the vagina.

nence is complained of), and should preferably have defaecated that morning. If urinary infection is suspected, a mid-stream specimen of urine may be obtained at this time.

The patient is asked to strain down, to enable detection of any evidence of prolapse after which a bivalve speculum is inserted and the cervix visualized. If the physician intends to take a cervical smear to examine the exfoliated cells, *no lubricant apart from water* should be used on the speculum. The vagina and cervix are inspected by opening the bivalve speculum *(Fig. 2.2)*. If the patient has a prolapse, the degree of the vaginal wall or uterine descent can best be assessed if a Sims speculum is used with the patient in the left lateral position *(Fig. 2.3)*.

Digital examination follows, one or two fingers of the gloved hand being introduced. In most countries, apart from the USA, it is usual to to use the right hand as the fingers of this hand in a right-handed person are more 'educated'. After the labia minora have been separated with the left hand to expose the vestibule, the fingers are introduced passing *upwards and backwards* to palpate the cervix. The left hand palpates the pelvis through the abdominal wall simultaneously so that the uterus and ovaries may be palpated. Normal oviducts are never palpable. As the intravaginal fingers push the cervix backwards, the abdominally located hand is placed just below the umbilicus and the fingers reach down into the pelvis, slowly and smoothly, until the fundus is caught between them and the fingers of the right hand in the anterior vaginal fornix *(Fig. 2.4)*.

The information obtained by bimanual examination includes:

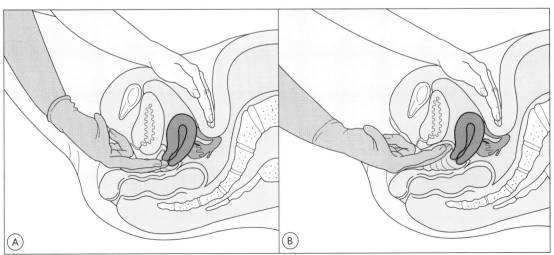

Fig 2.4 Bimanual examination of the uterus. Note that the bladder is empty, the patient having voided just before the pelvic examination. (A) The vaginal fingers push the cervix back and upward so that the fundus can be reached by the abdominal fingers; (B) The vaginal fingers now palpate the anterior surface of the uterus which is held in position by the abdominal fingers.

- *By palpation of the uterus.* Position, size, shape, consistency, mobility, tenderness, attachments. The normal uterus is either in the anterior or posterior position, and is about 9cm long. It is pear-shaped and of firm consistency, and can be moved in all directions. It is normally tender when squeezed between the two hands.
- *By palpation of the ovaries and oviducts.* The tips of the vaginal fingers are placed in each lateral fornix in turn and then pushed backwards and upwards as far as possible without causing pain. The abdominally located fingers simultaneously press backwards about 5cm (2in) medial and parallel to the superior iliac spine *(Fig. 2.5)*. The normal oviduct cannot be palpated, and the normal ovary may or may not be felt. If the latter is palpable, it is extremely tender on bimanual pressure.

RECTAL EXAMINATION

A rectal examination, or a recto-abdominal bimanual examination, may replace a vaginal examination in children and in virgin adults, but the examination is less efficient and more painful than the vaginal examination. A rectal examination is a useful adjunct to a vaginal examination, when either the outer parts of the broad ligaments, or the uterosacral ligaments, require to be palpated. On occasions, a rectovaginal examination, with the index finger in the vagina and the middle finger in the rectum, may help to determine if a lesion is in the bowel or between the rectum and the vagina.

TESTS

Appropriate tests may be required. For example if the woman complains of a vaginal discharge, swabs should be taken to determine the cause (see page 248). Urinary symptoms may require a specimen of mid-stream urine to reach a diagnosis.

Medical practitioners have a crucial role in encouraging sexually active women to have a cervical smear (pap smear) taken at regular intervals, to detect abnormal cells. At present fewer than one-third the number of women over the age of 40, who are at greatest risk of developing cervical carcinoma, have regular pap smears.

ANCILLARY GYNAECOLOGICAL INVESTIGATIONS

PELVIC ULTRASOUND

The development of pelvic ultrasound scanning enables doctors to identify many disorders in the genital tract with greater accuracy than with clinical examination. Ultrasound is particularly helpful in defining cystic benign and malignant tumours of the internal genital organs. The examination may be made transabdominally through a full bladder, or transvaginally when the bladder is empty.

COLPOSCOPE

The colposcope is a low-powered microscope for inspecting the cervix and vagina in some cases where abnormal cells have been detected in a pap smear. The cervix and vagina are exposed by introducing a Cusco vaginal speculum. The colposcope is placed in front of the vagina and its focal length is adjusted to examine the suspicious part of the lower genital tract.

COMPUTED TOMOGRAPHY AND MAGNETIC RESONANCE IMAGING

These technologies have a role in assessing the nature and spread of malignant disease of the genital

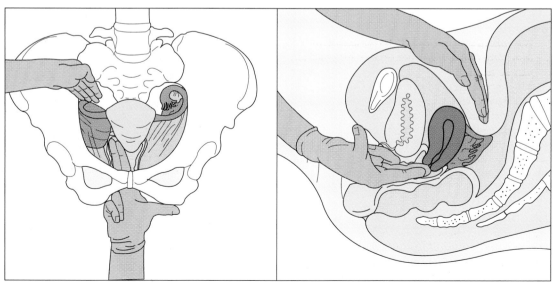

Fig 2.5 Bimanual palpation of the adnexal area. Note the position of the fingers; normally the ovary cannot be felt. In this case a cystic mass lying in the position of the ovary can be identified.

organs, but both are expensive and should only be used when they confer a real benefit.

LAPAROSCOPY

Inspection of the pelvic organs with a laparoscope inserted into the peritoneal cavity through a small sub-umbilical incision, may give valuable information about the state of the pelvic organs, particularly in cases of infertility, chronic pelvic pain and probable ectopic gestation. Techniques have been developed which enable operations to be conducted through a laparoscope, avoiding long hospital inpatient stay.

HYSTEROSALPINGOGRAPHY

The injection through the cervix of a radio-opaque substance and following its progress on a screen as it fills the uterus and Fallopian tubes provides information in cases of infertility.

HYSTEROSCOPY

A small fibre-optic telescope is inserted through the cervix into the uterine cavity, which is inspected. The procedure may help the doctor to reach a diagnosis in cases of menstrual disorders. Endometrial polyps can be removed and the endometrium ablated (see page 215) using this technique.

ENDOMETRIAL BIOPSY

This technique is used to obtain a sample of endometrium for histological examination, by introducing a small curette through the cervix without anaesthesia. Endometrial biopsy has a role in the investigation of infertility and in helping to reach a diagnosis in cases of postmenopausal bleeding.

THE OBSTETRIC PATIENT

Most women consulting a medical practitioner today have a good idea that they are pregnant. The woman:
- Has missed a menstrual period (has amenorrhoea).
- May have noticed that her breasts are fuller and may be tender.
- May have nausea and perhaps have vomited.
- May have frequency of micturition. Some women have purchased a 'Home Pregnancy Test' or have had the test made by their pharmacist.

The woman visits the doctor to confirm that she is pregnant and either to seek antenatal care from the doctor or to be referred to an obstetrician or to a hospital clinic.

HISTORY

At this first visit the doctor should take a history in the manner described earlier. The information includes more than that described for gynaecological examination. The history of previous pregnancies should be detailed and include information about:
- Spontaneous and induced abortions.

- Complications during pregnancy.
- The gestation period at delivery.
- The method of delivery (spontaneous vaginal birth, forceps, ventouse delivery, caesarean section).
- Complications in the puerperium.

The medical practitioner should enquire about any problems in the current (presumed) pregnancy.

CLINICAL EXAMINATION

Having taken a history the doctor should examine the woman as described earlier. The vaginal examination should include taking a pap smear if this has not been taken in the previous 12 months. The vaginal examination will usually reveal that the uterus is enlarged. If the woman first attends the doctor between 6 and 10 weeks after her last menstrual period (LMP), the uterus may feel as if it is separate from the cervix. This is because the cervix has softened, and the examiner's fingers seem to meet below the ball-shaped uterus (Hegar's sign) as shown in *Fig 2.6*.

In most cases the doctor will confirm the pregnancy either clinically or by an immunological pregnancy test. The test depends on the fact that human chorionic gonadotrophin (hCG) is secreted into the circulation within 10 days of conception. Using a sensitive monoclonal antibody test, small amounts of the beta fraction of hCG can be detected if the woman is pregnant.

Once the pregancy has been diagnosed the medical practitioner should ask if any close family member has hypertension or diabetes mellitus, as these may be pointers to the development of the condition in the pregnancy.

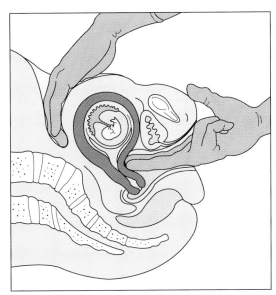

Fig 2.6 Hegar's sign.

A question invariably asked by the patient when the pregnancy has been confirmed is 'When can I expect my baby to be born?'. This can be determined by asking the woman if the length of her menstrual cycle falls into the normal range (22–35 days). The calculation is to add one year and 10 days to the first day of her LMP and then to subtract 3 months. This gives the estimated date of confinement (EDC). Thus if her LMP began on 14 November 1994 she may expect to give birth on 24 August 1995 (±14 days). Most doctors do not need to do the calculation as Obstetric Calculation Discs are supplied to doctors by some pharmaceutical manufacturers.

The calculation has to be altered if the woman's menstrual cycle is prolonged, or if she was taking oral contraceptives during the cycle before she became pregnant, as in the pregnancy cycle ovulation may have been delayed, and conception may have occurred up to 14 days later than expected. In these two circumstances, the EDC will be later than calculated, and to obtain greater accuracy of predicting the EDC an ultrasound examination at the 18th to 20th week of pregnancy may be needed.

Most women seek to have the pregnancy confirmed in the first 10 weeks of pregnancy. Some women delay until later in the pregnancy. In the second quarter the uterus becomes palpable on abdominal examination *(Fig 2.7)* and fetal heart sounds can be heard using an ultrasonic heart detector at this time. The woman feels her fetus moving from about 18 weeks' gestation.

earlier in multi

Once pregnancy has been diagnosed further investigations should be made. These are discussed in Chapter 7.

EVIDENCE OF A PREVIOUS PREGNANCY
In a few cases the woman may deny that she has been pregnant previously but the doctor is suspicious. This suspicion can grow stronger if
- The breasts show pigmentation of the areolae.
- The abdominal wall has silver-grey longitudinal lines (striae gravidarum).
- On inspection of the vulva, the perineum shows evidence of damage and repair. However, a firm diagnosis can not be given as these signs can be produced by other disorders.

PSEUDOCYESIS
Emotional disturbance such as an intense desire to have a baby or fear of loss of a lover, may lead some women to believe that they are pregnant, when they are not. The emotions stop the release of gonadotrophic hormones with resulting amenorrhoea. The woman's emotions cause her to complain of the symptoms of pregnancy, often in a bizarre order. The breasts become full and may secrete a cloudy fluid; the abdomen becomes enlarged because of fat or flatus. On superficial examination the woman appears to be pregnant; however, vaginal examination shows the uterus to be normal in size. It may be necessary to have an ultrasound examination to convince the woman that she is not pregnant. Once the absence of pregnancy has been confirmed, the woman should be given sympathetic psychiatric attention.

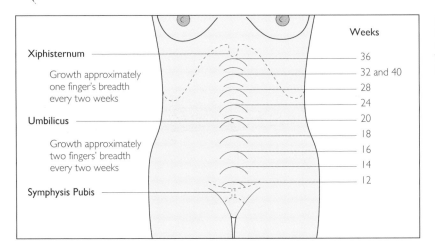

Fig 2.7 The abdominal markings of uterine growth related to the number of weeks after the last menstrual period..

Weeks

Xiphisternum

Growth approximately one finger's breadth every two weeks

Umbilicus

Growth approximately two fingers' breadth every two weeks

Symphysis Pubis

36
32 and 40
28
24
20
18
16
14
12

3

OVULATION AND THE MENSTRUAL CYCLE

The endocrinological changes which occur to transform a female child into an adolescent, who menstruates and ovulates and is capable of conceiving a child, begin several years before puberty, but the most marked changes occur in the 2 years before the girl's first menstrual period (menarche).

THE MENARCHE

The underlying major endocrinological change is that the hypothalamus begins to secrete releasing hormones. These in turn lead to the release into the circulation of adrenal androgens and pituitary human growth hormone (hGH). It is hGH which causes the growth spurt which begins 3–4 years before the menarche, and is maximal in the first 2 years *(Fig 3.1)*. The physical growth slows down as the first menstruation (menarche) approaches. This is because increasing quantities of oestrogen are secreted by the ovaries and feed back negatively, reducing hGH secretion. Shortly after the secretion of hGH starts, the hypothalamus begins to release gonadotrophin releasing hormone (GnRH) in an episodic pulsed manner. At first, the pulses are greater in amplitude during sleep, but after 2 years they occur by day and night at about 2-hour intervals. GnRH induces the release of follicle stimulating hormone (FSH) and luteinizing hormone (LH) from the pituitary gland, which in turn bind to receptors in the ovaries and induce the secretion and release of oestrogen and progesterone into the circulation. The quantity of FSH and LH increases as the girl matures.

Until the age of 8 years, only small quantities of oestrogen are secreted (and less of progesterone). After that age, oestrogen secretion begins to rise, slowly at first, but after the age of about 11 quite rapidly. The FSH levels reach a plateau when the girl is aged about 13. LH levels rise more slowly until one year before menarche, at which time a rapid rise occurs *(Fig 3.2)*. By this time, the GnRH pulses occur every 90 minutes. These hormonal changes persist until after the age of 40, when changes presaging the menopause begin (see Chapter 44).

It is thought that the rapid rise of LH induces onset of the menarche, but other factors are also involved. These include an increase in the fat:lean ratio of body composition, which in turn is related to good nutrition and the absence of debilitating diseases.

The age at which the menarche occurs has fallen from over 15 years a century ago, to about 12.5 years today. This reduction is believed to be due to better childhood nutrition. It is hypothesized that the greater amount of body fat in girls today, permits the greater aromatization of androgens to oestrogens. Rapidly rising levels of oestrogens feed back positively to the hypothalamus and pituitary gland leading to the LH surge, which precedes the menarche.

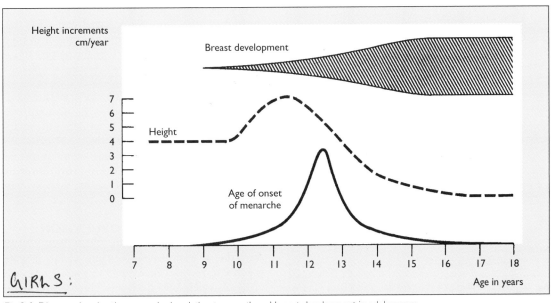

Fig 3.1 Diagram showing the menarche in relation to growth and breast development in adolescence.

The menarche may be delayed among women who are at low body-weight (such as ballet dancers and women who have anorexia nervosa) or who are compulsive exercisers.

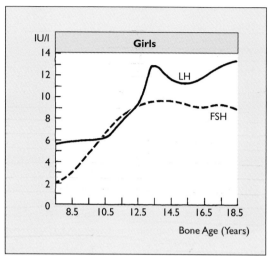

Fig 3.2 Pubertal changes in level of FSH and LH in girls. (Derived from Aptar, D. *et al. Acta Paediatric. Scand.* 1978, 67, 417.).

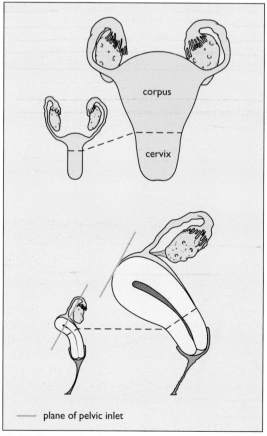

— plane of pelvic inlet

Fig 3.3 The prepubertal uterus compared with the adult uterus. Note particularly the change in ratio of the corpus and cervix.

THE EFFECTS OF OESTROGEN AND PROGESTERONE ON BODY TISSUES

More than 20 oestrogens have been isolated, the three considered the most important being oestrone, oestradiol and oestriol. Oestrone is a relatively weak oestrogen and inter-converts with 17-beta oestradiol, which is the most active and the predominant oestrogen in the reproductive years. Oestradiol is rapidly transported in the blood bound to albumin and binds to tissues which have specific receptor proteins. The tissues of the genital tract and the lobular elements of the breasts have the highest concentration of cells containing specific oestrogen-binding receptors and consequently are most affected by circulating oestradiol.

Once attached to the specific binding sites, oestradiol is transferred to the cell's nucleus, where it activates genes, leading to RNA synthesis. This process is regulated to some extent by progesterone, which blocks the formation of new receptors and induces intracellular enzyme production; these enzymes also regulate oestrogen metabolism.

Following nuclear gene activation, oestradiol is rapidly converted to the relatively inactive oestriol which is transported to the liver, where it is conjugated with glucuronic acid and excreted, mostly in the urine. This leaves the cell receptors free to bind more oestradiol.

Oestradiol stimulates the growth of the vulva and the vagina after the menarche, the hormone causing proliferation of both the epithelial and muscular layers. It also stimulates the formation of more blood vessels which supply the organs.

The uterus is particularly stimulated by oestradiol, which increases the vascularity of the organ. Oestradiol causes endometrial proliferation, stimulating the growth of the glands and stroma. It stimulates the growth of the muscular layers of the uterus, so that the uterus grows from its prepubertal size to its adult size in the perimenarchal years *(Fig 3.3)*. The great increase in circulating oestrogen in pregnancy causes the rapid growth of the uterus, and its lack after the menopause leads to uterine atrophy.

Progesterone acts on tissues which have oestrogen receptors, but only if they are first sensitized by oestrogen. Progesterone hinders the maturation of the vaginal epithelial cells. It renders the cervical mucus viscous. It increases the thickness and succulence of an oestrogen-primed endometrium, preparing it to accept a fertilized egg. It also aids in fat deposition and is thermogenic, raising the body temperature by 0.2–0.5°C.

MENSTRUATION AND OVULATION

At puberty each ovary contains about 200 000 oogonia surrounded by mantles of theca lutein cells, many of which have developed fluid-filled cavities (antra) to become primary follicles.

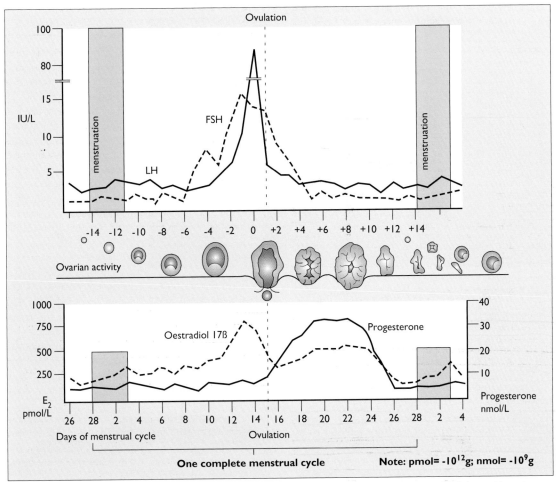

Fig 3.4 Hormone levels in the normal menstrual cycle – considerable variations are compatible, however, with normal menstrual function. In this figure the interrelationship of ovarian steroids and hypothalamic-pituitary gonadotrophins is shown. After menstruation , rising levels of oestrogen exert a negative feedback, reducing FSH release. Towards midcycle still higher oestrogen levels exert a positive feedback causing a sudden peak release of LH which induces ovulation. An increased release in FSH also occurs. Failure of this sequence will lead to anovulation and irregular cycles. In the luteal phase, LH levels must be sufficiently high to maintain the corpus luteum until the conceptus has implanted and commenced hCG secretion, which then maintains corpus luteum function. If conception fails to occur, the corpus luteum deteriorates after about 7 days, with the resulting falling levels of progesterone and oestrogen. As a consequence menstruation occurs, and FSH levels rise, initiating a new menstrual cycle.

From now on until their disappearance at the time of the menopause, in the absence of pregnancy, of severe weight loss or of certain other conditions, between 15 and 20 of these follicles are stimulated to grow each month by follicle stimulating hormone (FSH) and luteinizing hormone (LH) secreted by the anterior pituitary gland. One (occasionally more) of the follicles grows more rapidly than the others, and reaching the ovarian surface causes the release of an ovum. If an ovum is released and pregnancy does not occur, menstruation follows.

The control of this system is complex and reciprocating. The initial stimulus originates in the hypothalamus with the release of gonadotrophic-releasing hormone (GnRH) into the hypophyseal portal vessels. As mentioned, GnRH released in a pulsatile manner, reaches the pituitary gland where it stimulates the growth and maturation of gonadotrophs which secrete FSH and LH. FSH acts on 10–20 'selected' primary follicles, by binding on to the theca granulosa cells which surround them. The effect of the rising amounts of FSH is to cause fluid to be secreted into the cavity of the follicles, one of which grows more rapidly than the remainder. Simultaneously the theca granulosa cells which surround the selected follicles secrete increasing amounts of oestradiol, which enters the circulation.

The endocrinological effect of the rising levels of oestradiol is that it exerts a negative feedback on the anterior pituitary and the hypothalamus, with the result that the secretion of FSH falls whilst that of oestradiol rises to a peak *(Fig 3.4)*. Some 24 hours later a sudden large surge of LH and a smaller surge of FSH occurs. This positive feedback leads to the

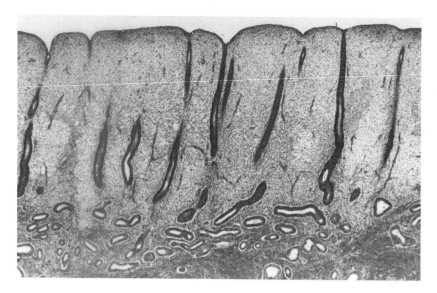

Fig 3.5 Endometrium – early proliferative phase. Note that the glands are straight, short and narrow. The surface epithelium is thin.

release of an ovum from the largest follicle. Ovulation has occurred. (If large amounts of FSH are produced by the anterior pituitary gland, or usually if FSH injections are given, superovulation occurs, seven or more follicles reaching maturity, a technique used in In Vitro Fertilization).

The collapse of the follicle from which the ovum has been released leads to a change in its nature. The theca granulosa cells proliferate and become yellow in colour (luteinized) and are referred to as theca-lutein cells. The collapsed follicle becomes a corpus luteum. The lutein cells of the corpus luteum secrete progesterone as well as oestrogen. Progesterone secretion reaches a plateau about four days after ovulation and then rises progressively should the fertilized ovum implant into the endometrium. The trophoblastic cells of the implanted embryo immediately secrete human chorionic gonadotrophin (hCG) which maintains the corpus luteum so that the secretion of oestradiol and progesterone continues. On the other hand if pregnancy fails to occur, the theca-lutein cells degenerate and produce less oestradiol and progesterone. This reduces the negative feedback on the gonadotrophs with a rise in the secretion of FSH. The falling circulating levels of oestradiol and progesterone cause changes in the endometrium (see page 14) which lead to menstruation.

THE ENDOMETRIAL CYCLE

Menstruation is the periodic discharge from the uterus of blood, tissue fluid and endometrial cellular debris, in varying amounts. The quantity of tissue fluid is the greatest variable. This means that some women who complain of heavy periods do not become anaemic as might be expected (see Chapter 30). The mean blood loss during menstruation is 30ml (range 10–80ml). Menstruation normally occurs at intervals of 22–35 days (counted from day one of one menstrual flow to day one of the next) and the menstrual discharge lasts from 1 to 8 days.

A convenient way to describe the endometrial menstrual cycle is to start just after menstruation

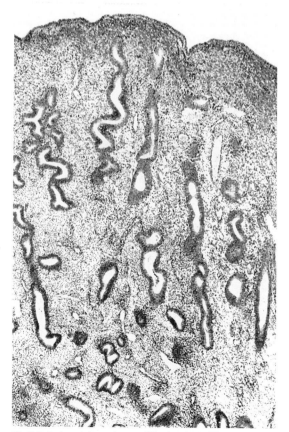

Fig 3.6 Endometrium – late proliferative phase. The glands have become longer and tortuous, and in a few, early secretory changes may be observed. The stroma remains dense.

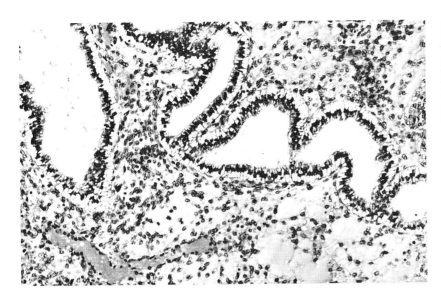

Fig 3.7 Endometrium – early luteal phase. The tortuosity of the glands, and the subnuclear vacuoles, can be seen. Note the gland in the lowest part of the picture has not been affected (×160). Reproduced with kind permission of Dr CH Buckley MD FRCPath.

ceases and follow the cycle to the next menstruation as it passes through the proliferative and secretory (luteal) phases.

THE PROLIFERATIVE PHASE

As each area of the endometrium is shed during menstruation, regenerative repairs begin, the endometrial surface being reformed by the metaplasia of stromal cells and by an outgrowth of epithelial cells of the endometrial glands. Within 3 days of menstruation ceasing, the repair of the entire endometrium is complete.

The endometrium in the early proliferative phase is thin, the glands few, narrow, straight and lined with cuboidal cells and the stroma is compact *(Fig 3.5)*. The early regenerative phase lasts from day 3 of the menstrual cycle to day 7, when proliferation speeds up. The epithelial glands increase in size and grow down perpendicular to the surface. Their cells become columnar with basal nuclei. The stromal cells proliferate, remaining compact and spindle shaped *(Fig 3.6)*. Mitoses are common in glands and stroma. The endometrium is supplied by basal arteries in the myometrium which send off branches at right angles to supply the endometrium. At first as each artery penetrates the basal endometrium it is straight, but in the middle and superficial layers it becomes spiral. The coiling permits the artery to supply the growing endometrium by becoming uncoiled. Each spiral artery supplies a defined area of endometrium.

THE LUTEAL PHASE

If ovulation occurs, as is usual, except at the extremes of the reproductive years, the endometrium undergoes marked changes. The changes start in the last 2 days of the proliferative phase, but increase dramatically after ovulation. Secretory vacuoles, rich in glycogen, appear in the cells lining the endometrial glands. At first the vacuoles are basal and displace the cell's nucleus superficially *(Fig 3.7)*. They rapidly increase in number and the glands become tortuous. By the 6th day after ovulation, the secretory phase is at its peak. The vacuoles have streamed past the nucleus. Some have discharged mucus into the cavity of the gland; others are full of mucus, leading to a saw-toothed appearance. *(Fig 3.8)*. The spiral arteries increase in length by uncoiling *(see Fig 3.9)*.

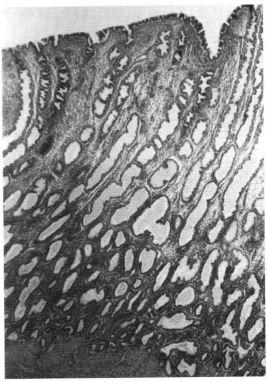

Fig 3.8 Endometrium – 6 days after ovulation. The glands are now very tortuous with secretion in the lumen and increasing fluid separating the stromal cells. In a fertile cycle this is the day the ovum reaches the uterine cavity (× 40).

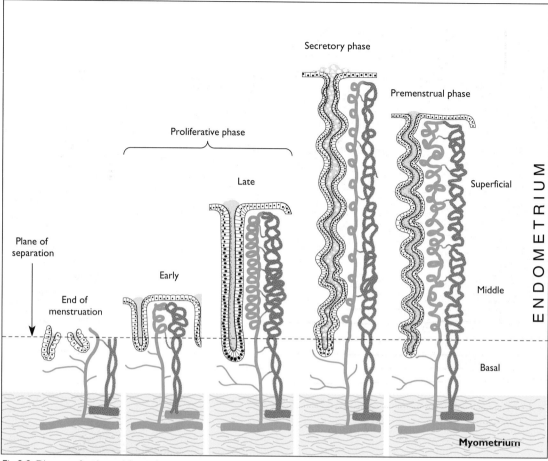

Fig 3.9 Diagram of endometrial vascular patterns.

In the absence of pregnancy, the secretion of oestrogen and progesterone fall as the corpus luteum ages. The fall leads to an increase in endometrial free arachidonic acid and endoperoxidases. These enzymes induce stromal cell lysosomes to synthesize and secrete prostaglandins ($PGE_{2\alpha}$ and PGE_2) and prostacyclin. $PGF_{2\alpha}$ is a powerful vasoconstrictor and causes uterine contractions; PGE_2 causes uterine contractions and some vasodilatation; prostacyclin is a vasodilator, causes muscle relaxation and inhibits platelet aggregation. During menstruation the ratio of $PGF_{2\alpha}$ to the other two prostaglandins increases. This change reduces the blood flow through the endometrial capillaries and leads to a shift of fluid from the endometrial tissues into the capillaries, with a resulting decrease in endometrial thickness. This leads to increased coiling of the spiral arteries with a further decrease in blood flow. The area of endometrium supplied by the spiral artery becomes hypoxic, and ischaemic necrosis occurs. The vasoconstriction occurs in different spiral arteries at different times, alternating with vasodilatation. The necrotic area of the endometrium is shed into the uterine cavity accompanied by blood and tissue fluid. Menstruation has begun.

THE MENSTRUAL PHASE

During menstruation the superficial and middle layers of the endometrium are shed, the deep basal layer being spared *(Fig 3.10)*. The shedding occurs in an irregular, haphazard manner, some areas being unaffected, others undergoing repair, whilst simultaneously other areas are being shed. The shed endometrium, with tissue fluid and blood, forms a coagulum in the uterine cavity. It is immediately liquefied by fibrinolysins and the liquid, which does not coagulate, is discharged through the cervix by uterine contractions. If the quantity of blood lost in the process is considerable, there may be insufficient fibrinolysins and the woman expels clots through her cervix.

The blood vessels supplying the area beneath the shed endometrium are sealed with a haemostatic plug consisting of aggregated platelets and by fibrin fibres which infiltrate the platelet aggregations to form a stable occlusive plug. In addition vasoconstriction occurs. The basal layer of the endometrium regenerates and new epithelium covers the denuded area. When regeneration exceeds necrosis and repair is complete or nearly complete, menstruation ceases and a new menstrual cycle begins.

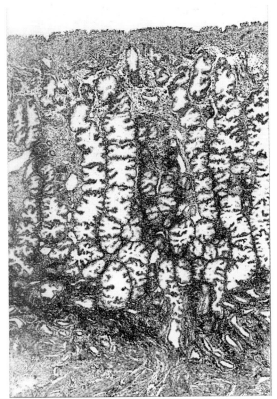

Fig 3.10 Endometrium – early menstrual phase. The section shows beginning of focal necrosis in the superficial zone of the endometrium with small areas of haemorrhage into the stroma and infiltration with neutrophils (× 40).

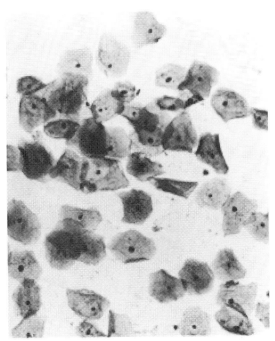

Fig 3.11 Vaginal exfoliative cytology – late proliferative phase. Note the discrete cells with small nuclei and the clear background (× 160).

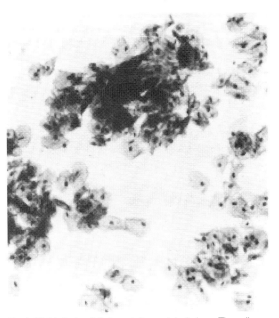

Fig 3.12 Vaginal exfoliative cytology – luteal phase. The cells have clumped and the background infiltration of leucocytes has begun (× 160).

THE CERVICAL CYCLE

During the follicular phase the glands lining the clefts of the cervical canal proliferate and secrete a thick mucus, which forms a complex mesh in the cervical canal. Just before ovulation, the sudden surge of oestrogen changes the character of the cervical mucus which becomes thin and forms long strands through which helical channels appear. Following ovulation, progesterone alters the nature of the cervical mucus which again becomes thick and impenetrable.

THE VAGINAL CYCLE

Cyclic changes occur in the vaginal epithelium, which are dependent on the ratio between oestrogen and progesterone. In the follicular phase, superficial and large intermediate cells predominate. As ovulation approaches, the proportion of superficial cells increases and few leukocytes can be seen *(Fig 3.11)*. Following ovulation a marked change occurs as progesterone is secreted. The superficial cells are replaced by intermediate cells, and leukocytes increase in number causing the smear to look dirty *(Fig 3.12)*.

PSYCHOSOMATIC DISTURBANCES DURING THE MENSTRUAL CYCLE

These are discussed in Chapter 31.

4

CONCEPTION AND PLACENTAL DEVELOPMENT

By the time a woman reaches puberty each of her ovaries contains about 200 000 primary oocytes, enclosed in primordial follicles. Each oocyte is separated from the cellular primordial follicle by a clear area, the perivitelline space and a thickened 'shell', the zona pellucida. Each primordial follicle is capable of growing under the influence of follicle stimulating hormone (FSH) to form a mature follicle. Each month from about the age of 15 to the age of 45, some 20 of the primordial follicles grow through the stage of vesicular follicles to become mature antral follicles.

In contrast to other body cells, the oocyte has only 23 chromosomes. At some stage of its growth the oocyte undergoes a meiotic division of its nucleus and an unequal division of its cytoplasm, to become a secondary oocyte. The smaller cell is expelled into the perivitelline space, and is termed a polar body *(Fig 4.1[B])*. The oocyte and its polar body both contain 23 chromosomes.

One of the 20 follicles (occasionally 2 or more, particularly if the ovaries are hyperstimulated in an IVF programme) outstrips the others, developing a large fluid-filled antrum and migrating to bulge through the thickened surface of the ovary *(Fig 4.2)*. With the release of luteinizing hormone (LH) surge by the pituitary, at mid-cycle, the follicle bursts expelling the ovum, which is gathered into the Fallopian tube by the fimbria which project from its proximal end. The ovum, surrounded by the perivitelline is contained in a condensed opaque substance

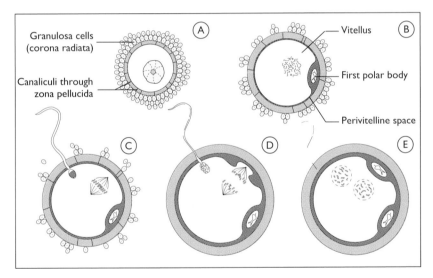

Fig 4.1 Formation of the ootid and fertilization; (A) primary oocyte; (B) secondary oocyte formed after first maturation division, first polar body pinched off. Both oocyte and polar body have undergone reduction division and now each has a haploid number of chromosomes (BC); (C) second maturation division stimulated by sperm penetrating into vitellus; (D) second polar body forming. The first polar body may also undergo a reduction division; (E) male and female pronuclei formed.

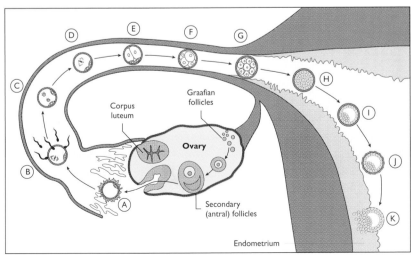

Fig 4.2 The development of the ovum and its passage through the Fallopian tube into the cavity of the uterus is shown diagrammatically; (A) unsegmented oocyte; (B) fertilization; (C) pronuclei formed; (D) first spindle division; (E) two cell stage; (F) four cell stage; (G) eight cell stage; (H) morula; (I) and (J) blastocyst formation; (K) zona pellucida lost, implantation occurs.

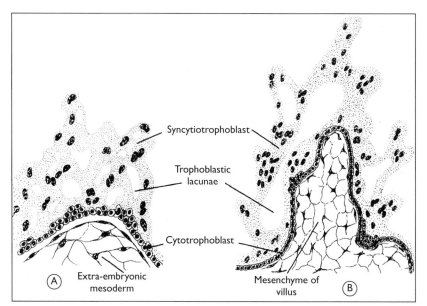

Fig 4.3 Early stage in development of chorionic villi. (A) The trophoblast projection has occurred with the development of lacunae, and much intermingling with maternal tissue, which for clarity is not shown. No mesoblastic core has yet entered the villus. (B) The mesoblastic core is now developing within the villus (redrawn from Patten. *Tend. Act. Gynecol. et Obstet.* 1959, Beauchemin, Montreal).

5–10μm thick, called the zona pellucida. Adherent to the zona pellucida are theca granulosa cells derived from the mature follicle.

Once the ovum has been expelled, the follicle collapses and turns yellow, forming the corpus luteum *(see Fig 4.2[D])*. The ovum is now ready to be fertilized should a sperm reach it.

Of the 60–100 million sperm ejaculated into a woman's vagina at the time she ovulated, several million will negotiate the helical channels in the cervical mucus to reach the uterine cavity. Several hundred sperm may pass through the narrow entrance to the Fallopian tubes, and a few will survive to reach the ovum in the fimbrial end of the Fallopian tube. One sperm may penetrate the zona

pellucida of the ovum, its head entering the substance of the ovary. When this occurs a chemical reaction prevents the entry of any other sperm. At the same time the oocyte undergoes another division of its chromosomes and a second polar body is formed *(see Fig 4.1[D])*.

Once inside the cytoplasm of the ovum, the sperm's nuclear membrane dissolves, leaving a naked male pronucleus. The ovum, having divided to produce a second polar body, also loses its nuclear membrane. The two naked nuclei approach each other and fuse *(see Fig 4.1[E])*. Fertilization and conception have occurred.

Within a few hours of fertilization, the fused nuclei divide to form two cells. *(see Fig 4.2[E])*.

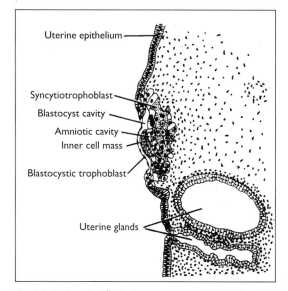

Fig 4.4 Section of a 7½ day human ovum partially implanted in secretory endometrium (× 100). The embryo is represented by the inner cell mass; the blastocyst has collapsed (by courtesy of Drs Rock and Hertig).

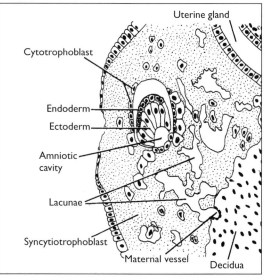

Fig 4.5 A section through the middle of the Hertig–Rock 9-day embryo (redrawn from Hertig, A. J. and Rock, J. *Contrib. Embry. Carnegie Inst.* 1941, 29, 127).

Once this event has occurred, further cell division proceeds rapidly until within 3 to 4 days a solid mass of cells (the morula) has formed *(see Fig 4.2[G,H])*.

IMPLANTATION

The morula is rapidly propelled along the Fallopian tube to enter the uterine cavity. During its passage, fluid passes through canaliculae in the zona pellucida to create a central fluid-filled cavity in the morula, forming a blastocyst *(see Fig 4.2[I])*. On reaching the uterine cavity the zona pellucida becomes distended and thin. It soon disappears leaving the surface cells of the blastocyst in contact with the endometrial stroma. About 50 per cent of blastocysts adhere to the endometrium. The surface trophoblastic cells of the adhering blastocyst, differentiate into an inner cellular layer, the cytotrophoblast, and an outer syn-cytiotrophoblast.

Knobs of trophoblast rapidly form, which invade the endometrial stroma in a controlled manner *(Fig 4.3)*. By the 10th day after fertilization, the knobs of trophoblastic tissue have developed a mesodermal core and have pushed deeply into the endometrial stroma *(Fig 4.4)*. The stromal cells react to the invasion by becoming polyhedral in shape and filled with glycogen and lipid, converting into a decidua, which supplies the energy needed by the invading trophoblast.

At the same time a number of deep cells at one pole of the blastocyst differentiate to become an inner cell mass, from which the embryo will develop.

By the 9th to 10th day after fertilization, the inner cell mass has differentiated into an ectodermal layer, a mesodermal layer and an endodermal layer in which a small fluid-filled cavity, the amniotic sac, has formed *(Fig 4.5)*. The further development of the amniotic sac, in which the fetus will float relatively weightless until it is born, is shown in *Fig 4.6*.

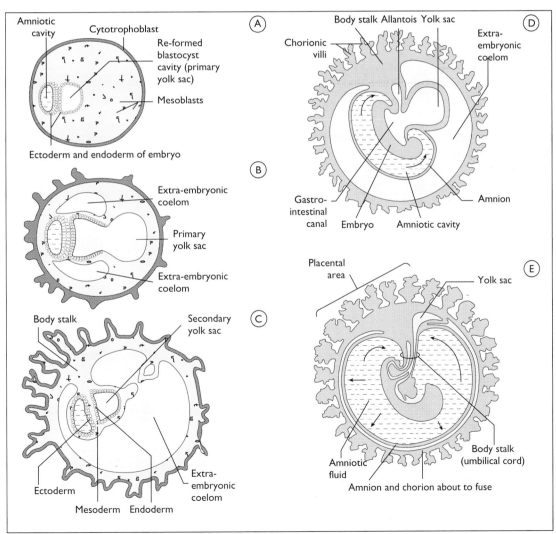

Fig 4.6 Formation of the amniotic cavity. (A) Formation of the inner cell mass, and the development of the amniotic cavity and the primary yolk sac. (B) Spaces appear in the mesoblast to form the extra-embryonic coelom. (C) The primary yolk sac diminishes in size as the extra-embryonic coelom enlarges. (D) The amniotic sac develops and begins to occupy the extra-embryonic coelom. (E) By the 45th day, the amniotic sac has surrounded the embryo which is suspended in the protective liquor amnii.

The inner cell mass projects into the original blastocystic cavity, the walls of which are formed from cytotrophoblast *(Fig 4.7)*. The cavity is filled with mesoderm. Quickly, the surface layer of ectoderm divides to surround a fluid-filled cavity in the mesoderm – the yolk sac *(Fig 4.6[A–C])*.

With further development the yolk sac shrinks in size and a second fluid-filled cavity, the amniotic sac, surrounds the growing embryo *(Fig 4.6 [D, E])*.

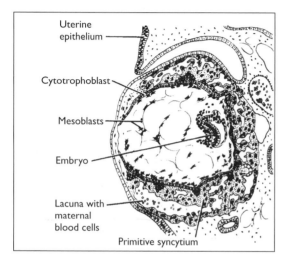

Fig 4.7 Section of an 11½-day human embryo (Barnes embryo). The blastocystic trophoblast has differentiated into primitive syncytium and cytotrophoblast. Mesoblast has differentiated from the inner surface of the latter and almost fills the original blastocyst cavity. Lacunae have appeared in the actively growing syncytium, and maternal blood cells have seeped into several of them. Buds appear at intervals on the syncitium; these are the forerunners of chorionic villi (redrawn from Hamilton, Boyd and Mossman. *Human Embryology*. Heffer, Cambridge, 1962).

THE FORMATION OF THE PLACENTA

Meanwhile the trophoblastic syncytium has penetrated more deeply into the decidua. As well as invading the endometrial stroma, the syncytium secretes human chorionic gonadotrophin (hCG), which aids in maintaining the function of the corpus luteum to secrete oestrogen and progesterone. In some areas of the decidua the syncytium has surrounded and invaded the walls of the interdecidual portions of the uterine spiral arteries to convert them from relatively thick walled arteries to thin walled vessels, permitting a greater flow of blood. These vessels are fragile and break to form small blood lakes or lacunae. In normal pregnancies the process is complete by 20–22 weeks' gestation. Failure of the process to occur normally may be a factor in the development of pregnancy-induced hypertension.

With further proliferation the knobs of trophoblast become finger-like and blood vessels appear in their mesodermal core. These vessels will soon link up with blood vessels forming in the embryonic mesoderm. The finger-like projections are termed chorionic villi. The chorionic villi proliferate and erode more vessels so that the lacunae increase in size. Blood flows under pressure into them to create large blood-filled spaces in which the proliferating chorionic villi float.

By the 19th day after fertilization, the entire conceptus is covered by growing chorionic villi, some attached to the decidua (anchoring villi) but most floating freely in the blood lakes. At this stage further penetration of the decidua ceases, by immunological or chemical mechanisms, and a collagen layer appears through which the spiral arteries and veins pass. As the blood supply to the chorionic villi is greatest on the deep surface of the conceptus, the villi grow profusely here, resembling

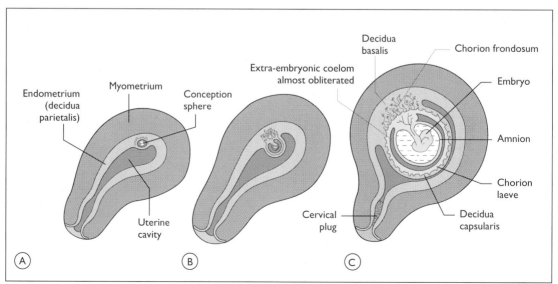

Fig 4.8 Diagram to show the relationship of the chorionic sac, amnion and developing embryo to the endometrium and uterine cavity at successive stages in early pregnancy. A: three weeks, B: five weeks and C: ten weeks after the last menstrual period.

leafy trees (chorion frondosum). The chorionic villi covering the remainder of the conceptus degenerate, forming the chorion laeve. The chorion frondosum forms the placenta, which is the functional union between the conceptus and the maternal tissues. By the 70th day after fertilization the placental development is complete *(Fig 4.8)*.

The placenta is composed of about 200 trunks, some large, some of medium size but most small, which divide into limbs, branches and twigs, covered with chorionic villi. Each of the main trunks forms a cotyledon, 10 being large, 40 medium and the rest small and of little functional significance *(Fig 4.9)* .

As the blood lakes coalesce a large blood-filled space is created in which the villi covering each fetal cotyledon float, moved by the motion of the blood. The roof of the space is formed by chorion (the chorionic plate) and its base by trophoblast and decidua (the decidual plate). Septa of varying heights and sizes grow from the decidual plate to separate each fetal cotyledon, each forming an intervillous space. Each intervillous space is supplied by a number of separate arteries, which enter the space at the base of the septa. During maternal systole, arterial blood spurts into the space like a fountain at a pressure of 80mmHg. The pressure of the blood pushes the villi aside and the blood hits the chorionic plate and then flows laterally and downwards, bathing the villi, to escape slowly through veins in the decidual plate *(Fig 4.10)*.

It has been estimated that the maternal blood flow through the placenta increases from 300ml per minute at 20 weeks' gestation to 600ml per minute at 40 weeks. The total surface area of the villi has been estimated to be $11m^2$, and the placenta at 40 weeks weighs one-seventh of the weight of the baby.

Each villus has a complex anastomosis of capillaries *(Fig 4.11)*, so there is ample opportunity for exchange of gases and nutrients. The exchange is enhanced by the vascular resistance in the vessels of the chorionic villi *(Fig 4.12)*.

The increasing blood flow as pregnancy advances compensates for ageing changes which occur in the placenta, and for the development of placental infarcts.

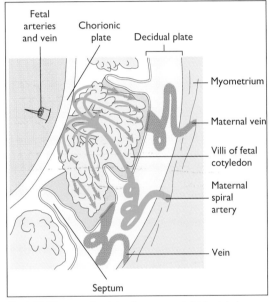

Fig 4.10 Diagram of an intervillous space. A fetal cotyledon can be seen, in which the fountain effect of the maternal arterial blood is demonstrated. The blood cascades over the tree-like villi to escape through the maternal veins.

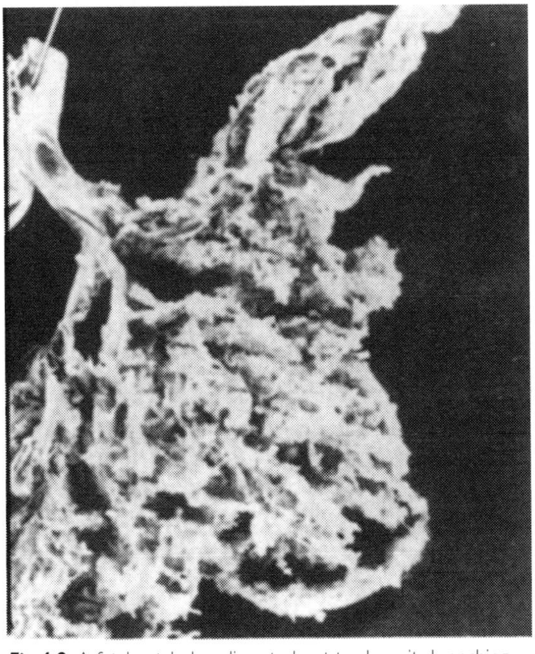

Fig 4.9 A fetal cotyledon dissected out to show its branching, tree-like form (from Crawford, J.M. *J. Obstet. Gynaecol. Brit. Emp.* 1956, 63, 542).

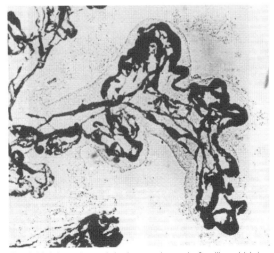

Fig 4.11 Injected vessels in the growing end of a villus which is 'budding off' daughter villi. The complex anastomosis of the vessels can be seen (Crawford, J.M. *J. Obstet. Gynaecol. Brit. Emp.* 1959, 66, 885).

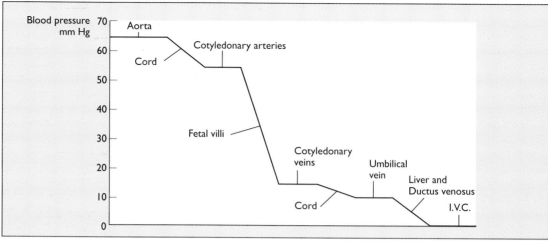

Fig 4.12 Diagram showing the fall in blood pressure from the aorta through the umbilical circulation and liver to the inferior vena cava in the mature fetal lamb (re-drawn from Dawes, G.S. *Amer. J. Obstet. Gynecol.* 1962, 84, 1643).

THE FUNCTION OF THE PLACENTA

The placenta acts for the fetus as:
- an organ of respiration.
- an organ of nutrient transfer and excretion.
- an organ of hormone synthesis.
- it may act as an immunological barrier protecting the fetus (formed from paternal as well as maternal genes) from rejection by the mother's immune system.

TRANSPORT MECHANISMS THROUGH THE PLACENTA

Transport of substances through the placenta takes place by:

1. Passive transport   a. simple diffusion
                      b. facilitated diffusion
2. Active transport   a. enzymatic reaction
                      b. pinocytosis

These mechanisms require the expenditure of energy and the rate of placental metabolism has been calculated as comparable to that of the liver or kidney. The transfer of substances is shown in *Table 4.1*.

RESPIRATORY FUNCTIONS OF THE PLACENTA

The extensive vasculature in the villi and the relatively slow passage of maternal blood through the intervillous space permits a good exchange of oxygen and carbon dioxide between the fetal and the maternal blood by passive diffusion. The exchange is further enhanced by the maternal blood entering the intervillous space having a 90–100 per cent saturation and a pO_2 of 90–100mmHg. After the metabolic needs of the placenta have been met, the fetal erythrocytes take up the oxygen, which is 70 per cent saturated and has a pO_2 of 30–40mmHg, sufficient to meet all fetal needs. Carbon dioxide, like oxygen, passively diffuses across the placenta *(Fig 4.13)*.

Transfer Of Substances Through the Placenta				
		Placental transfer methods		
Maternal blood	Intervillous space	Passive	Active	Pinocytosis
H_2O, O_2, CO_2, urea, Na, K	⟶	+		
Glucose	Facilitated by carrier molecule		+	
Polysaccharides	Mono- and di-saccharides		+	
Protein ⟶	Aminoacids		+	
Fat ⟶	Free fatty acids		+	
Vitamin A ⟶	Carotene	+		
Vitamin B complex Vitamin C	⟶		+	
Iron, phosphorus	⟶		+	
Antibodies	Only IgG	+		+
Erythrocytes	⟶	±		+

Table 4.1 Transfer of substances through the placenta.

Hydrogen ions, bicarbonate and lactic acid diffuse across the placenta, so that the acid–base status of mother and fetus are closely related. As the transfer takes place slowly, the fetus is able to buffer any additional acidity from its reserves, unless maternal acidosis is aggravated by dehydration or acidoketosis, as may occur in late labour, when fetal acidosis may result.

The efficiency of these exchanges depends on a good maternal blood supply to the spiral arteries and a well-functioning placenta. Should the maternal blood supply to the arteries be reduced, as may occur in severe hypertensive states (Chapter 16), placental ageing (Chapter 21), uterine hyperactivity or cord compression (Chapter 22), fetal acidoketosis may occur independently of maternal acidosis.

NUTRIENT TRANSFER

Most nutrients are transferred from mother to fetus by active transfer methods, involving enzyme processes. Complex nutrients are broken down into simple com-

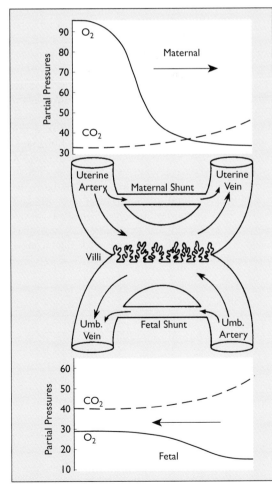

Fig 4.13 A schematic representation of the placental gas exchange. It can be seen that fetal blood has a much lower partial pressure of oxygen than that of the adult; the fetus in utero has been described as living in conditions of oxygenation resembling those of the top of Mount Everest.

ponents before transfer and are reconstituted in the fetal chorionic villi. Glucose is particularly important as it is the major source of energy for the growing fetus, supplying over 90 per cent of its requirements (10 per cent deriving from amino acids). The quantity of glucose transferred increases after the 30th gestational week. Towards the end of pregnancy about 10g of glucose per kilogram weight is retained daily and the excess over metabolic requirements is converted into glycogen and fat. The glycogen is stored in the liver and the fat is deposited around the heart and behind the scapula. In the last quarter of pregnancy, 2g of fat are synthesized daily, and thus by 40 weeks gestation, 15 per cent of the fetal body weight is fat. This provides an energy store of 21 000kJ and provides for the metabolic functions and the regulation of body temperature in the days after birth. In preterm and dysmature babies, the energy stores are lower, which may cause problems (see Chapter 21).

Oddly, lipids, as free fatty acids, are poorly transferred. Such as are transferred are resynthesized into phospho- and other lipids and are stored in fetal adipose stores until the 30th gestational week. After this time the fetal liver becomes capable of synthesizing lipids and now takes over.

DRUG TRANSFER THROUGH THE PLACENTA

The transfer of drugs through the placenta is no different from that of nutrients and all pass through to some extent. The rate is governed by the solubility of the ionized molecules in fat and the thickness of the trophoblast. In the second half of pregnancy the trophoblast becomes thinner, whilst the placental area increases in size; the drugs therefore pass through more rapidly.

Illegal drugs (narcotics, cocaine and marijuana) taken by the mother pass through the placenta and may affect fetal development. The extent of their effect is difficult to determine as most drug abusers also smoke and drink alcohol. The fetus tends to be growth retarded, may have a congenital abnormality, is likely to be born preterm and, if the mother takes narcotics, the infant may have withdrawal symptoms.

HORMONE SYNTHESIS

The placenta synthesizes a number of hormones, the function of which, in many cases, is not understood. The main hormones produced are **human chorionic gonadotrophin, human placental lactogen, oestrogen** and **progesterone**.

Human chorionic gonadotrophin

Human chorionic gonadotrophin (hCG) is synthesized from the early days of placentation. Its blood level reaches a peak between the 60th and 80th days of pregnancy when 500 000–1 000 000iu of hCG are secreted each day. The amount secreted then falls to between 80 000–120 000iu a day, a level which is maintained to term *(Fig 4.14)*. The peak is higher and lasts longer in multiple pregnancy and in gestational trophoblastic disease. After childbirth the level falls rapidly. Initially the function of hCG is to maintain the corpus luteum's secretion of progesterone and oestrogen. Once the placenta takes over this function, the level of hCG declines. HCG may also regulate oestrogen production by the placenta and suppress maternal immunological reactions directed against the fetus.

Oestrogen

In pregnancy the main source of oestrogen is the placenta. The synthesis of oestrogen requires the intervention of the fetus, as the placenta lacks specific enzymes (C17,20-desmolase and 16-hydroxylase) which are required in the synthesis of oestrogen from acetate and cholesterol. Of the three classical oestrogens, oestriol (E_3), oestradiol (E_2) and oestrone (E_1), the placenta produces more oestriol and retains it selectively. The result is that compared to a non-pregnant circulating E_3:E_2:E_1 ratio of 3:2:1, in pregnancy the ratio of E_3:E_2:E_1 is 30:2:1. This means that over 90 per cent of the oestrogen secreted in pregnancy is oestriol and the level rises progressively throughout pregnancy *(Fig 4.14)*.

Actions of oestrogen. At the cellular level, oestrogen, mainly in the form of oestradiol, enhances RNA and protein synthesis. Oestrogen alters the polymerization of acid mucopolysaccharides, which has the effect of increasing the hygroscopic properties and reducing the adherence of collagen fibres in connective tissue. This effect is most marked in the cervix, which becomes swollen and soft in pregnancy.

Oestrogen aids the growth of uterine muscle both by its enzymatic action on the muscle fibres and by increasing the blood flow.

In the breast, oestrogen increases the size and mobility of the nipple and causes duct and alveolar development. It may also play a part in causing water retention in pregnancy.

Progesterone

In pregnancy, progesterone is secreted initially by the corpus luteum but, by the 35th gestational day, the placental cytotrophoblast takes over all significant production from maternally supplied precursors, mainly cholesterol. At this stage of pregnancy the plasma progesterone level is 50ng/ml. From now on the level rises in a linear manner to reach 150ng/ml by term *(Fig 4.14)*.

Actions. In pregnancy the main action of progesterone is to cause muscle relaxation and because the uterus has a large number of progesterone receptors, its effect is most marked on the myometrium. Progesterone also relaxes the lower oesophageal sphincter, the stomach muscles, the intestines and the ureters. These effects account for some minor disturbances of pregnancy, for example, heartburn, delay in stomach emptying, reduced peristaltic activity leading to constipation and ureteric dilatation.

Progesterone regulates the storage of body fat to some extent and is hyperthermic, leading to a rise in body temperature of 0.5–1.0°C. It may have a hypnotic effect on brain cells and may be responsible for the placidity experienced by many pregnant women.

It is implicated in the hyperventilation some women experience.

Protein hormones

The placenta secretes a number of pregnancy-specific hormones, of which **human placental lactogen** (hPL) is the best understood. Its secretion is the reverse of that of hCG: when hCG falls from its peak, hPL continues to rise *(Fig 4.14)*. The most important pregnancy-preserving function of hPL is to mobilize free fatty acids from maternal body stores. This lipolytic effect reduces utilization of maternal glucose, which is then diverted for fetal energy needs. hPL also stimulates insulin secretion but inhibits its effects at peripheral sites, and aids in the transfer of amino acids to the fetus.

IMMUNOLOGY OF THE TROPHOBLAST

The fetus is an allograft, but paradoxically is not rejected by the maternal immune system. The explanation for this is unclear. One hypothesis is that the trophoblast secretes antigens which bind to sites on the trophoblast. Bound to these sites it induces the production of fetal immunosuppressor cells. A further mechanism may be that hCG partially blocks maternal immunological responses. These mechanisms prevent the 'foreign' cells of the conceptus from being recognized and rejected.

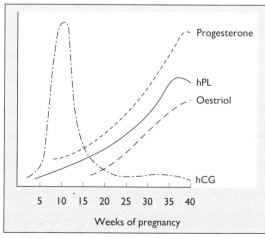

Fig 4.14 Oestriol, progesterone, hCG and hPL plasma levels in pregnancy.

5

THE EMBRYO AND FETUS

The embryo develops rapidly once implantation has occurred. A neural primitive streak develops in the second week after fertilization; during the third week the fetal heart develops and links up with a primitive vascular system; during the fourth week the gut has formed; and by the sixth week a urogenital sinus has formed.

By the seventh week after fertilization, most of the organs have formed and the embryo becomes a fetus. The early growth of the fetus is shown in *Table 5.1*.

FETAL NUTRITION

Fetal growth is determined by many factors, both genetic and environmental. Of the latter, adequate placental perfusion and placental function are crucial. Maternal nutrition is not a limiting factor except in cases of extreme starvation, although chronic undernutrition may be associated with anaemia and may lead to a low birth-weight baby.

The fetus, insulated in its protective amniotic sac and relatively weightless, has most of the energy supplied to it directed to growth. The energy is derived mainly from glucose. Only small amounts of lipids, as free fatty acids, cross the placenta until the fourth quarter of pregnancy. Any excess carbo-hydrate after the growth and metabolic energy needs of the fetus have been met is converted into lipids, and this conversion increases as term approaches.

From the 30th gestational week the fetal liver becomes increasingly efficient and converts glucose into glycogen, which is stored in the fetal heart muscle, the skeletal muscle and the placenta. Should fetal hypoxia occur the fetus is able to obtain energy from these stores (with the exception of skeletal muscle) for anaerobic glycolysis (Chapter 22).

Free fatty acids are formed and stored in brown and white adipose tissue. Brown fat is deposited around the fetal neck and behind the scapulae and the sternum and around the kidneys. It is metabo-lized to provide energy to maintain the infant's body temperature after birth. White adipose tissue forms the subcutaneous cover of the body of a term fetus, but in preterm babies the layer may be thin. It acts as an insulator and as a lipid store.

The fat stores of an 800g fetus (24–26 weeks' gestation) constitute 1 per cent of its body weight; by the 35th week fat constitutes 15 per cent of fetal body weight.

As the placenta clears the blood of bilirubin and other metabolic products which require a transferase activity, the fetal (and neonatal) liver is deficient in certain transferases. The result is that unless the

Characteristics Indicating Maturity of the Fetus By TV.u/S			
Period of gestation (in weeks from the first day of the last menstrual period	Period of gestation (in weeks from fertilization)	Length of fetus (crown of rump in centimetres)	Characteristics
8	6	2.3	Nose, external ears, fingers and toes are identifiable but featureless, head is flexed on the thorax
12	10	6.0	External ears show main features, eyelids fused, neck has formed, external genitals formed but undifferentiated
16	14	12.0	External genitals can be differentiated, skin transparent red
20	18	15.0	Skin becoming opaque, fine hair (lanugo) covers the body
24	22	21.0	Eyelids separated, eyebrows, eyelashes and fingernails present, skin wrinkled due to lack of subcutaneous fat
28	26	25.0	Eyes open, scalp hair growing

Table 5.1 Characteristics indicating maturity of the fetus. Length of the fetus determined by transvaginal ultrasound.

deficiencies are corrected in the early neonatal period, bilirubin may accumulate in the neonate's blood, which is of some consequence in haemolytic disease of the newborn (page 128).

Amino acids cross the placenta by active transfer and are converted into protein. Protein synthesis exceeds protein breakdown, and the fetus uses some of the breakdown amino acids for resynthesis.

The fetus also synthesizes a specific protein, alphafetoprotein (AFP) in its liver. The peak of AFP is reached between the 12th and 16th gestational week, after which a decline occurs to term. The protein is secreted in the fetal urine and swallowed by the fetus to be degraded in its gut. If the fetus is unable to swallow, as in cases of anencephaly, the level of AFP in the amniotic fluid rises.

THE CARDIOVASCULAR SYSTEM

The circulatory pattern of the fetus is shown diagramatically in *Fig 5.1*. It should be noted that over 50 per cent of the cardiac output passes through the umbilical arteries to perfuse the placenta. The cardiac output increases to term, at which time about 200ml/kg/min is usual. The heart rate lies between 110 and 150 beats per minute to maintain this output. The fetal blood pressure also increases though the pregnancy and after the 36th week has a mean of 75 mmHg systolic, 55 mmHg diastolic.

The red-cell count, the haemoglobin level and the packed cell volume increase as pregnancy advances. Most of the erythrocytes contain fetal haemoglobin (HbF). At 15 weeks' gestation all the

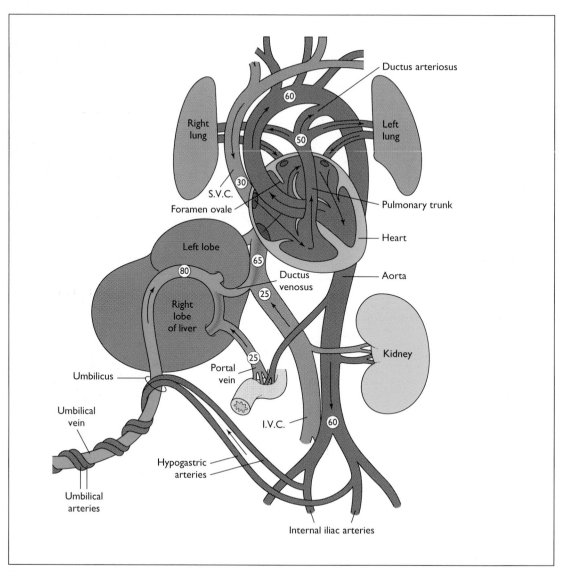

Fig 5.1 Normal circulation in the fetus in utero. IVC = inferior vena cava; SVC = superior vena cava. The figures give the approximate oxygen saturation of the blood at given points in the circulatory system.

cells contain HbF; by the 36th week 70 per cent of the erythrocytes contain HbF, and 30 per cent adult haemoglobin, but there are wide variations. Cells containing HbF are able to absorb more oxygen at a given pO_2. They are more resistant to haemolysis but less resistant to trauma than cells containing adult haemoglobin.

THE FETAL LUNGS

In the early embryo the lungs are made up of epithelial tubes surrounded by mesoderm. With further development the epithelium becomes folded and glandular to form primitive alveoli. By the 22nd gestational week a capillary system has developed and the lungs are capable of gas exchange. By term, three or four generations of alveoli have developed and been replaced. Their epithelium, which has a cuboidal appearance, becomes flattened with the first breath. By the 24th week, fluid fills the alveoli and the passages. By this stage the lungs begin to secrete a surface-active lipoprotein which facilitates lung expansion at birth and helps the air-containing lung to maintain its normal volume. However, until the 35th week the amount of surfactant may be insufficient for some babies to expand their lungs after birth and hyaline membrane disease may develop.

The fetus makes respiratory movements (breathing) from early in pregnancy. In early pregnancy they are sporadic, but by mid pregnancy become regular and increase in frequency as the pregnancy advances. Respiratory activity results in the inspiration of amniotic fluid into the bronchioles but no further, as the fluid secreted into the alveoli is under higher pressure. Episodes of hypoxia in late pregnancy or during the birth may stimulate gasping and amniotic fluid, often meconium-contaminated, is inhaled deeper into the lungs.

THE GASTROINTESTINAL TRACT

In the uterus the intestinal tract is relatively quiet. Some of the swallowed amniotic fluid, and the cellular material contained therein, enters the gut, where it is acted upon by enzymes and bacteria to produce meconium. The meconium remains in the gut unless an episode of severe hypoxia leads to contractions of the gut, at which time the meconium is expelled to mix with the amniotic fluid.

THE FETAL RENAL SYSTEM

The fetal kidney develops from the metanephros, and new glomeruli continue to be formed until the 36th gestational week. Urine is secreted and expelled into the amniotic fluid from the 16th week and probably earlier. Its rate of flow increases as term approaches.

THE FETAL IMMUNE SYSTEM

In early pregnancy the fetus has a poor capacity to produce antibodies in response to invasion by maternal antigens or by bacteria. From the 20th week (perhaps earlier) it becomes able to mount an immune response to a challenge. The fetal response is supplemented by the transfer of maternal antibody molecules (provided that they are not too large in size) to the fetus which provide it with passive protection which may persist for some weeks after birth.

THE FETAL MUSCULAR SYSTEM

Almost weightless in its amniotic capsule, the fetus makes movements from an early age. As the pregnancy advances the fetal movements become stronger, and occur more often. Bouts of activity are followed by periods when the fetus seems to be sleeping. Fetal movements strengthen the fetal muscles and a count of them gives an indication of fetal well-being (see page 149).

FETAL ENDOCRINE ACTIVITY

As noted earlier, the fetus is involved in the production of oestrogen. In addition, the fetus produces thyroid stimulating hormone from about the 14th week of pregnancy, which leads to the release of T_3 and T_4. The quantity of T_3 is small but a relatively large amount of reverse T_3 is secreted. Immediately after birth a surge of TSH is released, causing a surge in T_3 and T_4 and a fall in reverse T_3.

6

THE PHYSIOLOGICAL AND ANATOMICAL CHANGES IN PREGNANCY

HORMONAL CHANGES

Most of the anatomical changes which occur in pregnancy are due to the hormones secreted by the placenta. These hormones and their effects on the female body are described in Chapter 4. In addition, other endocrine glands synthesize hormones, in different quantities during pregnancy compared with the non pregnant state. These changes will now briefly be described.

THE PITUITARY GLAND

In pregnancy the secretion of FSH and LH falls to low levels, whilst the secretion of ACTH, thyrotrophin, melanocyte hormone and prolactin increases. Prolactin levels, for example, increase to the 30th gestational week and then more slowly to term. Prolactin may be a factor in the fall of FSH and LH to very low levels by the 8th week of pregnancy.

ADRENAL GLAND

Total corticosteroids increase progressively to term. This could account to some extent for a pregnant woman's tendency to develop abdominal striae, glycosuria, and hypertension.

THYROID GLAND

The thyroid gland enlarges during pregnancy, occasionally to twice its normal size. This enlargement is mainly due to colloid deposition caused by a lower plasma level of iodine, consequent on the increased ability of the kidneys in pregnancy to excrete. Oestrogen stimulates an increased secretion of thyroxin binding globulin. In consequence both T_3 and T_4 levels rise. The raised levels do not indicate hyperthyroidism as both the TSH and the free thyroxin levels are in the normal range. When tests are made to determine thyroid function these changes should be taken into account.

CHANGES IN THE GENITAL TRACT

UTERUS

The effect of the hormonal stimulation is most marked upon the tissues of the genital tract, and the uterine muscle fibres grow to 15 times their prepregnant length during pregnancy, whilst uterine weight increases from 50g before pregnancy to 950g at term *(Fig. 6.1)*. In the early weeks of pregnancy the growth is by hyperplasia and more particularly by hypertrophy of the muscle fibres so that the uterus

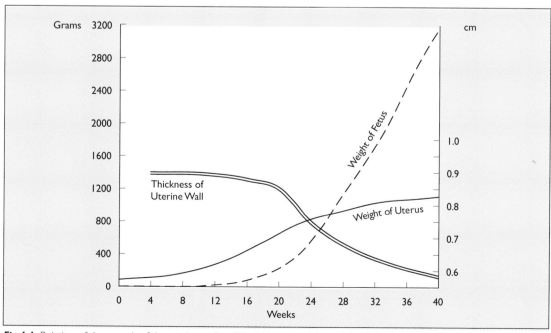

Fig 6.1 Relation of the growth of the uterine wall and its thickness and the weight of the fetus at varying times in normal pregnancy.

becomes a thick-walled spherical organ. From the 20th week, growth almost ceases and the uterus expands by distension, the stretching of the muscle fibres being due to the mechanical effect of the growing fetus. With distension the wall of the uterus becomes thinner and the shape cylindrical *(Fig. 6.2)*. The uterine blood vessels also undergo hypertrophy and become increasingly coiled in the first half of pregnancy, but no further growth occurs after this, and the additional length required to match the continuing uterine distension is obtained by uncoiling the vessels.

The uterus is derived from the two Mullerian ducts and the myometrium is made up of a thin external, largely longitudinal, layer; a thin inner, largely circular, layer and a thick, intricately interlaced middle layer, which comprises two spiral systems of interdigitating muscles derived from the two Mullerian ducts. The proportion of muscle to connective tissue is greatest in the fundal area and diminishes as the lower segment of the uterus and cervix is approached, the lower half of the cervix having no more than 10 per cent of muscle tissue.

The effect of the uterine distension is to stretch both interdigitating spiral systems, and the angle of crossing of the fibres, in the thinner lower segment area where the fibres cross at an angle of about 160° and are less stretched. Incision of the myometrium in this zone is anatomically more suitable, and experience of lower segment caesarean section confirms that healing is better *(Fig. 6.3)*.

The lower uterine segment is that part of the lower uterus and upper cervix lying between the line of attachment of the peritoneum of the uterovesical pouch superiorly and the histological internal os inferiorly. It is that part of the uterus where the proportion of muscle diminishes, being replaced increasingly by connective tissue (mainly collagen fibres) which forms 90 per cent of the cervical tissues *(Fig. 6.4)*. Because of this it becomes stretched in late pregnancy as the thickly muscled fundus draws it up from the relatively fixed cervix.

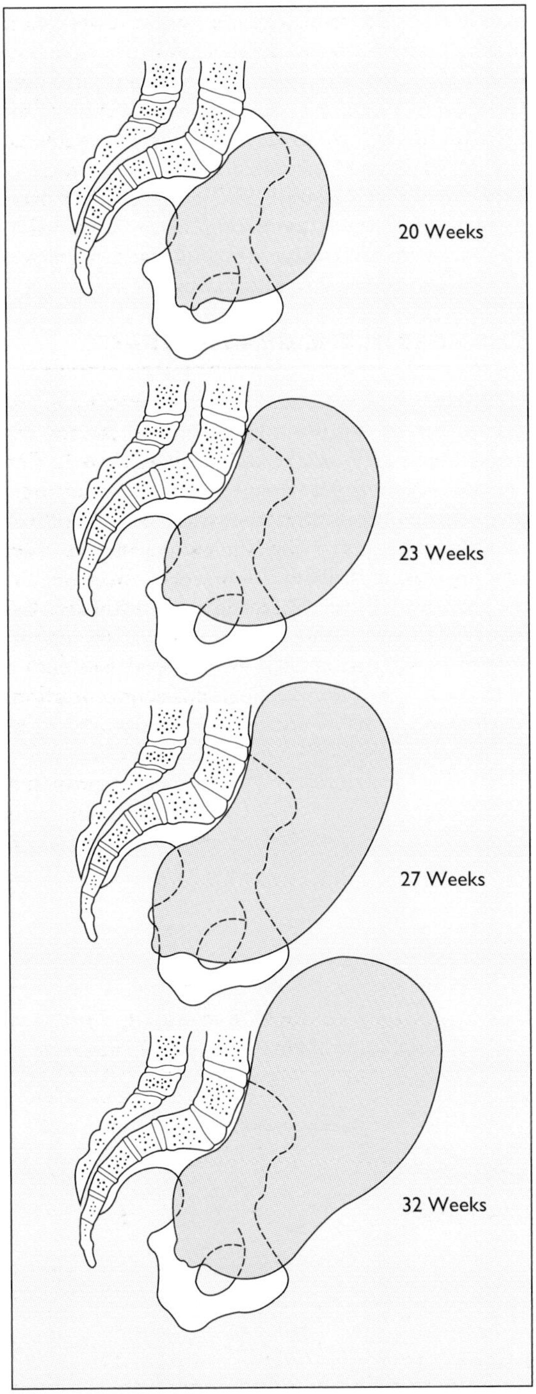

20 Weeks

23 Weeks

27 Weeks

32 Weeks

Fig 6.2 The enlargement of the uterus in normal pregnancy, drawn from radiographs.

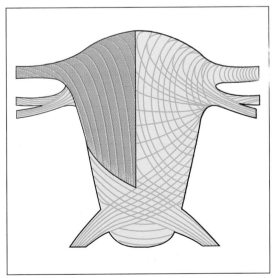

Fig 6.3 Representation of the obliquity of decussation and interweaving of myometrial fibres. The obtuse angle of decussation in the lower segment can be seen.

CERVIX

The cervix becomes softer and swollen in pregnancy so that the columnar epithelium lining the cervical canal becomes exposed to the vaginal secretions. This change in the cervix is due to oestradiol which increases the hygroscopic properties of the cervical connective tissue and loosens the acid mucopolysaccharides (glycosaminoglycans) of the collagen-binding ground substance.

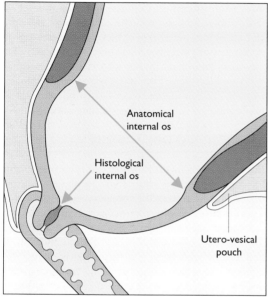

Fig 6.4 The lower uterine segment in late pregnancy (see also **Fig 8.7**).

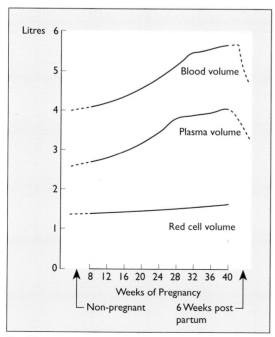

Fig 6.5 Blood changes in pregnancy (information obtained from Hytten and Leitch).

In addition, prostaglandins act on the collagen fibres, especially in the last weeks of pregnancy. The cervix becomes softer and more easily dilatable, the so-called 'ripening' of the cervix. In this way the cervix is more easily able to dilate in labour.

VAGINA

The vaginal mucosa becomes thicker, the vaginal muscle hypertrophies and there is an alteration in the composition of the surrounding connective tissue, with the result that the vagina dilates more easily to accommodate the fetus in parturition. The changes, initiated by oestrogen, occur early in pregnancy and there is an increased desquamation of the superficial vaginal mucosal cells with increased vaginal discharge in pregnancy. Should pathogens, whether bacterial, fungal (such as candida) or parasitic (such as trichomonads) enter the vagina they can more easily establish themselves, and vaginitis is consequently more frequently found.

THE CARDIOVASCULAR SYSTEM

The changes which occur during pregnancy to the blood volume, the plasma volume, and the red cell mass are shown in *Fig 6.5.* and *Table 6.1.* The plasma volume increases to fill the additional intravascular space created by the placenta and the blood vessels. The red cell mass increases to meet the increased demand for oxygen. Because the increase in the red cell mass is proportionately less than the increase in the plasma volume, the concentration of the erythrocytes in the blood falls with a reduction in the haemoglobin concentration. Although the haemoglobin concentration falls to about 120g/l at the 32nd week, the woman has a larger total haemoglobin than when not pregnant. Concurrently the number of white blood cells increases (to about 10 500 per ml) as does the blood platelet count.

Plasma Volume, Red Cell Volume, Total Blood Volume and Hematocrit in Pregnancy				
	Non-pregnant	Weeks of pregnancy		
		20	30	40
Plasma volume (ml)	2600	3150	3750	3850
Red cell mass (ml)	1400	1450	1550	1650
Total blood volume (ml)	4000	4600	5300	5500
Body hematocrit (%)	35.0	32.0	29.0	30.0
Venous hematocrit (%)	39.8	36.4	33.0	34.1

Table 6.1 Plasma volume, red cell volume, total blood volume and hematocrit in pregnancy.

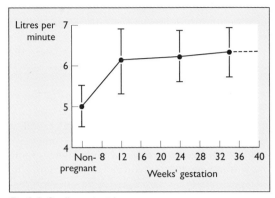

Fig 6.6 Cardiac output in pregnancy.

CARDIOVASCULAR DYNAMICS

To deal with the increased blood volume and the additional demand for oxygen, the cardiac output increases by 30–50 per cent in pregnancy, a rise from 5l/min at 8 weeks gestation to 6.5l/min at the 25th week *(Fig 6.6)*. Most of the increased cardiac output is due to an increased stroke volume, but the heart rate increases by about 15 per cent. The increased cardiac output is balanced by a decrease in the peripheral resistance *(Fig 6.7)*. For these reasons the woman's blood pressure is altered only minimally in the first three-quarters of pregnancy, unless pregnancy-induced hypertension occurs. After the 30th week of pregancy, there is a tendency for the blood pressure to rise.

In common with other blood vessels, the veins of the legs become distended. The leg veins are affected particularly in late pregnancy because of the obstruction to venous return caused by the higher pressure of

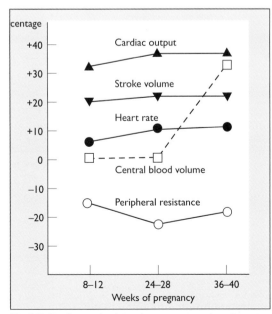

Fig 6.7 Cardiovascular dynamics: percentage alterations over non-pregnant levels occurring in pregnancy.

the venous blood returning from the uterus and the mechanical pressure of the uterus on the vena cava. This may lead to varicosities in the leg veins (and occasionally the vulval veins) of susceptible women.

THE REGIONAL DISTRIBUTION OF THE BLOOD

The uterus receives the greatest proportion of the blood flow, which is vital to perfuse the placenta properly. Renal blood and plasma flow increase to 400ml/min above non-pregnant levels by the 16th week of pregnancy and remain at this high level to term. Blood flow through the capillaries of the skin and mucous membranes increases, reaching a maximum of 500ml/min by the 36th week. The increased skin blood flow is associated with peripheral vasodilatation . This is the reason why pregnant women 'feel the heat', sweat easily and often profusely and may complain of nasal congestion.

THE RESPIRATORY SYSTEM

Breathing remains diaphragmatic during pregnancy, but because of the restricted movement of the diaphragm after the 30th week, pregnant women breathe more deeply, increasing tidal volume and ventilation rate, thus permitting an increased mixing of gases and an increased oxygen consumption of 20 per cent. It is thought that this effect is due to the increased secretion of progesterone. It may lead to overbreathing and a lower arterial pO_2. In late pregnancy the lower rib cage flares out to some extent, and may not return to its prepregnancy state, causing some concern to figure-conscious women.

THE ALIMENTARY SYSTEM

In the mouth, the gums may become 'spongy', probably induced by intracellular fluid retention, a possible progesterone effect. The lower oesophageal sphincter is relaxed, which may permit regurgitation of gastric contents and cause heartburn. Gastric secretion is reduced and food remains longer in the stomach. The intestinal musculature is relaxed, with lower motility. This permits a greater absorption of nutrients, but may lead to constipation.

THE RENAL SYSTEM

The smooth muscle of the renal pelvis and ureters relax, causing their dilatation. This increases the capacity of the renal pelvis and ureters from 12ml to 75ml and increases the chance of urinary stasis. The bladder musculature relaxes, which also encourages urinary stasis. The consequence is that urinary tract infection is more common in pregnancy. The muscles of the internal urethral sphincter relax and this, together with the pressure of the uterus on the bladder, may cause some degree of incontinence.

The renal blood flow increases to the 16th week of pregnancy and then levels off. The glomerular filtration rate increases by 60 per cent in early pregnancy and remains at the new level until the last 4 weeks of pregnancy when it falls. As tubular re-absorption is unaltered, the clearance of many solutes is increased. The increased glomerular filtration rate together with the natruretic effect of progesterone would cause an increased loss of sodium were it not for increased production of renal renin and, in consequence, angiotensin.

THE IMMUNE SYSTEM

Human chorionic gonadotrophin may reduce the immune response of pregnant women. In addition, serum levels of IgG, IgA, and IgM decrease from the 10th week of pregnancy, reaching their lowest level at the 30th week and remaining at this level to term. These changes may account for the anecdotal increase in the risk of infection among pregnant women.

WEIGHT GAIN IN PREGNANCY

The better absorption of nutrients from the gut, the reduction of muscle tone, and a reduction in thyroid activity produces a quiescence in the maternal metabolism. The female adapts to preserve and nourish the growing fetus.

During pregnancy a woman inevitably gains weight. A healthy woman may expect to gain 12.5kg (range 9–15kg) in pregnancy, of which 9kg is gained in the last 20 weeks. The 'ideal' weight gain is only a guide and individual variations within the weight range should be allowed for. However, a woman whose prepregnancy weight is in the normal range (body mass index or BMI 19–24.9) or who is overweight (BMI 25–29.9) should avoid excessive weight gain (>15kg) as she may find it difficult to regain her prepregnancy weight after the birth. This is of concern to many women who want to be reassured that they will regain their body shape and prepregnancy weight as soon as possible after the baby has been born.

After the birth there is a great variability in weight loss. Six weeks after the birth, an average woman weighs 3kg more than her prepregnancy weight. Six months after the birth, she will weigh about 1kg more than she weighed before she became pregnant.

The situation is different for obese and underweight women, both during pregnancy and after birth. An obese women (BMI >30) should be encouraged to limit her weight gain during pregnancy as she has an increased risk that pregnancy-induced hypertension may occur and that she will have a large baby. She should be advised to eat a prudent but not a very low calorie diet as such a diet does not confer any benefit on mother or fetus. An underweight woman (BMI <19) should avoid becoming pregnant until she has gained weight as she has a 20 percent of giving birth to a low birth-weight baby.

THE COMPONENTS OF WEIGHT GAIN IN PREGNANCY

Weight gain in pregnancy applies to several components:

- The products of conception – the fetus, placenta and amniotic fluid
- The maternal components – the uterus and breasts, the increased blood volume, the increased stores of fat, water retention.

The fetus, placenta and amniotic fluid

In the first 20 weeks of pregnancy, the fetal weight-gain is slow; in the second 20 weeks, it increases more rapidly. The weight gain of the placenta shows the reverse of that of the fetus *(Fig 6.8)*. The amniotic fluid increases rapidly from the 10th week, being 300ml at 20 weeks, 600ml at 30 weeks, and peaking at 1000ml at 35 weeks. After this a small decline in the total quantity of amniotic fluid occurs.

The maternal components

The weight of the *uterus* increases throughout pregnancy. It is more rapid in the first 20 weeks, when myohyperplasia is occurring, than in the second 20 weeks when most of the enlargement is due to stretching of the muscle fibres. The *breasts* increase in weight throughout pregnancy due to deposition of fat, increased retention of fluid and growth of the glandular elements. The *blood volume* increases throughout the pregnancy (Fig 6.5 on page 31). The amount of fat deposited in adipose tissues depends

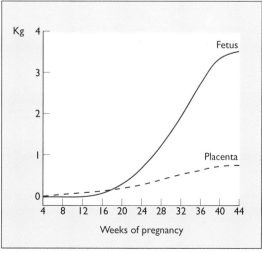

Fig 6.8 Fetal and placental weight curves compared at various gestation periods.

on the amount of fat and carbohydrate in the diet. A gain of 2.5–3.0kg of fat is usual, of which 90 percent is deposited in the first 30 weeks of pregnancy. The fat contains 90–105MJ of energy, which can be released after birth for various activities, including breast feeding. In normal pregnancy, the *total body fluid* increases by 6–8 litres, of which 2–4 litres is extracellular. Most of the fluid is retained before the 30th week but a pregnant woman who has no clinical oedema, retains 2–3 litres of extracellular fluid in the last 10 weeks of pregnancy.

The components and their weight at 40 weeks are shown in *Table 6.2*).

ENERGY

The resting metabolic rate in pregnancy is 10–15 per cent higher than in non-pregnant women. The extra energy required in the 40 weeks of pregnancy for the increased RMR, the growth of the fetus and placenta, the increase in size of the uterus and breasts, and the extra fat is about 250MJ. This works out at about 0.9MJ a day – an amount provided by two slices of bread and 100ml of milk. A pregnant woman does not need to eat for two!

There are exceptions to this statement. Poor women in developing countries, particularly where starvation is not uncommon, benefit by having food supplements during pregnancy. These supplements aid modestly in increasing the birth-weight of the baby, and giving her or him a greater chance of survival.

The Components of the Weight Gain in Pregnancy	
Fetus	3300g
Placenta	600g
Uterus	900g
Breasts (glandular tissue)	400g
Blood	1200g
Fat deposited	2500g
Fluid (extracellular)	2600g
	11 000g

Table 6.2 The components of the weight gain in pregnancy.

7

ANTENATAL CARE

The aims of antenatal care are to ensure that:
- The mother reaches the end of the pregnancy as healthy as, or even heathier than she was before she became pregnant.
- Any physical or psychological problems arising during the pregnancy are detected and treated.
- Any complication of pregnancy is either prevented or detected early and managed adequately.
- The mother gives birth to a healthy baby.
- The mother has the opportunity to discuss her anxieties and fears about the pregnancy.
- The mother is informed about any proposed procedures, the reason for the procedure and the probable outcome.
- The couple are prepared for the birth and for child rearing, including receiving information about diet, child care and family planning.

The provider of antenatal care may be a general practitioner or an obstetrician, working in conjunction with nurse–midwives. Shared antenatal care is becoming increasingly common. Antenatal care may take place in a doctor's rooms, in a hospital clinic or in a clinic conducted by a nurse–midwife. The opportunity should be available for an expectant mother to choose which facility she would prefer, but she should know that if a complication arose, she would be transferred if necessary, quickly and efficiently, to a facility staffed by experienced obstetricians.

Whichever facility a pregnant women has chosen she should have the opportunity to talk to a health professional about matters which concern her during the pregnancy in an unhurried way and have her questions answered by an informed, communicative doctor or nurse–midwife.

PSYCHOLOGICAL PREPARATION FOR MOTHERHOOD

Some women appear confident that their pregnancy will proceed normally and that the birth of the baby will be easy. Most women have concerns about the pregnancy and the process of childbirth. In the early weeks of pregnancy many women fear that the pregnancy may terminate as a miscarriage. Later in pregnancy many women fear that the baby will be malformed or retarded, or that childbirth will be dangerous and painful. A few women are concerned that after the birth they will not be able to regain their prepregnancy body shape. These fears may not be expressed unless the woman feels confident that she is able to ask her doctor about them and may expect to receive a reasoned answer. Fears about the difficulty and pain of childbirth can be reduced by simple explanations of the nature and course of labour.

Studies have shown that women who obtain social and psychological support during pregnancy are less likely than women who do not, to have negative feelings about their pregnancy and the forthcoming birth. They are more likely to feel that they are 'in control' during the pregnancy, to have a worry-free childbirth, to communicate more effectively with their doctor or nursing staff, and to be more satisfied with the care they receive.

Many women are helped by antenatal classes run in conjunction with antenatal clinics, or privately. Other women are helped by reading books written for women (one of which is *Everywoman. A Gynaecological Guide for Life*, published by Penguin Books).

DIET IN PREGNANCY

Many pregnant women are confused about what they should eat during pregnancy to make sure that the fetus is properly nourished. What should a pregnant woman eat? To a large extent this will depend on her cultural background, her eating behaviour and her income level. As a general principle, a woman should be advised to eat more fruits and vegetables, and less fatty foods including confectionery and cakes. This is termed a prudent diet *(Fig. 7.1)*. However, the woman should be able to choose and should follow a diet which is similar to that of her family.

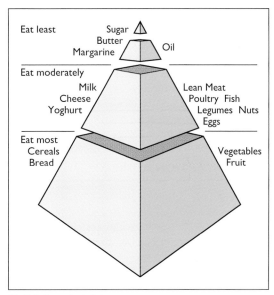

Fig 7.1 A prudent diet.

In terms of nutrients a woman should try to obtain each day the amounts listed below:

Kilojoules	9 000kJ (2200 kcal)
Protein	51g
Calcium	1g
Iron	30mg
Vitamin A	750μg
Vitamin D	10μg
Thiamin	1mg
Riboflavin	1.5mg
Niacin	1.5mg
Ascorbic acid	50mg
Folate	400 μg

Folate

If this is translated into the foods a housewife buys, a pregnant woman should try to eat the following each day:

Fish or meat 120g and an egg.
Milk 500ml or cheese 30g.
An orange, an apple or some other fruit.
Green leafy vegetables at least three times a week.

When the woman has complied with the above, she can eat any other foods to satisfy her hunger as long as this is in agreement with the earlier suggestions for a prudent diet.

Most pregnant women who eat a prudent diet do not need vitamin supplements, with the exception of women carrying a multiple pregnancy, who need extra folate. It should be noted that if a pregnant woman ingests excessive amounts of retinol (vitamin A) from dairy foods, oily fish and, particularly, liver, the fetus may develop abnormalities. The current recommendation is that pregnant women should avoid eating liver.

Healthy women living in the industrialized countries, whose haemoglobin is within the normal range, and who eat a good diet, do not need iron supplements. However, some women in the developed countries, particularly if poor and single, and most women living in the developing countries, require iron supplementation. This is discussed in Chapter 17.

Often pregnant women are prescribed additional calcium. Most women in the developed countries obtain all the calcium they need from the diet suggested above, as 75 per cent of the dietary calcium is absorbed when a woman is pregnant (compared with 58 per cent in non-pregnant women).

PRECONCEPTION ADVICE

In recent years clinics have been established to provide preconception advice (the cost benefits of such clinics have not been determined). Women who have a history of disease, diabetes for example, are advised that they should make sure that the diabetes is under control before trying to become pregnant. This is discussed on page 130.

Other women who probably benefit from the advice given by such clinics are those who have given birth to a baby with spina bifida or anencephaly. There is evidence that if these women increase their intake of folate in the weeks before becoming pregnant and for the first 10 weeks of pregnancy the risk of a second affected baby is considerably reduced. Folate intake can be increased if the woman eats more green leafy vegetables, but these should be eaten raw or lightly cooked as folate dissolves in boiling water. Doctors may prefer to prescribe folate 5mg a day during the prepregnancy weeks.

ANTENATAL SCREENING

A great deal of prenatal care is spent in detecting potentially dangerous conditions early; screening is one strategy used. In its simplest form blood pressure measurement is a screening strategy, as is discussed later. Currently, much interest is being shown in screening for congenital defects, such as Down's syndrome, neural tube defects and single gene defects, using DNA probes (Table 7.1).

SCREENING FOR GENETIC DEFECTS

Screening for Down's syndrome and certain other genetic defects (e.g. cystic fibrosis, thalassaemia, haemophilia, Huntington's disease, some muscular dystrophies) can be carried out by chorionic villus sampling or amniocentesis.

Chorionic villus sampling (CVS)

A sample of chorionic tissue is removed from the placental edge between the 9th and 11th week of pregnancy, by introducing a small catheter though the cervix and advancing it to the edge of the placenta under ultrasonic guidance (Fig. 7.2). About 20mg of chorionic tissue is sucked into a syringe. The karyotype of the sample is determined within 24 hours.

Amniocentesis

The procedure is carried out at about the 15th week of pregnancy. A needle is thrust through the abdominal wall and into the amniotic sac, guided by ultrasound to avoid the placenta and fetus, and a sample of amniotic fluid is removed. This is centrifuged and the fetal cells obtained are cultured for 3 weeks. They are then harvested and a karyotype is made.

CVS or amniocentesis?

The choice between chorionic villus sampling and amniocentesis is controversial. CVS is performed in the first quarter of pregnancy, and the karyotype is obtained within 24 hours, so the parental anxiety about the result is reduced. However, compared with amniocentesis, the karyotyping is slightly less accurate, and the risk of an abortion following CVS is claimed to be slightly higher (1 per cent above the background rate compared with 0.5 per cent following amniocentesis). There is also a suggestion that in

Possible Indications for Diagnostic Tests in First Half of Pregnancy
• Pregnancies in women over 35 years of age ✓
• Pregnancies at increased risk for fetal neural tube defects (i.e. previously affected child)
• History of Down's syndrome or other chromosomal abnormality in the family
• Previous pregnancy resulting in the birth of a chromosomally abnormal child, or one with multiple malformations
• Known chromosomal abnormality in either parent
• History of sex-linked disease (e.g. thalassaemia, haemophilia, Duchenne muscular dystrophy)
• Couples at risk for detectable inborn errors of metabolism

Table 7.1 Possible indications for diagnostic tests in first half of pregnancy.

[Handwritten note:] TRIPLE TEST on — Maternal Serum AFP, Unconj oestriol, Free β HCG.

late pregnancy oligohydramnios (and fetal limb-reduction defects) may be more common than after amniocentesis. On the other hand the karyotype is only obtained 3 weeks after amniocentesis, which increases the psychological stress on the parents, and if the fetus is abnormal and termination of pregnancy is suggested, the process is more painful and psychologically disturbing.

Down's syndrome

At present screening for Down's syndrome is only made in women over the age of 35, or who have had a previously affected baby. As this misses over half of all affected babies, a new strategy is under investigation. This is to measure, in all pregnant women at the 14th–16th week of pregnancy the following: alpha fetoprotein (AFP), unconjugated oestriol, and free beta HCG. If the serum levels of AFP and unconju-

gated oestriol are low and that of free beta HCG is high, Down's syndrome may be suspected and an amniocentesis made. There is some concern that if this strategy is adopted and all pregnant women are offered screening, although more babies with Down's syndrome will be detected, more women will require an amniocentesis, which may increase the miscarriage rate. In addition more women will be caused anxiety whilst waiting for the results.

Screening for open neural tube defects

Open neural tube defects (NTD) occur in 2–5 pregnancies per 1000. The Clinical Genetics Society in Britain has recommended that all pregnant women should be offered prenatal screening by measuring the AFP level at the 16th gestational week, but the cost effectiveness of this strategy has been questioned.

A blood sample is taken at about the 16 week of pregnancy. If the serum AFP level is more than 2.5 times the median for the week of pregnancy, the test is repeated. If it is raised in this sample an ultrasound examination is made to check the gestation period and exclude the presence of a multiple pregnancy. If this is excluded, an amniocentesis is made to measure the amniotic AFP. If the latter is raised (×3 the mean for the gestational week), 99.5 per cent of the fetuses will have an NTD. The parents may choose to have the pregnancy terminated.

[Handwritten note:] AMNIOCENTESIS FOR NTD

MEDICAL IMAGING IN PREGNANCY

The development of ultrasound imaging, particularly using newer technologies, for example real-time ultrasound and colour Doppler imaging, has made a considerable impact on the care of the pregnant women.

The role of ultrasound examination in obstetrics is shown in *Table 7.2*. Examples of ultrasound

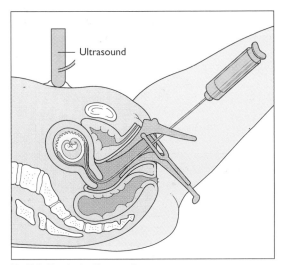

Ultrasound

Fig 7.2 Chorionic villus sampling.

	Some Indications for Ultrasound Imaging in Pregnancy
Weeks 0–10	Do not use ultrasound to diagnose pregnancy, but scan if there is any doubt about gestational age, particularly if chorionic villus sampling is considered. **Threatened abortion.** Scan at time of bleeding. Repeat scan only if fetal heart sounds are undetectable. **Recurrent abortion.** Scan at 6–10 weeks. **Ectopic gestation.** If suspected clinically, but not confirmed. **Hyperemesis gravidarum.** If admission required, scan to exclude hydatidiform mole and multiple pregnancy.
11–20	Many obstetricians routinely scan women at 18–20 weeks' gestation. In addition scanning may be used to: **Estimate fetal maturity,** if suspected from a uterus smaller (by 4 weeks) or larger than dates. **Detect multiple pregnancy,** if suspected clinically. **Exclude a fetal malformation,** if a previous malformation reported.
21–30	Detection of multiple pregnancy. Diagnosis of fetal death. Antepartum haemorrhage. Clinical polyhydramnios.
31–40	**Placental localization,** particularly if a low-lying placenta is detected at 18th week scan Antepartum haemorrhage. Moderate or severe Pregnancy Induced Hypertension. Diabetes. Severe renal disease. **Malpresentation** suspected at or after 36 weeks. **Multiple pregnancy,** repeat scan at 34 weeks gestation.

Table 7.2 Some indications for ultrasound imaging in pregnancy.

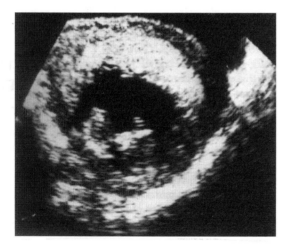

imaging are shown in *Figs 7.3 to Fig. 7.14.* Ultrasound imaging has reduced the need for radiology, the place of which in obstetrics is limited to determine the pelvic dimensions in a few cases of breech presentation at term and in some cases of 'trial of labour'. In these cases a single lateral x-ray is taken.

The one controversial issue about ultrasound use in obstetrics is whether a woman should be screened routinely at about the 18th week of pregnancy. The supporters of routine imaging claim that the information gained, such as the age of the fetus and the presence or absence of some fetal malformations, is

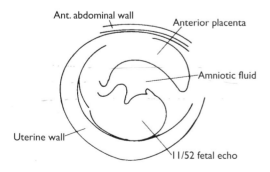

Fig 7.3 Transverse scan showing normal fetus at 11 weeks gestation. Line drawing shows the relevant identifying points.

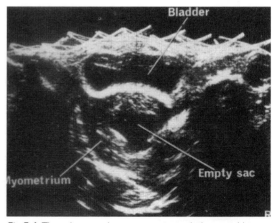

Fig 7.4 The echogram shows an empty amniotic sac at 11 weeks gestation. The patient aborted one week later.

valuable. The parents can be reassured that the fetus is healthy and normal, and can obtain a photograph for their Baby Book! The opponents of routine imaging point out that it is costly and that some fetal malformations may be missed (one British study showed that 10 per cent were misdiagnosed or missed). If this occurs and the parents are wrongly informed that the fetus is normal, it may cause great distress and may have unpleasant legal consequences.

THE CARE OF THE PREGNANT WOMAN

With this background information it is now possible to discuss the care of a pregnant woman. As mentioned in Chapter 2, most women have a good idea that they are pregnant when they visit a medical practitioner to confirm the diagnosis. At this visit the doctor will inquire about the present pregnancy, the history of previous pregnancies, family history,

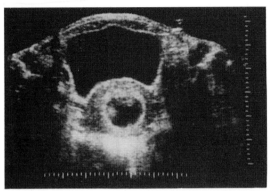
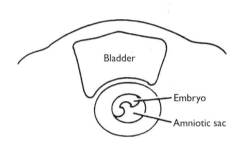

Fig 7.5 Early intra-uterine pregnancy (9 weeks) (transverse scan). Line drawing shows identification of relevant points.

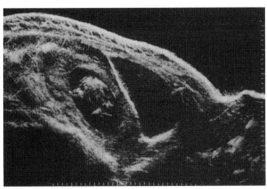
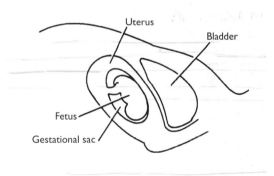

Fig 7.6 Twelve-week fetus (sagittal scan). Line drawing shows identification of relevant points.

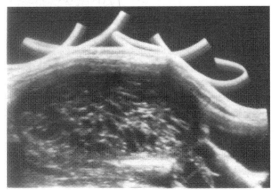
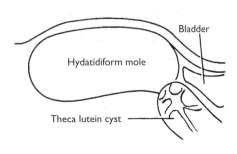

Fig 7.7 Benign trophoblastic disease (hydatidiform mole), 24 weeks' gestation. The honeycomb appearance is found using grey-scale ultrasound. Line drawing shows identification of relevant points.

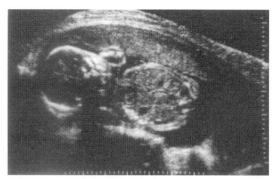

Fig 7.8 Breech at 24 weeks' gestation (sagittal scan).

and other matters, and will examine the woman (including her breasts) as already described.

Two examinations require further discussion. These are the (1) blood pressure and (2) weight; whether the patient should be weighed at each antenatal visit.

BLOOD PRESSURE

A significant rise in blood pressure from the base-line in early pregnancy, provides an early warning that the patient may develop pregnancy-induced hypertension (also known as pre-eclampsia or pre-eclamptic toxaemia). For this reason the woman's blood pressure should be measured at each antenatal visit.

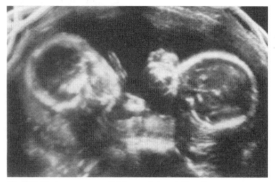

Fig 7.9 Twin pregnancy, 26½-weeks' gestation (transverse scan).

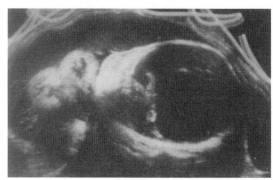

Fig 7.10 Hydrocephaly with distended cerebral ventricles and disturbances of the midline structures. The placenta is anterior (transverse scan).

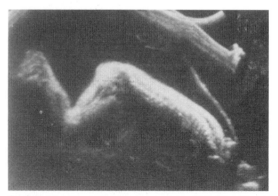

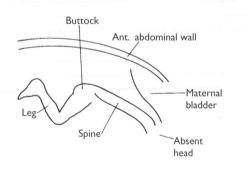

Fig 7.11 Ultrasound scan showing an anencephalic fetus. Line drawing indicates relevant landmarks.

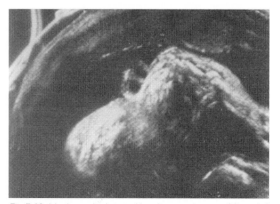

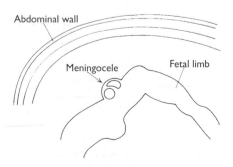

Fig 7.12 Meningocele detected by ultrasound scan at 30 weeks' gestation. Line drawing shows relevant landmarks.

In a normal pregnancy the blood pressure tends to remain at a constant level until the last quarter when a rise of less than 10mmHg may occur. By convention a systolic pressure of >140 and a diastolic pressure of >90 are considered to indicate hypertension. However, a rise from the baseline measurement of >30mmHg systolic pressure and >15mmHg diastolic pressure should be noted and a further reading made a few days later.

Problems in recording blood pressure which may make the readings erroneous occur in pregnant as well as in non-pregnant patients. These include the posture of the woman, the size of the cuff, the accuracy of the sphygmomanometer, the time of day and the emotional state of the patient ('White Coat' hypertension).

To reduce these variables, blood pressure recording equipment should be calibrated regularly, cuffs checked and the blood pressure taken with the patient seated or reclining with her arm at heart level. The brachial artery should be palpated and an appropriately sized cuff inflated until the pulsation disappears. Elevations of 2mmHg should be recorded, and if the rise is significantly above the baseline, a further estimation should be made after an interval.

The systolic pressure is easy to record. The diastolic pressure should be recorded when the beats change from a hard to a muffled thumping (Korotkoff IV). The use of Korotkoff IV to identify the diastolic pressure in hyperkinetic states such as pregnancy is recommended by the British and US Hypertension Societies. The disappearance of sounds may also be recorded.

WEIGHING THE PREGNANT PATIENT

It is customary to weigh a pregnant patient at each antenatal visit as it is believed that a small weight gain (or no gain) between visits is associated with retarded fetal growth, a weight gain of >1kg a week in the second half of pregnancy is an early marker for the possible development of pregnancy-induced hypertension. Careful studies show that the measurement of weight gain is of minimal value as a sign that the problems will develop and the medical indications for regular weighing can be abandoned. When the doctor chooses to continue to weigh the patient, a weight gain of <4kg may be expected before the 20th week of pregnancy; after that a gain of not more than 0.5kg a week should occur. Many pregnant women are concerned about their weight and wish to be weighed (or will weigh themselves). In such cases the doctor should offer to weigh the patient and offer sensible advice if the weight gain is 'abnormal'.

[handwritten margin note: wt. gain & wt. loss]

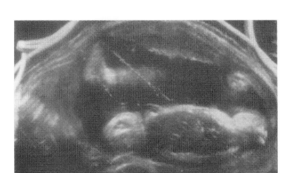

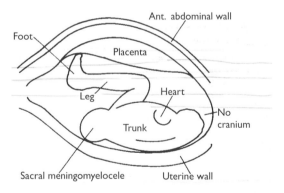

Fig 7.13 Anencephalic fetus with large sacral meningomyelocele detected by ultrasound scan. Line drawing shows relevant landmarks.

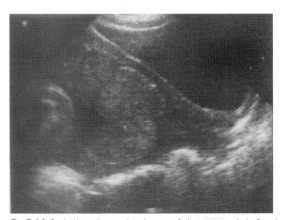

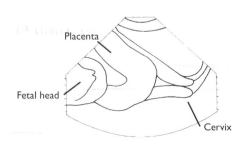

Fig 7.14 Sagittal section, major degree of placenta previa in fourth quarter of pregnancy. Cervix and vagina on right.

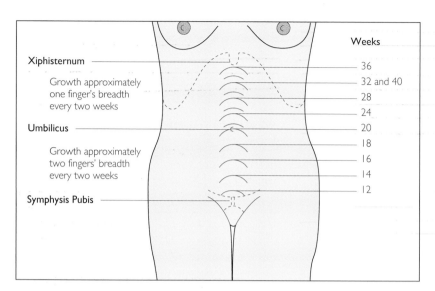

Xiphisternum

Growth approximately one finger's breadth every two weeks

Umbilicus

Growth approximately two fingers' breadth every two weeks

Symphysis Pubis

Weeks

36
32 and 40
28
24
20
18
16
14
12

Fig 7.15 The abdominal markings of uterine growth related to the number of weeks after the last menstrual period.

LABORATORY TESTS

Several laboratory tests are made at the first antenatal visit, either by the doctor consulted or, if the woman is referred to a hospital antenatal clinic or to an obstetrician as a private patient, at the referral visit (*Table 7.3*).

FREQUENCY OF ANTENATAL VISITS

There was in 1929 in Britain increasing concern that the maternal mortality rate had not fallen since 1880 (when it was 5 per 1000 live births). This led to the formation of a committee which recommended that a pregnant woman should visit an antenatal clinic every 4 weeks to the 28th week of pregnancy, then every 2 weeks to the 36th week, and thereafter weekly until delivered. Much discussion has arisen recently regarding whether this 65-year-old recom-

mendation is appropriate today. One suggestion is that whilst a primigravida should be seen according to this schedule, a 'normal' multigravida need only be seen once in the first 10 weeks of pregnancy, then at the 22 week and again at the 30th week before entering the later schedule of visits.

Whatever schedule is adopted, a pregnant woman should be asked at each antenatal visit if she has any problems she wishes to discuss and if she is feeling fetal movements. She should have her blood pressure measured, her urine tested for protein, the height of her fundus estimated *(Fig. 7.15)* or measured with a tape measure *(Fig. 7.16)* to evaluate the growth of the fetus. Some medical practitioners listen for fetal heart sounds after 'quickening' (fetal movements) has occurred. Quickening is usually noticed by an expectant mother between 16 and 24 weeks of preg-

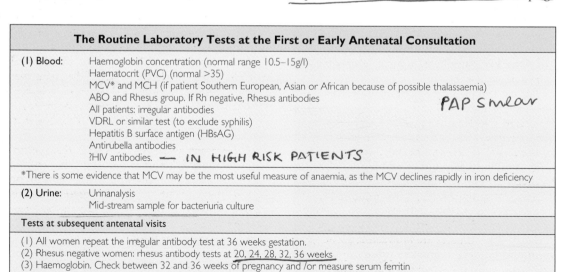

The Routine Laboratory Tests at the First or Early Antenatal Consultation	
(1) Blood:	Haemoglobin concentration (normal range 10.5–15g/l) Haematocrit (PVC) (normal >35) MCV* and MCH (if patient Southern European, Asian or African because of possible thalassaemia) ABO and Rhesus group. If Rh negative, Rhesus antibodies All patients: irregular antibodies *PAP smear* VDRL or similar test (to exclude syphilis) Hepatitis B surface antigen (HBsAG) Antirubella antibodies ?HIV antibodies. — *IN HIGH RISK PATIENTS*
*There is some evidence that MCV may be the most useful measure of anaemia, as the MCV declines rapidly in iron deficiency	
(2) Urine:	Urinanalysis Mid-stream sample for bacteriuria culture
Tests at subsequent antenatal visits	
(1) All women repeat the irregular antibody test at 36 weeks gestation. (2) Rhesus negative women: rhesus antibody tests at 20, 24, 28, 32, 36 weeks (3) Haemoglobin. Check between 32 and 36 weeks of pregnancy and /or measure serum ferritin (4) Random blood sugar when 'booking' or at about 28 weeks	

Table 7.3 The routine laboratory tests at the first or early antenatal consultation.

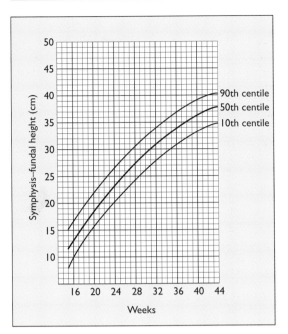

Fig 7.16 Gestational age estimated from symphysis–fundal height.

DOPPLER

nancy. Other doctors apply a fetal heart sound machine so that both doctor and patient can listen to the fetal heart sounds.

In addition, after the 28th week the doctor customarily palpates the woman's abdomen to determine the growth, presentation and position of the fetus in the uterus. The technique used is discussed later in this chapter.

PREPARATION FOR BREAST-FEEDING

During pregnancy the medical practitioner should ask the patient if she wishes to breast-feed her infant. If she intends to breast-feed, her wish should be positively reinforced. The benefits of breast-feeding should be discussed:

- Breast milk provides the ideal nutrition for infants and contributes to their healthy growth and development.
- For most women breast-feeding provides a sense of satisfaction and pleasure.
- Among poorer women, particularly in the developing countries, exclusive breast-feeding contributes to a woman's health by increasing the space between pregnancies.
- Breast-feeding reduces the chance that the baby will develop infections, particularly gastrointestinal infections, thereby lowering infant mortality.

The doctor should examine the woman's breasts and note if her nipples are protractile, pseudoprotractile or inverted. Inverted nipples may be made protractile if, in the second half of pregnancy, the woman places her thumbs on the opposite sides of the base of her nipples and draws her thumbs apart in both the vertical and horizontal planes, to break

INSTRUCTIONS ON BREAST CARE:

supposed adhesions which are preventing the nipples from everting. Some doctors advise the woman to wear nipple shields, but the benefit of these is uncertain.

Nipple care should be discussed. The nipples should be washed daily with water to remove any crusts which have formed, and if the woman wishes she may apply anhydrous lanolin. It also helps to expose the nipples to the air.

The medical practitioner may provide the woman with a pamphlet about the breast-feeding groups which are available in the area.

Should the woman choose not to breast feed, for whatever reason, the doctor should avoid making her feel guilty and should discuss the importance of preparing the breast milk substitute according to the manufacturer's directions.

THE GROWTH OF THE FETUS DURING PREGNANCY

As mentioned in the previous paragraphs, fetal growth can be determined roughly by the height of the fundus or the distance between the symphysis pubis to the top of the uterus. A more accurate assessment of the fetal growth and weight can be obtained by ultrasound imaging *(see Fig. 7.17)*, but this is only required in some pregnancies, for example, if the doctor suspects that the fetus is growth retarded. It was also mentioned that until about the 28th week of pregnancy the fetal head (or buttocks) related to the mother's pelvis was of little clinical importance. After that time it becomes increasingly important, and should be monitored by the doctor. For the purposes of communication descriptive terms are used.

These are as follows:

The **lie** of the fetus refers to the relationship of its long axis to the mother. By the 38th week the fetus may have a longitudinal lie (cephalic or breech) or an oblique or a transverse lie *(see Fig. 7.18)*.

The **presentation** of the fetus relates to the fetal part which occupies the lower part of the uterus over the pelvic brim. If the fetal head presents it is termed a cephalic presentation; if the buttocks present it is a breech presentation; if a shoulder presents it termed a shoulder presentation.

The **presenting part of the fetus** is that portion of the fetus which is presenting against the cervix in the first stage of labour, or against the vagina in the second stage of labour. If the presentation is cephalic, the presenting part is usually the posterior part of the fetal head, the vertex or occiput, but it may be the face or the brow.

The **attitude** of the fetus is defined as the relation of various fetal parts to other parts. Normally the fetus lies with all its joints flexed, but in some breech presentations the fetal legs are extended along its body.

43

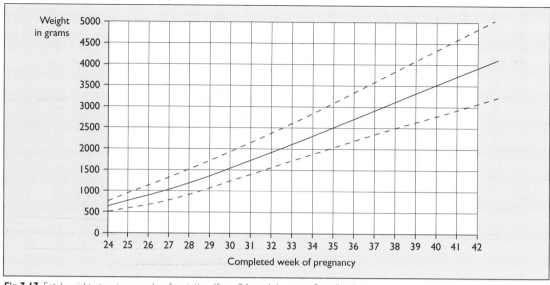

Fig 7.17 Fetal weight at various weeks of gestation (from 24 weeks) among Scandinavian woman as determined by ultrasound.

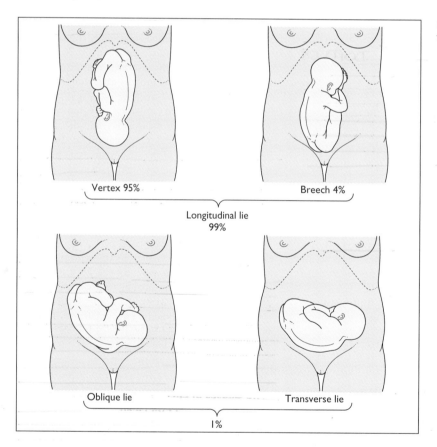

Fig 7.18 The presentation of the fetus.

The **position of the presenting part** of the fetus is of little clinical significance until labour is established. It refers to the relationship of the presenting part to the bony pelvic walls, and will be discussed in Chapter 10.

THE TECHNIQUE OF ABDOMINAL EXAMINATION

The patient assumes a reclining position having emptied her bladder. The abdominal examination to determine the lie, the presentation and position of the fetus is made by four 'manoeuvres' which are shown in *(Figs 7.19-22)* The information is recorded in the patient's antenatal records.

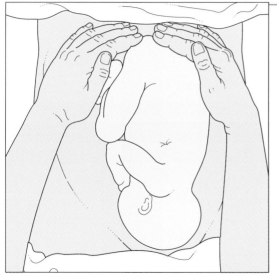

Fig 7.19 First manoeuvre – Fundal palpation. The height of the fundus is estimated and the fundal area gently palpated in an attempt to identify which pole of the fetus (breech or head) is occupying the fundus.

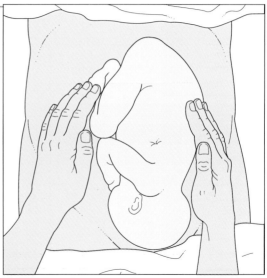

Fig 7.20 Second manoeuvre – Lateral palpation. The examiner's hands gently slip down the sides of the uterus with quick palpation to try to identify on which side the firm back of the fetus or the soft belly and knobbly limbs can be detected.

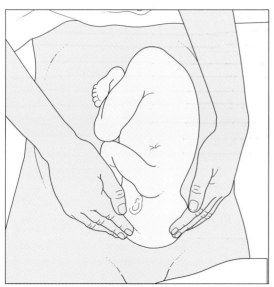

Fig 7.21 Pelvic manoeuvre. The examiner turns to face the patient's feet and slides his hands gently on the lower part of the uterus, pressing down on each side to determine the presenting part. If it is the fetal head it can be ballotted between the fingers.

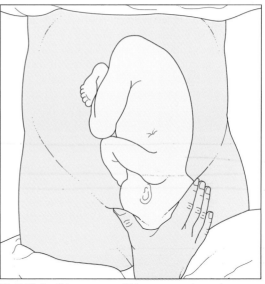

Fig 7.22 Pawlik's manoeuvre. This manoeuvre is not always necessary and must be performed gently. The presenting part is moved between the fingers and thumb of the examiner's hand, to determine whether it is the fetal head or breech and the degree of descent into the maternal pelvis.

ASSESSMENT OF THE SHAPE AND SIZE OF THE MATERNAL PELVIS

This procedure should be delayed until the 38th week of pregnancy because firstly it is then more comfortable for the patient, and secondly the fetal presenting part may be expected to have descended into the pelvis to some degree in most primigravidae. In multigravidae the fetal presenting part may not descend into the pelvis until labour supervenes. Possible reasons for non descent in primigravidae are shown in *Table 7.4*. In most cases, pelvic assessment is only required in primigravidae, as the history of previous labours will give information about the pelvis.

The Causes of Lack of Engagement of the Fetal Head
(1) Lack of adequate formation of the lower uterine segment
(2) Malposition of the fetal head
(3) Cephalopelvic disproportion or contracted pelvis
(4) Tumours in the pelvis obstructing the entry of the fetal head
(5) Placenta praevia
(6) Incorrect estimation of the period of gestation

Table 7.4 The causes of lack of engagement of the fetal head.

[handwritten margin note: Causes FETAL Maternal placenta]

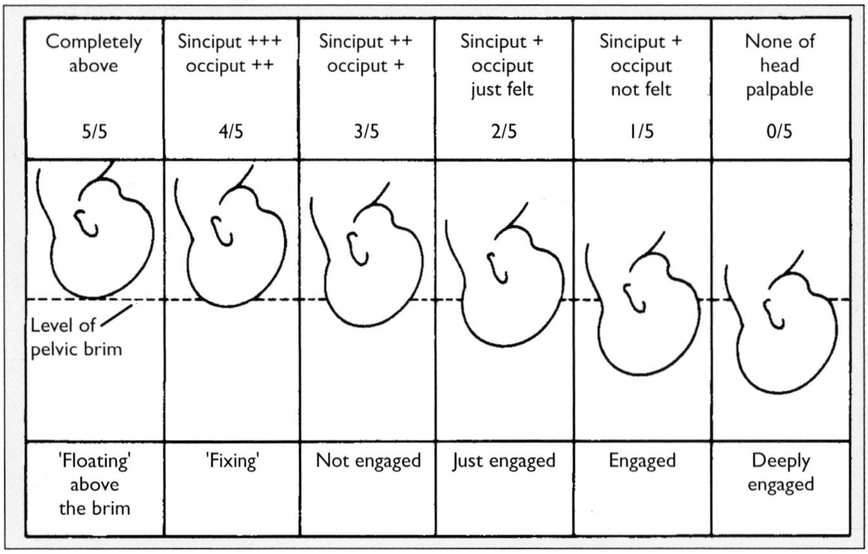

Completely above 5/5	Sinciput +++ occiput ++ 4/5	Sinciput ++ occiput + 3/5	Sinciput + occiput just felt 2/5	Sinciput + occiput not felt 1/5	None of head palpable 0/5
Level of pelvic brim					
'Floating' above the brim	'Fixing'	Not engaged	Just engaged	Engaged	Deeply engaged

Fig 7.23 Descent of the fetal head

The patient lies in a reclining position, with her legs flexed and her bladder empty. The doctor inserts two gloved fingers, lubricated with chlorhexidine cream, into the vagina. The condition of the vaginal walls and the cervix is noted. The degree of engagement of the fetal presenting part is recorded *(Fig. 7.23)*. If the fetal head presents and has not descended into the pelvis, a test can be made to determine if it will descend. This test estimates the relative sizes of fetal head and maternal pelvis *(Fig. 7.24)*.

The architecture of the pelvis is explored by the fingers reaching diagonally upwards and backwards to determine if the sacral promontory can be reached. The curve of the sacrum is next palpated, and the prominence of the ischial spines noted. The sacrospinous ligament is palpated and should accommodate two of the examiner's fingers. Finally the distance between the two sacral tuberosities is measured by the clenched fist.

AGE AND REPRODUCTIVE PERFORMANCE

TEENAGED PREGNANCY

More teenaged women are becoming sexually active at an earlier age than in previous decades. Studies in Northern Europe and in North America have shown that by the age of 17, 50 per cent of teenaged women have had sexual intercourse and that by the age of 20, the proportion has risen to 70 per cent. Only one woman in four uses contraceptives in the first 4–6 months of starting sexual intercourse. These two facts account for the increasing numbers of young women who become pregnant. In Australia and Britain, 5 per cent of teenaged women, and in the USA 9 per cent of teenaged women become pregnant each year. Of these woman, 35–45 per cent obtain an induced abortion; 5 per cent miscarry; and the remainder continue the pregnancy and give birth.

Pregnant women under the age of 18 have an increased risk of developing complications of pregnancy and childbirth. The woman is more likely to develop pregnancy-induced hypertension or anaemia and to give birth to a low birth weight baby. The reasons appear to be:

- Low socioeconomic status.
- A nutritionally poor diet.
- Substance and/or drug abuse.
- A lack of antenatal care.

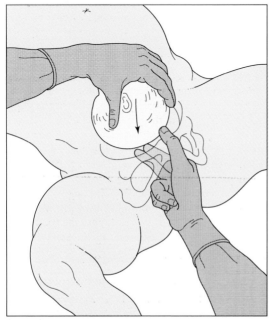

Fig 7.24 Estimating the relative size of the fetal head and the maternal pelvis by Muller-Kerr 'head fitting' test

The problems can be avoided if the adolescent woman accepts the need for and receives antenatal care from helpful medical attendants and social workers. If this occurs the proportion of adolescent pregnant woman developing complications in pregnancy is no greater than among women aged 20–35.

PREGNANCY IN OLDER WOMEN

In the past decade the proportion of women choosing to delay their first pregnancy until they are in their thirties has increased in most developed countries. The women tend to belong to the upper socioeconomic group, to be well educated and to have a career. Births to women aged over 30 now account for between 25 and 35 per cent of all births, (and the proportion of all births to women over the age of 35 is between 5 and 15 per cent). Births to primigravidae aged 35 or more account for about 3 per cent of all births. These 'older primigravidae' have an increased risk of having essential hypertension, of developing pregnancy-induced hypertension, gestational diabetes and antepartum haemorrhage. They are also more likely to have a baby with Down's syndrome, but they have no increased risk of a preterm birth or of fetal growth retardation.

They have an increased chance of having a caesarean section or a vaginal operative delivery, but this may be due to concern by the obstetrician that the woman's fecundity is reduced and the desire to obtain a 'perfect baby', as much as to a medical or obstetric complication.

Provided pregnant women over the age of 35 attend antenatal care early in pregnancy and receive sound genetic diagnosis and counselling, the outcome in terms of a live healthy mother and a live healthy child is excellent.

PREPARING FOR CHILDBIRTH

A woman who knows what to expect in childbirth, is better able to cooperate and to find the experience less painful. Antenatal classes are available in many hospitals and are provided by private obstetric physiotherapists for childbirth training. Childbirth training has broadened in recent years along with the expansion of the original technique of psychoprophylaxis first developed in Russia. It is based on the belief that fear and anxiety about pain and danger in childbirth, learned before the woman becomes pregnant and during pregnancy, sink deeply into her memory and produce a 'conditioned reflex'. Because of this reflex, every time a woman thinks of childbirth a mental image of pain and danger is conjured up, so that she enters labour anxious and tense. The tension and fear may increase the pain and delay the birth of the baby. Psychoprophylaxis seeks to eliminate the 'conditioned reflex' and to replace the negative image of childbirth with a more positive one. This is achieved by education during pregnancy in the hope that knowledge and insight will change the woman's perceptions of labour. Psychoprophylaxis also seeks to alter the brain's perception of pain and to convert it into a sensation of discomfort, which can be relieved by muscular activity. This is based on the concept of 'pain dissociation'. Pain becomes less intense if the woman keeps her mind busy by concentrating on something else. The suggested mental activity usually involves concentrating on a learned pattern of breathing, counting breaths, focusing on a particular point in the room or consciously commanding the body to release its tension. However, it is very difficult for most women to maintain control and remain in a calm state during the particularly painful stages of labour. The distraction techniques of psychoprophylaxis are therefore unrealistic and unsatisfactory for many women during childbirth.

As anthropologists, psychologists, physiotherapists and midwives have become increasingly active in the development of prepared childbirth, new strategies for pain management have been developed which offer more than the original psychoprophylaxis concept.

The social enviornment in which the baby will be born, and its effect on the woman, is now becoming an important consideration. Many women want their partner or some other 'support person' to be with them during childbirth. The presence of an informed loved one during labour gives the woman familiar and personal support to reduce the clinical environment of a delivery ward.

The discomfort and pain of childbirth is decreased if the attending nursing and medical staff treat the woman as an intelligent individual, who has needs and who can make choices, and who is perceived as a woman having a baby, rather than as a patient requiring medical attention. Some hospitals are trying to make the place of birth as non-clinical as possible by providing a supportive environment with floor mattresses, functional beds, soft fabrics and colours, and a shower. These innovations decrease a woman's anxiety and enable her to cope more efficiently with the process of childbirth.

Techniques of auditory and visual imagery provide an additional means of managing pain in labour. Instead of dissociating from her pain (as in psychoprophylaxis) the woman uses the sensations of labour to assist her in creating an image of what is happening inside her body. For example, she may visualize her cervix opening each time she has a contraction; the baby's head moving deeper into her pelvis; or the baby opening her vagina in the second stage of labour.

Another development has been the use of relaxation techniques. In psychoprophylaxis, relaxation was taught as a method of 'control'. The woman used quiet, controlled breathing to convince herself that she was not experiencing pain. More recently, relaxation has been used by the woman as a method os 'letting go' and so reducing the pain. She may move and rock to achieve relaxation; she may stamp her feet, or bang her fists to release stress and diffuse the pain. She may discover that for her, the most effective form of pain control is a combination of floor positions, rhythmic groaning and belly rocking.

The proponents of active involvement in childbirth believe that the woman, if possible, should be given a free choice in the position she wishes to adopt and the movements she wishes to make during labour and the birth of the baby. The woman may choose to lie on her side, to squat, or to position herself on her hands and knees. She may prefer to be supported in a nearly upright position, with her partner in front of her or behind her. In this technique there is much less focus on breathing as an 'exercise' or 'pattern', and more focus on breathing as a method which helps the woman 'go with the flow'.

A current approach used by many obstetric physiotherapists is to stress women's differences, rather than adopting a rigid technique. Attempts are made to find out the woman's most preferred mode of behaviour, and to encourage her to use these in childbirth. A woman who is 'tactile', for example, will probably respond well to massage, hot packs applied to her back, and showers and will tend to move about a good deal during labour. Other women prefer 'visualization', eye to eye focusing, or respond to key words such as 'relax', 'go soft', 'let go'. A third group of women are able to relieve the pain of labour more effectively by using auditory strategies. They respond to their support person 'pacing' them during a contraction and to giving themselves positive messages.

When a woman responds to the pain in a way she naturally prefers, her behaviour ceases to be due to a technique or a method. This reduces the anxiety that comes from having to perform a technique with which she is not comfortable, and which she fears she may not perform well.

The philosophy adopted by numbers of childbirth educators is to provide information and to give permission to the woman to be herself. Some women prefer not to attend class or to employ a private childbirth educator. For them, training videotapes are available which enable the woman and her partner to learn at home. One such videotape is *Preparing for Childbirth with Julia Sundin*.

SIGNS THAT LABOUR IS ABOUT TO START

The signs which indicate that labour is soon to start or has started are described on p 69. An expectant mother should have these signs described to her or have access to a book which describes them, so that she can be comfortable knowing when probably she is in labour. A question asked by many women during an antenatal visit concerns whether they will be given drugs to relieve the pain of labour. They should be reassured that analgesics are readily available should they request them. This matter is discussed on pp 82–84.

Many women are fearful that they will be left alone during the course of childbirth. Today, many women want their husband or partner or a 'significant other person' to be with them through the childbirth process, and most hospitals agree to this.

ANTENATAL INFORMATION

Certain matters affecting the mother during pregnancy should be discussed at the early visits.

ALCOHOL

Heavy alcohol consumption in pregnancy (> 120g or 12 standard drinks a day) is associated with fetal growth retardation, developmental delay and neurological complications in the baby. There is some evidence that moderate alcohol consumption (> 100–120g a day) may be associated with an increased risk of spontaneous abortion, and a smaller fetal head circumference. A consumption of 20g a day or less does not appear to have any damaging effects on the fetus or mother. Nevertheless, a pregnant woman should be advised to limit her consumption of alcohol during pregnancy.

CLOTHING

In general, the patient should wear the clothes she prefers and which enhance her attractiveness. These clothes should be comfortable and non-constricting. Unless she is accustomed to wearing a girdle or has abdominal muscles stretched by previous pregnancies, a maternity support is not needed. She may wear what shoes she likes, but should be told that as pregnancy advances and her centre of balance alters, she should avoid high heels except on special occasions.

DENTAL CARE

An early visit to the dentist is advised, so that any dental care required can be carried out in the first half of pregnancy.

EMPLOYMENT

In current economic conditions many pregnant women choose to or have to work. Provided the woman does not become too tired, and that her enlarging abdomen does not interfere with the job, and provided that industrial conditions in the office, factory or store are appropriate, work during pregnancy will harm neither the mother nor the fetus. In most developed countries paid maternity leave is granted for 6 weeks before the expected date of the childbirth.

EXERCISE

Exercise is to be encouraged if this is the usual habit of the patient, but need not be insisted upon if the patient is usually sedentary. She should take walks, and may play ball games if she wishes. She should neither become a fanatic for exercise nor become a vegetable. If she enjoys swimming, she may continue to swim. In general, she should not alter her regimen of exercise just because she is pregnant, unless the exercise regimen is very strenuous and may raise the woman's body temperature significantly.

IMMUNIZATION

If about to travel overseas, anti-typhoid or cholera inoculations may be given. All pregnant women who have not been immunized against poliomyelitis, or whose immunity has lapsed, should be immunized in early pregnancy.

Anti typhoid   Polio
cholera   ✱ Malaria

SEXUALITY DURING PREGNANCY

Many doctors fail to discuss sexuality during pregnancy, and many women feel inhibited about asking. Because of this many couples are inadequately informed, and have considerable misconceptions.

Studies have shown that many women have reduced sexual desire and activity, especially in the early weeks of pregnancy and after the 30th week. The reason for this decline in libido is unclear. Some women find sexual intercourse uncomfortable, others fear that coitus and orgasm may damage the fetus or bring on premature labour. Others see themselves as unattractive; or find the physical awkwardness of coitus in late pregnancy inhibiting.

It is appropriate to talk with the couple. There is no evidence that coitus, cunnilingus or masturbation, whether leading to orgasm or not, have any damaging effect on the fetus, or induce labour prematurely. All forms of sexual enjoyment are permissible in pregnancy, with the proviso that, during cunnilingus, the man should be warned not to blow, forcing air into the woman's vagina, as this has led to air embolism in pregnancy.

other drugs of addiction :

Many pregnant women want additional closeness from their partner, and he should be supportive and gentle at all times. In late pregnancy, coitus with the man on top may be uncomfortable, but other coital positions are not, and non-coital sexual satisfaction may be preferred. Coitus can continue, if the couple wish, up to term without any damage to mother or baby.

SMOKING

Pregnant women should be advised not to smoke cigarettes, or if they are unable to break the habit, to restrict smoking to one cigarette after a main meal. This advice is given because cigarette smokers (especially women who smoke more than 20 cigarettes a day) have a slightly greater chance of aborting, or their baby's weight, at all stages of gestation, is between 150 and 300g less than the weight of a baby of a non-smoker, and the perinatal death rate, may be slightly higher. One reason for the damaging effect of smoking in pregnancy is that smokers have a reduced intervillous blood flow and higher blood levels of carbon monoxide. Smoking is associated with a 3-fold risk of the baby having a cleft palate. These findings suggest that if the adverse effects of cigarette smoking are to be minimized, smoking should be avoided from the time of conception. However, smoking behaviour is affected by many psycho-social factors, and the woman may find smoking an appropriate method for her to reduce stress and tension, so that the success of a non-smoking campaign in pregnancy may be limited. This is important to know as fortunately there is no evidence that smoking during pregnancy has any effect on the long-term mental or motor development of the child.

TRAVELLING

Provided the journey can be made in a leisurely and comfortable way, there need be no restriction on travelling during pregnancy.

8

THE MECHANICAL FACTORS IN CHILDBIRTH

To be born, the fetus has to negotiate the birth canal propelled by contractions of the uterus. Factors which can delay or prevent this are:

P • The shape and size of the bony and soft tissues of the woman's pelvis (the passages).
P • The size of the fetus (the passenger).
P • The quality and frequency of the uterine contractions (the powers).

THE PASSAGES

THE BONY PELVIS

The bony pelvis is made up of four bones, i.e. the two innominate bones, the sacrum and the coccyx,

united at three joints. When a woman stands erect, the pelvis is tilted forward. The pelvic inlet makes an angle of about 55° with the horizontal, so that the ischial spines are at the same horizontal level as the lower border of the pubic symphysis. The angle varies among individuals and between races; for example, black Africans have a lesser angle. An angle of >55° may make the descent of the fetal head into the pelvis difficult *(Fig. 8.1)*.

The 'true' pelvis is bounded by the pubic crest, the iliopectineal line and the sacral promontory. An 'ideal obstetric' pelvis is described in *Table 8.1* and the brim is shown in *Figure 8.2*. The true pelvis is cylindrical in shape, with a bluntly curved lower end and is slightly

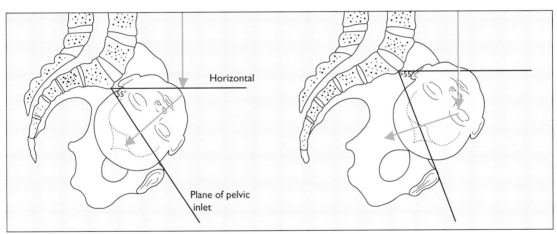

Fig 8.1 Diagram showing the effect of the inclination of the pelvic brim on the engagement of the fetal head.

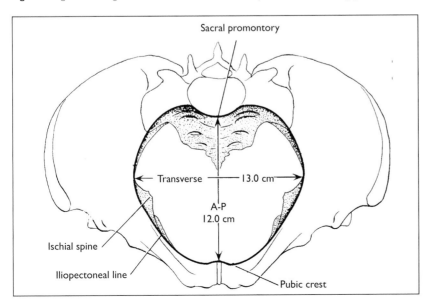

Fig 8.2 The 'ideal' obstetric pelvis: pelvic inlet..

The Ideal Obstetric Pelvis	
Brim	Round or oval transversely No undue projection of the sacral promontory Anterior posterior diameter 12cm Transverse diameter 13cm The plane of the pelvic inlet not less than 55°
Cavity	Shallow with straight side-walls No great projection of the ischial spines Smooth sacral curve Sacrospinous ligament at least 3.5 cm
Outlet	Pubic arch rounded Subpubic angle >80° Inter tuberous diameter at least 10cm

Table 8.1 The ideal obstetric pelvis.

curved anteriorly. Anteriorly the pubic bones form its boundary, measuring 4.5cm. Posteriorly, the curve of the sacrum forms its boundary, measuring 12cm. Laterally its walls narrow slightly distally *(Fig. 8.3)*. The walls are penetrated by the obturator foramen anteriorly, and the sciatic foramen laterally which is divided into two parts by the sacrospinous and sacro-tuberous ligaments.

For descriptive purposes the true pelvis can be divided into four zones. These are shown in Fig. 8.4. The measurements of the *zone of the inlet* are shown in *Fig. 8.2. The zone of the cavity* is wedge-shaped in profile and almost round in section. It is the most roomy part of the true pelvis, the anterior posterior diameter measuring 13.5cm and the transverse diameter 12.5cm.

The *zone of the midpelvis* passes through the apex of the pubic arch, the spines of the ischia, the

sacrospinous ligament and the tip of the sacrum. It is the smallest zone and its most important diameter is the ischial bispinous diameter which measures 10.5cm. If this zone is contracted the fetal presenting part may not be able to rotate and may become arrested.

The *zone of the outlet (Fig. 8.5)* does not usually interfere with the birth unless the pubic rami are narrow, which reduces the intertuberous diameter. In these cases delay may occur and the soft tissues of the perineum may be torn and damaged.

The axis of the birth canal corresponds to the direction the fetal presenting part, usually the head, takes during its passage through the birth canal *(Fig. 8.6)*.

FACTORS INFLUENCING PELVIC SHAPE AND SIZE

Minor alterations in pelvic shape were found when many women had routine radiological pelvimetry, but only in a few instances did the abnormality delay the birth. Smaller women tend to have a smaller bony pelvis but also tend to have smaller babies. More severe alterations occur among populations where rickets or osteomalacia is found but are uncommon in the developed countries today.

THE SOFT TISSUES OF THE FEMALE PELVIS

These include the uterus, the muscular pelvic floor and the perineum.

THE UTERUS
The uterus in pregnancy can be divided in three parts:
* The upper uterine segment.
* The lower uterine segment.
* The uterine cervix.

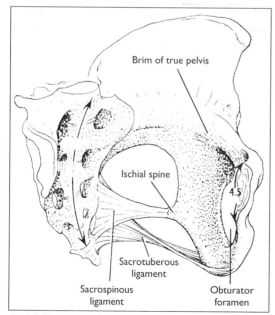

Fig 8.3 The pelvic cavity. The right innominate bone has been removed in order to show the extent of the cavity.

Brim of true pelvis

Ischial spine

Sacrotuberous ligament

Sacrospinous ligament

Obturator foramen

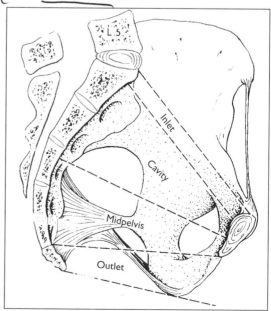

Fig 8.4 The 'zones' of the pelvis.

L.5

Inlet

Cavity

Midpelvis

Outlet

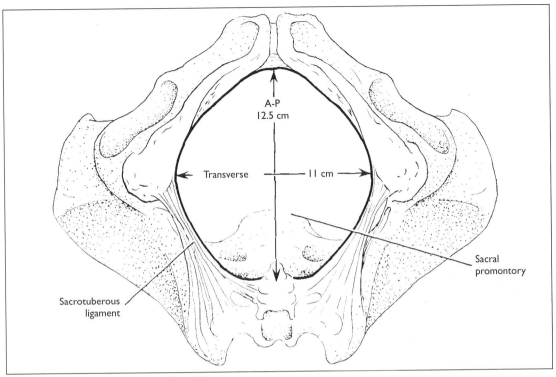

Fig 8.5 The female pelvic outlet viewed from below.

The upper uterine segment

This portion of the uterus consists of the fundus and that part the uterus lying above the reflection of the vesico-uterine fold of peritoneum. During pregnancy it undergoes the greatest degree of myometrial hyperplasia and hypertrophy. In labour it provides the strong contractions which push the fetus along the birth canal.

The lower uterine segment

This portion of the uterus lies between the vesico-uterine fold of peritoneum superiorly and the cervix inferiorly. During pregnancy the upper part of the cervix is incorporated into the lower uterine segment, which stretches to accommodate the fetal presenting part *(Fig. 8.7)*. In late pregnancy, as the upper segment muscle contractions increase in frequency and strength, the lower uterine segment develops more rapidly and is stretched radially to permit the fetal presenting part to descend *(Fig. 8.8)*. In labour the entire cervix becomes incorporated into the stretched lower uterine segment.

The cervix uteri

The cervix uteri is that part of the uterus which extends from the fibromuscular junction superiorly to the external cervical os inferiorly. The upper margin is not a fixed point, as most of the myometrial fibres end as a cone of muscle which protrudes into the collagenous tissue which comprises 90 per cent of the cervix. Some attenuated muscle fibres are present between the collagenous bundles and form 10 per cent of the cervical tissue. The endometrium ceases at the level of the muscular cone and becomes a single layer of cubical endocervical cells which are folded into clefts. In late pregnancy the cervix becomes softer because of chemical changes in the collagen fibres, and shorter as it is incorporated into the lower uterine segment. It also undergoes a variable degree

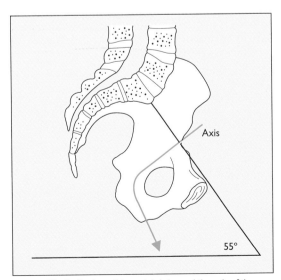

Fig 8.6 The inclination of the pelvic brim and the axis of the birth canal. The plane of the pelvic brim makes an angle of about 55° with the horizontal in the erect patient, and the plane of the outlet about 10° with the horizontal. The axis of the birth canal is angled, the alteration in direction occurring at the pelvic floor.

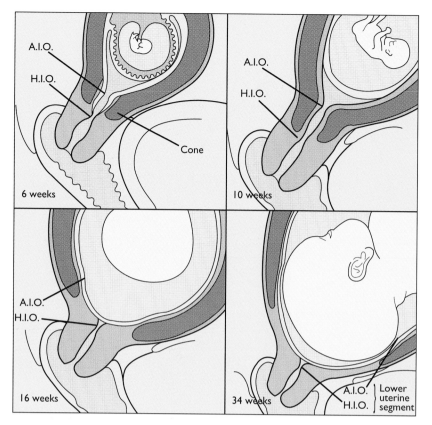

Fig 8.7 The formation of the lower uterine segment based on the observations of C. P. Wendell-Smith. Cone = the condensation of muscle at the junction of the body of the uterus and the cervix; A.I.O. = anatomical internal os; H.I.O. = histological internal os.

of dilatation. These changes collectively are termed cervical 'ripening'. The changes may occur abruptly or gradually at any time after the 34th week of pregnancy, but usually occur nearer term, especially in primigravidae. At the 34th gestational week the cervix is 2cm or more dilated in 20 per cent of primigravidae and in 40 per cent of multigravidae; and the proportion increases towards term *(Fig. 8.9)*.

At the onset of labour, the cervix of a primigravida is ripe, and is either partly, or not, effaced (i.e. incorporated into the lower uterine segment).

THE PELVIC FLOOR

The pelvic floor consists of the levator ani group of muscles, which arise on each side of the pelvis from the posterior surface of the pubis, from a condensation of fascia (the white line) which covers the obturator internus muscle, and from the pelvic aspect of the ischial spine *(Fig. 8.10)*. The muscle has several designated parts – the pubococcygeus muscle, the levator ani muscle and the coccygeus muscle as shown in *Fig. 8.11*. The fibres of these muscles slope downwards and forwards and interdigitate with

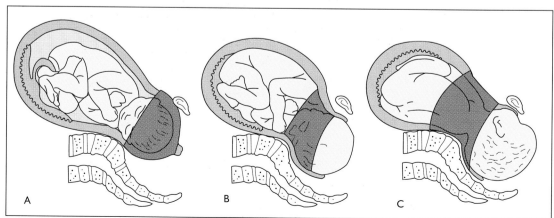

Fig 8.8 A. The lower uterine segment in late pregnancy. B. The lower uterine segment in late labour. It is dilated circumferentially and has thinned but is shorter. C. In obstructed labour the dilated and thinned lower uterine segment stretches and is in danger of rupture. Redrawn from Danforth, D. N. and Ivy, A. C. *Amer J. Obstet. Gynecol.* 1949, 57, 831.

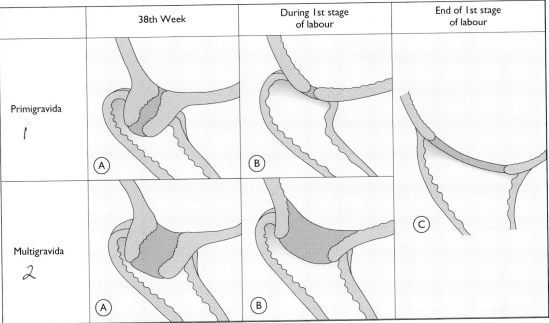

Fig 8.9 Diagram showing how the cervix progressively becomes effaced and dilated in late pregnancy and labour.
1. Primigravida. A 38th week of pregnancy. Little or no effacement or dilatation has occurred. B First stage of labour. Effacement has occurred but dilatation is not yet marked. C End of first stage of labour. The cervix is fully effaced and dilated.

2. Multigravida. A 38th week of pregnancy. Dilatation has begun but no effacement has yet occurred. B First stage of labour. Effacement and dilatation are occurring simultaneously.

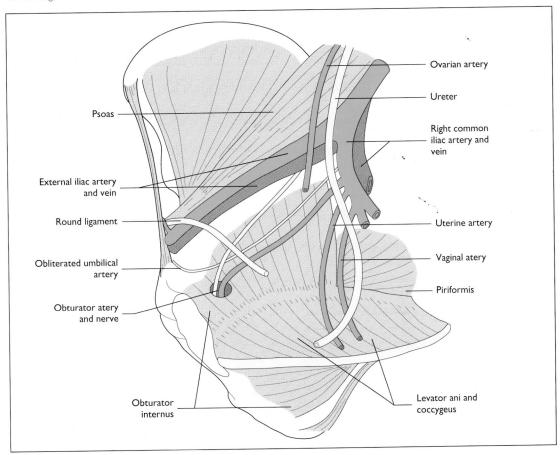

Fig 8.10 The lateral wall.

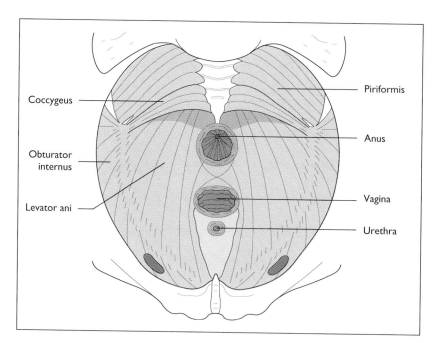

Fig 8.11 The muscles which form the pelvic floor viewed from above.

Coccygeus

Obturator internus

Levator ani

Piriformis

Anus

Vagina

Urethra

muscle fibres of the opposite levator ani group to form a muscular sling through which the urethra, the vagina and the rectum pass. The muscles enclosed in fascia form the pelvic diaphragm *(Fig. 8.12)*.

THE PERINEUM

The perineum (perineal body) is the tissue which lies distal to the pelvic diaphragm. It is pyramid shaped and is bounded superiorly by the lower surface of the pelvic diaphragm; laterally by the bones and ligaments of the pelvic outlet and below by the vulva and the anus. It can be subdivided into the urogenital triangle anteriorly and the anal triangle posteriorly by the transverse perineal muscles *(Fig. 8.13)*. The perineum contains a number of superficial muscles, is very vascular and is filled with fatty tissue. (Additional details of the perineum are given on p 79). Its importance in childbirth is that it is frequently damaged as the fetus is born.

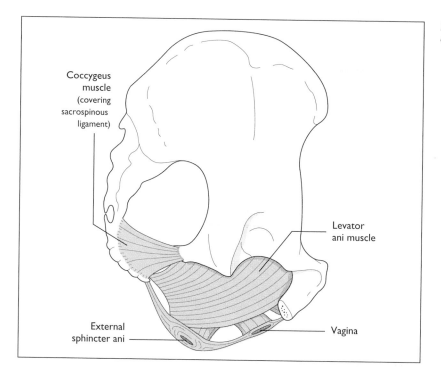

Fig 8.12 The pelvic diaphragm: lateral view.

Coccygeus muscle (covering sacrospinous ligament)

Levator ani muscle

External sphincter ani

Vagina

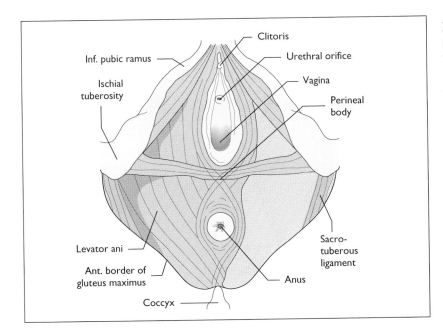

Fig 8.13 The muscles of the female perineum. In the left half of the diagram the fat pad which fills the space has been removed to show the lower surface of the levator ani which forms the roof of the space .

Clitoris

Inf. pubic ramus

Urethral orifice

Ischial tuberosity

Vagina

Perineal body

Levator ani

Sacro-tuberous ligament

Ant. border of gluteus maximus

Anus

Coccyx

THE FORMATION OF THE BIRTH CANAL DURING LABOUR (FIG. 8.14)

When myometrial contraction and retraction has led to full dilatation of the cervix the fetal head descends into the vagina which expands to encompass it. Normally an apparent space, the vaginal muscle has hypertrophied and the epithelium become folded during pregnancy so that it can accommodate the fetus without damage. As the fetal head descends it encounters the pelvic floor and the leading point is directed forwards by the gutter formed by the leva-tores ani. The fetus must now pass through the uro-genital diaphragm. The levator muscles stretch and are displaced downwards and backwards so that the anus receives the full force of the descending head and, dilating, gapes widely to expose the anterior rectal wall. Pressure is also exerted on the lower part of the vagina, and the central portion of the perineum, and as the head is born the tissues may tear.

The descent of the fetus from the uterus and out into the world is straight to the level of the ischial spines; it then moves in an anterior curve around the lower border of the symphysis pubis. If the pubic

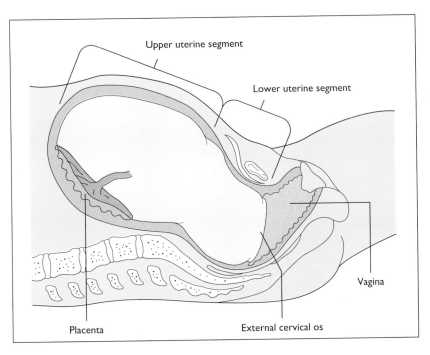

Fig 8.14 The birth canal of a patient in the second stage of labour.

Upper uterine segment

Lower uterine segment

Vagina

Placenta

External cervical os

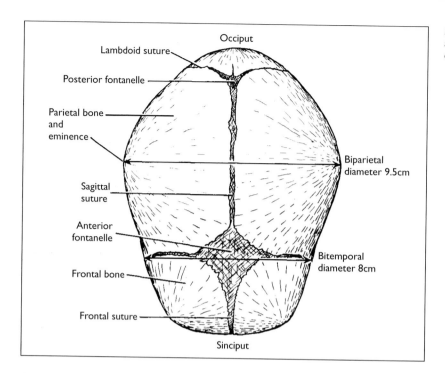

Fig 8.15 The fetal skull from above showing important obstetrical diameters.

arch is wide, the head will stem close behind the symphysis, and the perineum will not be so stretched. If the angle is narrow, the head is forced back, the direction of the curve is more obtuse and perineal damage likely.

THE PASSENGER

The fetus may influence the progress of childbirth by its size and its presentation. Of all the fetal parts, the fetal head is the least compressible and pliant. However, because of the ability of the skull bones to override each other, the fetus is able to negotiate the birth canal provided that the fetus is not too big and provided that the uterine contractions are sufficiently strong.

THE ANATOMY OF THE FETAL SKULL

The face of the term fetus is relatively small in relation to the cranium, which makes up most of the head. The cranium is made up of five bones held together by a membrane which permits their movement during birth and in early childhood. The bones are the two *parietal* bones, the two *frontal bones*, and the *occipital* bone *(Fig. 8.15)*. The membranous areas between the bones are called sutures. The *coronal suture* separates the frontal bones from the parietal bones. The *sagittal suture* separates the two parietal bones, and the *lambdoid suture* separates the occipital bone from the parietal bones *(Fig. 8.16)*. The *anterior fontanelle* is the diamond-shaped area at the junction of the sagittal and the two coronal sutures. The *posterior fontanelle* is a smaller Y-shaped

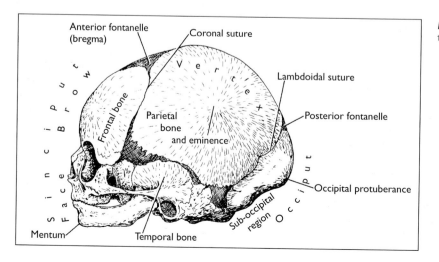

Fig 8.16 The fetal skull from the side, showing landmarks.

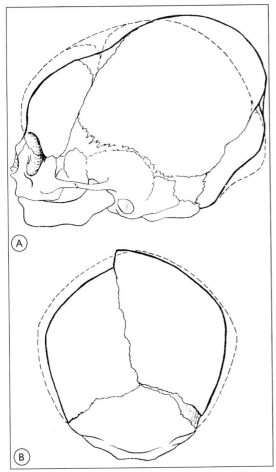

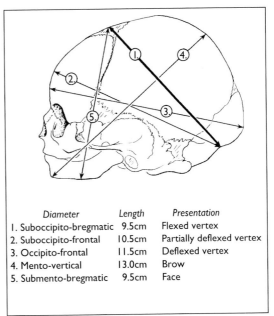

Diameter	Length	Presentation
1. Suboccipito-bregmatic	9.5cm	Flexed vertex
2. Suboccipito-frontal	10.5cm	Partially deflexed vertex
3. Occipito-frontal	11.5cm	Deflexed vertex
4. Mento-vertical	13.0cm	Brow
5. Submento-bregmatic	9.5cm	Face

Fig 8.18 The diameters of the fetal skull.

Fig 8.17 Moulding of the fetal skull. (A) lateral view; (B) posterior view. The dotted line shows the shape before moulding.

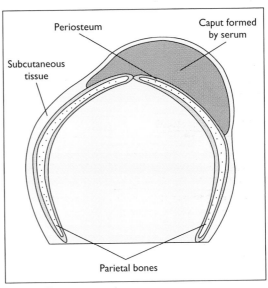

Fig 8.19 The caput succedaneum.

area at the junction between the sagittal suture and the two lambdoidal sutures. The configuration of the posterior fontanelle permits the occipital bone to be displaced under the two parietal bones during childbirth, thus reducing the volume of the fetal skull.

This is called *moulding*. During moulding, the parietal bones may also slip under each other *(Fig. 8.17)*.

Regions of the fetal skull have been designated to aid in the description of the presenting part felt at vaginal examination during labour. The *occiput* is the area lying behind the posterior fontanelle. The *vertex* is the area of the skull lying between the anterior and posterior fontanelle and between the parietal eminences. The *bregma* is the area around the anterior fontanelle. The *sinciput* is the area lying in front of the anterior fontanelle: it can be divided into two parts, the *brow* which is the area between the anterior fontanelle and the root of the nose, and the *face*, which is the area below the root of the nose.

The region of the skull which presents in labour depends on the degree of flexion of the head. The diameters are shown in *Fig. 8.18;* the diameter which is presented to the maternal pelvis in various degrees of flexion or deflexion of the head is shown in the caption.

In labour after the amniotic sac has ruptured releasing amniotic fluid, the dilating cervix may press firmly on the fetal scalp reducing both lymphatic and venous return from the fetal scalp. This causes a tissue swelling beneath the skin and is called a *caput succedaneum (Fig. 8.19)* It is soft and boggy to the touch and disappears within a few days of birth.

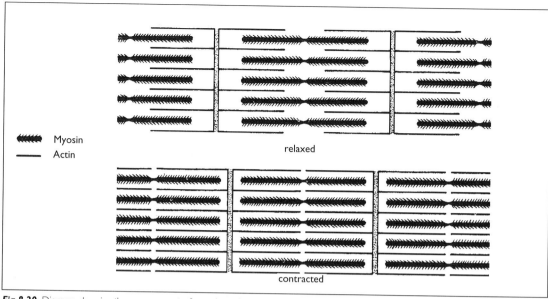

Myosin
Actin

relaxed

contracted

Fig 8.20 Diagram showing the arrangement of myosin and actin in a muscle fibre.

THE POWERS

The myometrium is formed from interdigitating muscle fibres of the two Mullerian ducts. The middle parts, of the ducts adhere and the central septum is lost to form a single hollow organ – the uterus. The myometrium has three layers:

- An outer longitudinal thin layer.
- A thick middle spiral layer, the size of which diminishes towards the cervix and occupies only 10 per cent of the cervical tissue.
- A thin circular inner layer. Each muscle fibre is made up of bunches of fibrils, which in turn are made up of spindle-shaped cells averaging 200mm in length and 7mm in diameter. These cells are composed of smaller contractile fibres comprising of interdigitating chains of actin and myosin, surrounded by a permeable membrane *(Fig. 8.20)*.

THE CHARACTERISTICS OF MYOMETRIAL CONTRACTIONS

The uterus, although composed of many individual muscle fibres, functions as a single hollow muscular organ. The myometrium is never completely relaxed. It has a resting tone of between 6 and 12mmHg. From early pregnancy the uterus contracts at intervals. Until late in pregnancy the contractions (Braxton Hicks contractions) are painless. Each contraction causes a rise in intra-uterine pressure of varying amplitude or intensity. This has two elements: a rapid rise to a peak and a slower return to the resting tone. For descriptive purposes the intensity of the contraction multiplied by the frequency of the contractions (per 10 minutes) provides

a measure of uterine activity, which is expressed in Montevideo Units *(Fig. 8.21)*. With the development of tocography, a different measure of uterine activity can be obtained. With a cardiotocograph linked to a computer, the area under the contraction can be measured and expressed in kilopascals per 15 minutes. These two methods of measuring uterine activity relate fairly closely to each other.

THE SPREAD OF UTERINE CONTRACTIONS

A uterine contraction starts from a pacemaker located at the junction of the Fallopian tube and the uterus on one side. The contractile wave passes inwards and downwards from the pacemaker at a rate of 2cm per second to involve the entire uterus in

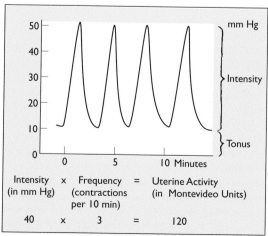

Intensity (in mm Hg)	x	Frequency (contractions per 10 min)	=	Uterine Activity (in Montevideo Units)
40	x	3	=	120

Fig 8.21 Quantitative measurements of tracings of uterine contractions (redrawn from Caldeyro-Barcia, R. and Poseiro, J. J.).

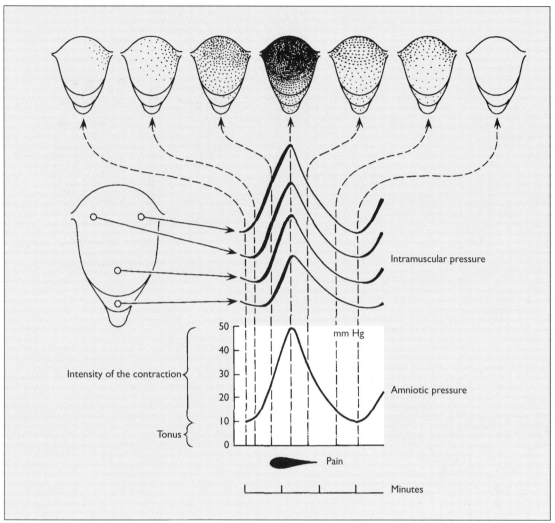

Fig 8.22 The normal wave of contraction passing over the uterus shown diagrammatically. The small uteri show how the wave starts and spreads, finally fading. The large uterus shows the four points at which the intramyometrial pressure was recorded with microballoons. The contraction phase is shown by the thick ascending line. Note how the peak of contraction occurs in all parts of the uterus simultaneously (redrawn from Caldeyro-Barcia, R. *Trans. Cong. Int. Gynecol. et Obstet.* 1958. Librairie Beauchemin, Montreal, 1959).

the contraction. In a normal labour the intensity and incremental phase of the contraction is greater in the upper uterine segment as the muscle is thicker and there is a greater amount of actinomyosin to contract. This permits the contraction to be coordinated, the maximal intensity occurring in the upper part of the uterus, with a reducing intensity as the wave passes down towards the cervix; the peak of the contraction occurs simultaneously in all parts of the uterus. The phenomenon is known as the *triple descending gradient (Fig. 8.22)*.

The intensity and frequency of the uterine contractions varies during labour, increasing as labour progresses. It has been found that uterine activity is greater if the woman walks about during early labour.

MYOMETRIAL ACTIVITY IN PREGNANCY AND LABOUR

Pregnancy

Up to the 30th week of pregnancy uterine activity is slight, small localized contractions of no more than 5mmHg occurring at intervals of 1 minute. Every 30 to 60 minutes a contraction of higher amplitude (10–15mmHg) arises which spreads to a wider area of the uterus and may be palpated *(Fig. 8.23A)*. These palpable contractions occur with increasing frequency and intensity after the 30th week and are referred to as Braxton Hicks contractions *(Fig. 8.22B)*. After the 36th week of pregnancy, uterine activity increases progressively until at a point in time labour starts *(Fig. 8.23C)*.

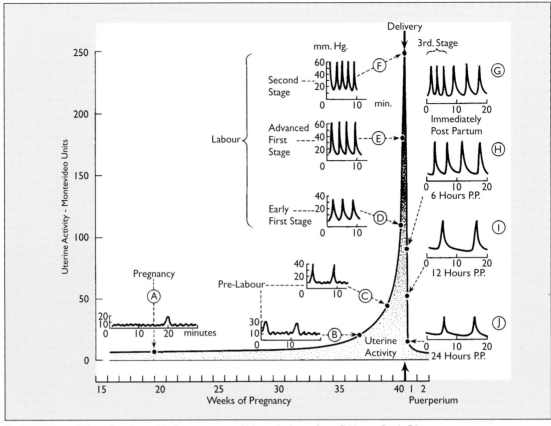

Fig 8.23 The evolution of uterine activity in pregnancy and labour (redrawn from Caldeyro- Barcia R.).

The onset of labour

This is difficult to determine with accuracy, and consequently difficult to define. At the most it can be said to be the time after which uterine contractions cause the progressive dilatation of the cervix beyond 2cm, and painful contractions usually occur at least every 10 minutes *(Fig. 8.23D)*.

Labour

In true normal labour the intensity and frequency of the contractions increase, but there is no rise in the resting tone. The *intensity* increases in late labour to 60mmHg and the *frequency* to 2–4 contractions every 10 minutes, or 150–200 Montevideo Units. The *duration* of the contraction also increases from about 20 seconds in early labour to 40–90 seconds at the end of the first stage, and in second stage *(Fig. 8.23E)*. Contractions are most effective when they are co-ordinated, with fundal dominance, have a maximum intensity of 40–60mmHg, last 60–90 seconds, recur with a 2- to 4-minute interval between the peaks of consecutive contractions, and the uterus has a resting tone of less than 12mmHg. More frequent contractions of higher intensity diminish the oxygen exchange in the placental bed

and may lead to fetal hypoxia and clinical signs of fetal distress. The efficiency of contractions is greater when the mother walks about or lies on her side during the first stage of labour, and this position also improves the placental blood supply.

The co-ordinated contractions of labour cause a permanent shortening of the muscle fibres and since this is maximal in the upper part of the uterus a distending tension is placed upon the less muscular lower part, and more particularly upon the scantily muscled cervix. The cervix therefore dilates circumferentially with each contraction, closing in at the end of the contraction; but because of the retraction of the muscle in the upper uterus, a permanent but slight dilatation occurs with each contraction.

In the second stage of labour, voluntary contraction of the diaphragm and abdominal muscles, added to the uterine contraction, propels the baby downwards through the dilated vagina and overcomes the resistance of perineal muscles to its advance *(Fig. 8.23F)*. At the height of each bearing-down effort the total force exerted on the fetus is approximately 8000g and this is resolved into two components: one, a force propelling the head downwards, and the other, a dilating force, which stretches the birth canal against the resistance of the pelvic and perineal muscles. (If the membranes are intact the resultant propelling force is less, as the amniotic fluid balances part of it.) Since the pelvic floor muscles form an inclined groove, and since the head is ovoid, the additional pressure leads to the rotation of the occiput through 90° to lie anteriorly.

Uterine activity continues unaltered after expulsion of the fetus and leads to the expulsion of the placenta from the upper uterine segment, between 2 and 6 minutes after the birth of the baby. Once the placenta has left the upper uterine segment, uterine activity diminishes, but contractions of an intensity of about 60–80mmHg still occur regularly for 48 hours after delivery, the frequency decreasing as time passes *(Fig. 8.23G)*. These contractions and those of the third stage are usually painless, but painful contractions disturb some patients. Further painful contractions may occur with suckling, due to a reflex release of oxytocin.

THE INNERVATION OF THE UTERUS

The sensory nerve fibres from the uterus, together with sensory nerve fibres from the upper vagina, pass through the 'felted' plexus of nerve ganglia which lie adjacent to the lateral aspect of the cervix on each side (the juxtacervical, or Frankenhauser's plexus). The sensory fibres then pass to the hypogastric plexus, and the lumbar and thoracic chains to reach the spinal cord at T11, T12 and T13.

A few sympathetic nerve fibres derive from the lumbar sympathetic nerves. The function of these nerves seems to be limited to regulating vasodilatation. Uterine activity can continue without interruption in the absence of any nerve connection. Whether parasympathetic nerves supply the uterus has not been determined.

Motor nerves to the uterus leave the spinal cord at T6 and T7. They pass through the hypogastric plexuses and the juxtacervical plexus to reach and spread through the entire uterus. The uterus can contract without motor nerve stimulation as occurs in labour among paraplegic women.

THE PAIN OF UTERINE CONTRACTIONS

The pain of uterine contractions is in part due to ischaemia developing in a myometrial fibre. Since there are more fibres and the contractions are stronger in the upper uterine segment, pain is felt

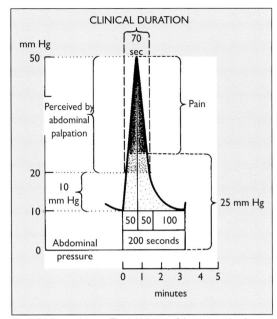

Fig 8.24 Pain in labour. The initial part of the contraction is painless and not perceived by abdominal palpation. The duration of the contraction observed clinically (70 sec) is shorter than the duration of myometrial activity (200 sec).

more strongly in the cutaneous distribution of cutaneous nerves T12 and L1. At the beginning of the contraction only slight pain is felt. This increases as the contraction grows stronger *(Fig. 8.24)*.

Many women in labour complain of backache, which may be severe. It occurs during cervical dilatation when the lower uterine segment contracts more strongly than usual, or when the triple descending gradient fails to arise. In the second stage of labour the pain is due to uterine contractions and to the stretching of the vaginal, the pelvic and the perineal tissues. This pain is felt in the back, in the pelvis and down the thighs.

The perception of pain during labour is increased if the woman is apprehensive and has little knowledge of the process of childbirth. One of the reasons for childbirth training (see page 47) is to reduce fear and improve the mother's understanding of childbirth.

9

THE PHYSIOLOGICAL CHANGES DURING CHILDBIRTH

Labour or childbirth is the process whereby the fetus and placenta are expelled from the uterus by coordinated myometrial contractions. The reason why labour starts remains obscure in spite of much research and many theories. If the information was available, it might be possible to prevent premature labour with its increased perinatal mortality.

Currently the roles of oxytocin and prostaglandins in initiating labour are being explored. There is evidence that in late pregnancy increasing numbers of oxytocin receptors appear in the decidua and myometrial cells. Oxytocin binds to these receptors and induces the release of prostaglandins, particularly PGE_2. Oxytocin may also enhance the passage of calcium ions which activate actin and myosin to produce contractions of the fibrils. It is also suggested that decidual prolactin is involved in modulating the effects of oxytocin. This remains a theory, and the statement made in 1965 that labour begins, 'as the gradual accelerating convergence of a number of factors, structural, humoral, nervous, nutritional and circulatory which, at a specific time in each species, and adapted to morphological conditions present in each, are so associated that they lead to the evacuation of the uterus of its contents', still represents most of our knowledge on the subject.

THE EFFECT OF CHILDBIRTH ON THE MOTHER

ENERGY EXPENDITURE

Labour is appropriately named, for it is a period of considerable expenditure of energy , mainly for the contractions of the uterus, but to some extent for increased cardiac activity. The energy is provided initially from metabolism of glycogen from the glycogen–water pool in muscles. In current obstetric practice, women in labour are denied food, and thus the pool is rapidly depleted and energy is obtained by the oxidization of stored body fat. This may lead to the accumulation of ketones in the blood, predominantly D-3 hydroxybuteric acid and to a lesser extent lactic and pyruvic acids. In consequence, a mild metabolic acidosis develops. This is most marked in the expulsive stage of labour when a fall in the blood pH is usual, although it remains in the normal range of 7.3–7.4. It is compensated for by a mild respiratory alkalosis, resulting from hyperventilation which is common during this time.

The mild acidoketosis is of little practical importance, provided that the women enters labour in a good nutritional condition and the birth occurs in <12 hours.

The extra expenditure of energy leads to increased heat production, and sweating occurs with a loss of body fluid.

BODY TEMPERATURE

The body temperature rises slightly during childbirth, but remains lower than 37.8°C, unless the woman becomes acidoketotic, at which point it may rise above this.

CARDIOVASCULAR CHANGES

The cardiac output increases by 12 per cent over the prelabour readings between contractions and by 30 per cent during contractions. The increased cardiac output is effected by an increase in stroke volume and heart rate. The mean arterial pressure rises by about 10 per cent and in the expulsive stage of labour the rise may be greater. These changes further increase cardiac work in response to a uterine contraction. The right atrial pressure rises and may reach 40–50mmHg in late labour, and the cardiopulmonary blood volume increases at the same time. Following the birth a further rise in cardiac output occurs. Since bradycardia is usual at this time, the rise is due to an increase in stroke volume. The effect lasts for 3–4 days.

For these reasons childbirth may pose a hazard to a woman who has uncompensated heart disease or who is severely anaemic.

GASTROINTESTINAL TRACT

In labour gastric emptying is delayed and partly digested food may remain in the stomach for >12 hours. Intestinal motility is also delayed.

TRAUMA TO THE TISSUES

Vaginal birth is always associated with some lacerations of the cervix, which usually cause no problems, the round cervical os becoming a slit. In some cases the damage is greater (Chapter 25). The vagina may suffer lacerations and the perineum is often torn, particularly among primigravidae, for these reasons an episiotomy is deliberately made.

Because of damage to the pubococcygeal muscle by the pressure of the fetus in late labour, retention of urine may occur after delivery.

BLOOD LOSS DURING CHILDBIRTH

Clinical estimates of blood loss during birth show that a mean of 300–500ml occurs. This may be an underestimate. In a healthy woman this loss is of no clinical significance, as it is less than the increased blood volume which occurs in pregnancy.

THE EFFECT OF CHILDBIRTH ON THE FETUS

The entry of a child into the world is not gentle. Unlike other mammals, humans have developed a large head which has to traverse a bony birth canal, propelled by uterine contractions. During a contraction the uterus exerts a force on the fetus of 1kg per cm^2 and during the expulsive stage the force doubles when voluntary expulsive efforts are added to the uterine contractions.

The effect of this force is mainly on the fetal head and so moulding of the fetal skull may occur. Normally the force does the baby no harm but if moulding is great, because of cephalopelvic disproportion, if the baby is delivered inexpertly by forceps or vacuum extraction, intracranial oedema or damage may occur.

During childbirth the fetus suffers some degree of hypoxia. If the fetus has obtained a good supply of glucose during pregnancy the hypoxia causes few problems. But if the fetus is growth retarded because of insufficient supplies of nutrients from the mother, it may enter labour with diminished glycogen reserves and may be unable to compensate for the reduction of glucose and oxygen during an abnormal or prolonged labour. This means that it may have to use anaerobic methods of obtaining energy, with resulting fetal acidaemia, which may affect the fetal heart rate as it attempts to compensate for the relative hypoxia. The fetal heart rate is the result of a balance between the tachycardia produced by sympathetic nerve stimulation and the bradycardia produced by vagal nerve stimulation. Normally the vagus is dominant and exerts a slowing effect on the fetal heart which beats at a rate of 140±20 times a minute. If fetal hypoxia occurs, the altered composition of the blood leads to a rise in sympathetic and vagal tones which differ in effect. The sympathetic effect becomes dominant in mild hypoxia. Its onset is delayed, but if the hypoxia persists it leads to fetal tachycardia. This persists for 10–30 minutes after the cause of the hypoxia has ceased. Vagal stimulation occurs if hypoxia is moderate or severe in degree. Bradycardia occurs rapidly, lasts as long as the hypoxia and does then resolves rapidly.

10

THE COURSE AND MANAGEMENT OF CHILDBIRTH

CHOICES IN CHILDBIRTH

In most developed countries nearly all women give birth in hospital. In contrast, in the developing countries, particularly in the rural areas where 75 per cent of the population live, most women have their babies at home. Health authorities attempt to select those women who would be more safely delivered in hospital and arrange for the transfer of other women to hospital should problems arise. To attend to emergencies occurring at home births, 'obstetric flying squads' are set up. The flying squad consists of an ambulance staffed by a doctor and nurse-midwife and is equipped to deal with haemorrhage, delay in birth and to rescusitation of the newborn.

With the almost universal trend towards hospital birth in the developed countries, some groups of women are questioning if this is always appropriate, claiming that on admission to hospital a pregnant woman loses her autonomy, often is not told about proposed procedures, and may be treated impersonally by busy attending staff. In other words, childbirth has been medicalized. Some of the women want a return to home births, despite potential dangers; others seek birth in a hospital-based, but home birth oriented, birth centre; others accept the benefits of hospital birth, but want some of the attitudes of the attending staff and some of the procedures changed.

Several international organizations have addressed this issue and have made recommendations, which are paraphrased as follows:
- A pregnant woman should have access to a family member during labour and childbirth, who will remain with her throughout the process if she wishes and if the doctor in charge agrees.
- A pregnant woman should participate in decisions regarding the birth experience, and the need for procedures (including episiotomy). Their technique should be explained to her.
- Routine pubic and perineal shaving and routine enema should be abandoned.
- Induction of labour by amniotomy or use of prostaglandins should be reserved for strictly medical reasons. Routine rupture of the amniotic sac early in labour is not justified.
- Analgesia and anaesthesia should be provided at the patient's request.
- During labour the pregnant woman should be able to walk about, lie, squat or sit to find the position most comfortable for her, unless medical reasons demand that she remain in bed. In this case she should be able to recline. The dorsal lithotomy position during delivery should only be adopted if a forceps delivery or other operative procedure is needed.
- The mother and the baby should have facilities for 'rooming-in'.
- Breast-feeding should be encouraged and the mother should have immediate access to her new-born baby, when this is practicable.

The criticisms advanced by women's groups have had an effect on obstetric practice and choices in childbirth are now provided in many places. These choices are:
- Prepared participatory childbirth.
- Conventional childbirth.
- Actively managed childbirth.

PREPARED PARTICIPATORY CHILDBIRTH

In this approach the parents undertake childbirth training, learning about the processes of childbirth and how to accept the pains of uterine contractions. This has been discussed on pp 47–48. Labour is supervised by trained staff, and the principles mentioned earlier are accepted by staff and patients. The birth takes place in a quiet environment and the baby is at once given to the mother so that she may suckle and celebrate the birth.

Woman can have a prepared participatory childbirth in a normal hospital delivery room, but it is more satisfactory if there is a Birthing Centre.

Birthing Centre

A Birthing Centre is usually attached to a hospital so that the patient can be transferred or treated by an experienced obstetrician should complications arise. The Birth Centre is furnished like a bedroom, containing a firm double bed, chairs and furnishings, with the necessary equipment for medical care and infant resuscitation discreetly hidden. The father of the child or a 'significant other person' remains with the labouring woman, providing support. The woman may have hired her own nurse-midwife (accredited by the hospital) or is looked after by a hospital nurse-midwife or a doctor. After the birth the baby remains with its parents so that 'bonding' and celebration may take place. Early discharge is usual and the mother is followed up at home by district nurse-midwives. Experience with established Birth Centres shows that women choosing this form of childbirth have fewer inductions of labour, require less analgesia, have more spontaneous deliveries, fewer episiotomies and fewer hypoxic babies than women delivering in conventional delivery units.

They are carefully selected, of course. About 5 per cent of women choosing a Birthing Centre require medical intervention, and most are transferred to the Delivery Floor.

CONVENTIONAL CHILDBIRTH

The woman gives birth in a Delivery Suite. She is generally content to leave the process of childbirth to be managed by the attending staff, and accepts their

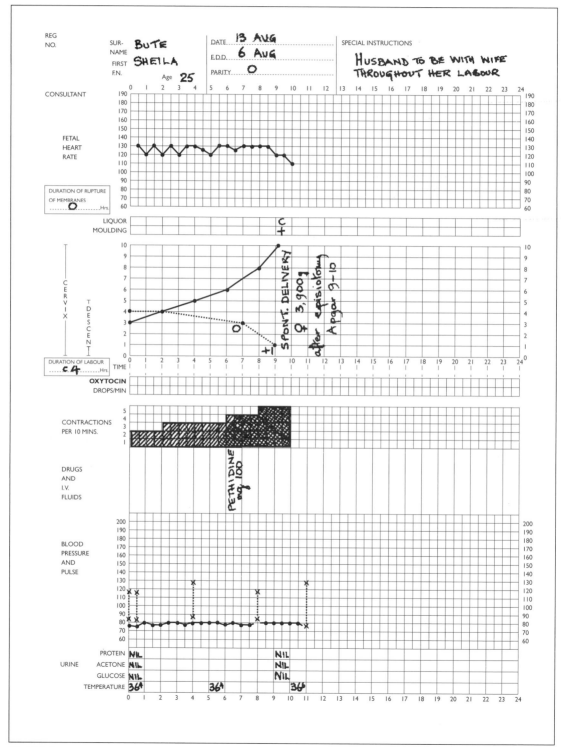

Fig 10.1 A partogram.

decisions about management. Although her partner is often present, he or a 'significant other person' may not always be in attendance. She is cared for with skill and does not participate overmuch in the process of childbirth.

ACTIVELY MANAGED CHILDBIRTH

The development of the partogram and the appreciation that most women have delivered within 12 hours of admission to hospital has led to another approach: actively managed labour.

On admission to the delivery unit, the diagnosis of labour is either confirmed or rejected. If the woman is in labour, the time of admission is designated as the start of labour. A partogram is started and the progress of labour is marked on it *(Fig. 10.1)*. Vaginal examinations are made every 2 hours and the cervical dilatation is recorded on the partogram. Action lines, printed on transparent plastic, are superimposed on the partogram *(Fig. 10.2)*. In the active stage of labour the slowest acceptable rate of cervical dilatation is 1cm/hr. If the cervical dilatation lies to the right of the appropriate action line, the membranes are ruptured and an incremental dilute oxytocin infusion is established in nulliparous women (and some multiparous women), provided that a single fetus presents as a vertex and there are no signs of 'fetal distress'. If the first stage of labour lasts longer than 10 hours a caesarean section is performed.

Progress in the second stage of labour is judged by the descent of the fetal head and its rotation. One hour is allowed for the fetal head to reach the pelvic floor (the first phase) and a further hour for the birth to be completed (the second phase). If these targets are not met, either a caesarean section is performed (in phase 1) or a forceps delivery is attempted.

Proponents of actively managed labour claim that the incidence of a labour lasting >12 hours is <3 per cent; the caesarean section rate is 7–12 per cent and the forceps rate is 8 per cent.

THE ONSET OF LABOUR

In the weeks before labour starts, the painless uterine contractions which have been becoming increasingly frequent merge into a prodromal stage of labour which may last up to 4 weeks.

During this time the lower segment expands to accept the fetal head, which enters the upper pelvis. This relieves the pressure on the upper part of the abdomen ('lightening') but increases the pressure in the pelvis. Consequently constipation and urinary frequency become apparent, and some patients complain of increased pressure in the pelvis and an increased mucoid vaginal discharge.

'FALSE LABOUR'

As term approaches, many women complain of painful uterine contractions, which may seem to indicate the onset of labour. However, despite the contractions, progressive dilatation of the cervix fails to occur. The condition is termed *false labour*.

In it, the triple descending gradient of uterine activity fails to become established. A reverse gradient of uterine activity is present, the lower part of the uterus contracting nearly as strongly as the upper part. Because of this, cervical dilatation fails to occur and the pain of the uterine contraction is often felt as low backache.

Clinically, the painful contractions occur more often at night, but their frequency and intensity do not increase as time passes.

A woman who complains of this pattern of uterine activity needs an explanation and, if the pains are distressing, treatment with analgesics, and perhaps a hypnotic so that she may enjoy a good night's sleep.

Often the pains of false labour recur on a number of days, and in some cases, the reverse gradient of activity changes and true labour starts.

THE ONSET OF TRUE LABOUR

True labour may start and progress rapidly, or the start may be slow, with contractions only occurring at long intervals, the so-called 'sluggish uterus', or in a more modern idiom – prolongation of the quiet (latent) phase of labour.

If the woman is becoming distressed that labour is not progressing, a more effective pattern of uterine activity can be obtained by performing an amniotomy and by starting an intravenous infusion of oxytocin. This regimen should only be instituted if there is no cephalopelvic disproportion and if the cervix is partly or wholly effaced, 2cm dilated and soft.

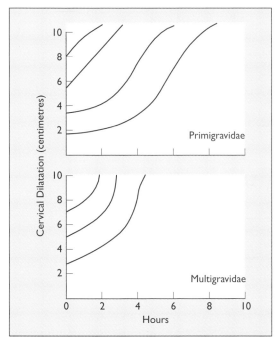

Fig 10.2 Action lines for the partogram.

The onset of labour is difficult to time with any degree of accuracy, and may be heralded by several signs: (1) the false labour pains may become co-ordinate and regular, or painful contractions may alert the patient that labour has started; (2) a discharge of mucus mixed with some blood may occur. This is due to the effacement and dilatation of the cervix allowing the 'plug' which previously filled it to be released. The blood comes from minute lacerations in the cervical mucosa. The passage of the mucus and blood is known as the 'show'.

The transition into labour is gradual but labour may be said to have begun when the cervix is at least 2cm dilated and contractions become painful and regular with diminishing intervals between each contraction.

Because of the difficulty in establishing the time of onset of labour with any degree of accuracy, many obstetricians mark the onset of labour from the time the woman is admitted to hospital. This has advantages if the graphic method of recording the progress of labour (the partogram) is adopted.

DURATION OF LABOUR

The duration of labour is not easy to determine precisely as its onset is often indefinite and subjective. In studies of informed women, whose labour started spontaneously, there was a wide variation in the duration of labour as can be seen in *Table 10.1*.

Labour is usually shorter when the patient knows something of the physiology of normal labour, is in good health at the onset of labour, has confidence in her attendants and is well adjusted.

Several factors influence the duration of labour. These include the age of the woman, her parity, her knowledge of the process of childbirth, the size of the fetus and its position in the uterus. Labour seems to last longer amongst nulliparous women, particularly older primigravidae, and if the baby presents in the occipito-posterior position.

Ninety per cent of nulliparous women (para 0) may be expected to deliver within 16 hours, and the same proportion of multiparous women (para 1+) will deliver within 12 hours.

THE PROGRESS AND MANAGEMENT OF LABOUR AND BIRTH

The management of labour begins when the woman seeks admission to hospital. She does this when she believes or knows that she is in labour. As labour is a time of anxiety and stress, the attitude of the member of staff who admits her is most important.

THE ADMISSION

On admission the woman may be offered a shower. During the time she takes it, her antenatal record is obtained and scrutinized for any past medical or

The Duration of Labour

	Para 0	Multiparae
1st stage	$8\frac{1}{4}(2–12)$h	$5\frac{1}{2}(1–9)$h
2nd stage	$1(\frac{1}{4}–1\frac{1}{2})$h	$\frac{1}{4}(0–\frac{3}{4})$h
3rd stage	$\frac{1}{4}(0–1)$h	$\frac{1}{4}(0–\frac{1}{2})$h
	$9\frac{1}{2}(2\frac{1}{4}–14)$h	$6(1–10\frac{1}{4})$h

Table 10.1 The duration of labour.

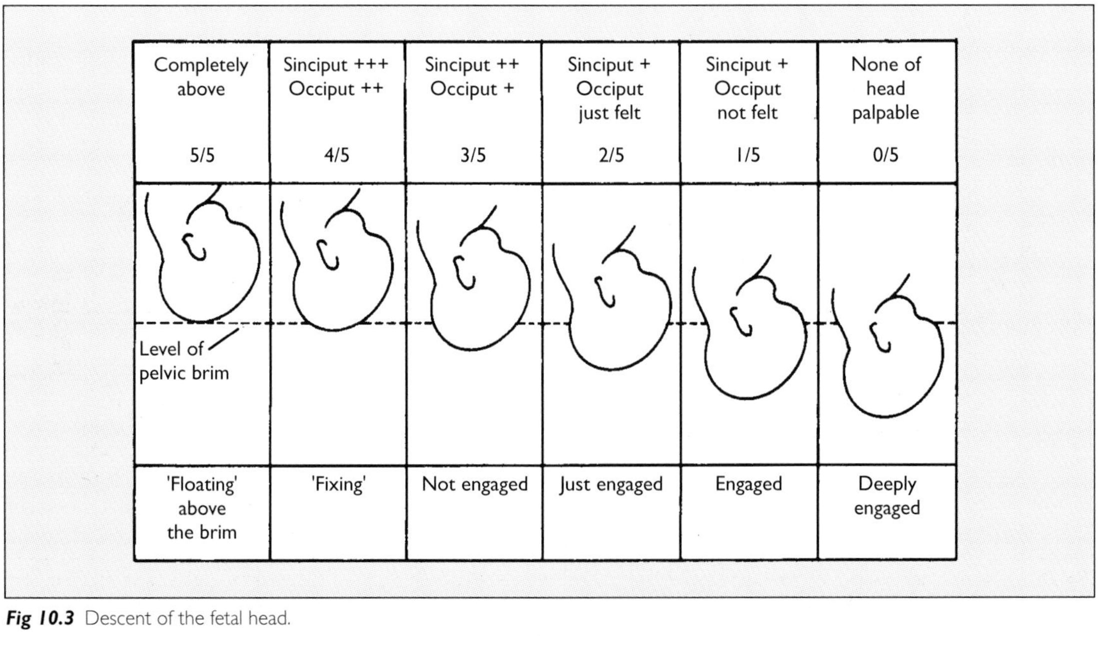

Completely above
5/5
Sinciput +++ Occiput ++
4/5
Sinciput ++ Occiput +
3/5
Sinciput + Occiput just felt
2/5
Sinciput + Occiput not felt
1/5
None of head palpable
0/5
Level of pelvic brim
'Floating' above the brim
'Fixing'
Not engaged
Just engaged
Engaged
Deeply engaged

Fig 10.3 Descent of the fetal head.

obstetrical problems, to check the history of the current pregnancy and to make sure that the appropriate laboratory tests have been made.

Pudendal shaving is no longer performed, but the hairs surrounding the vaginal entrance may be trimmed.

During these procedures the history of the present labour is obtained, the frequency and strength of the uterine contractions being noted, and information obtained about a 'show' of blood or mucus and whether or not the membranes have broken.

A general examination is made by a nurse–midwife or a doctor, the blood pressure, pulse and temperature being recorded. The abdomen is palpated to determine the presentation of the fetus and the position of the presenting part in relation to the pelvic brim *(Fig. 10.3)*.

A vaginal examination is made, with aseptic precautions, to determine the effacement and dilatation of the cervix and the position and station of the presenting part. The *station* of the presenting part is the level of the lowest fetal bony part (head or breech) in relation to an imaginary line joining the mother's ischial spines. It is measured in finger-breadths (1.6cm) above or below the ischial spines *(Fig. 10.4)*. If the amniotic sac (the membranes) has ruptured this is noted.

The woman is transferred from the admission room to a bed in a delivery room (if she has not already been admitted to it) and a partogram is started, which visually shows the progress of labour at a glance.

THE FIRST STAGE OF LABOUR

The first stage of labour begins, as mentioned earlier, at an imprecise time. For convenience it is estimated to start when the patient says that the pains are becoming regular, or on her admission to hospital when the signs of labour are evident. It ends with the full dilatation of the cervix.

At the beginning of the first stage of labour the fetal presenting part (usually it is the head, so this will be used in the rest of this chapter in place of the presenting part) has descended into the true pelvis to some extent. In a normally shaped pelvis the position of the occiput is in the transverse diameter of the pelvis in 75 per cent of cases, in the oblique diameter in 14 per cent of cases, in the direct anterior position in 3 per cent of cases and in a posterior diameter in 8 per cent of cases *(Fig. 10.5)*.

The first stage of labour can be divided into a latent (quiet) phase and an active phase. In the early part of the latent phase the uterine contractions are relatively painless and occur at intervals of 5–10 minutes. They do not distress the patient. As the latent phase progresses the contractions become stronger and more frequent but dilation of the cervix is relatively slow. Towards the end of the phase the membranes may rupture spontaneously.

The active phase starts when the cervix is 4–5cm dilated. The cervix dilates more rapidly in the active phase and its progress is considered to be normal if it dilates at a rate of 0.5–1.0cm/hr. Towards the end of the active phase, when the cervix is 9cm dilated, many women complain of very painful contractions and may have a desire to push. As it is unwise to push at this stage, a vaginal examination should be made to establish whether the cervix is fully dilated. ⟶

The duration of the latent and active phases is shown in *Fig. 10.6*. If they last for >12 hours in a nulliparous women or >9 hours in a multiparous woman the cause should be investigated (see Chapter 24).

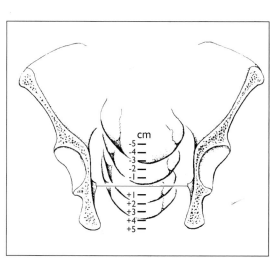

Fig 10.4 Station of the head (redrawn from Greenhill, *Obstetrics*, 13th edition. Saunders, 1965).

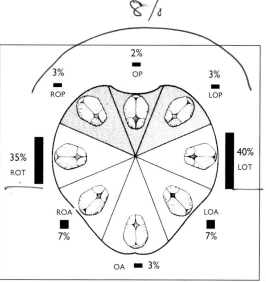

Fig 10.5 The positions of the vertex at the onset of labour and their relative frequency; the shaded positions are the pessimal ones.

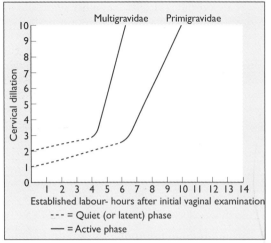

Fig 10.6 The phases of labour.

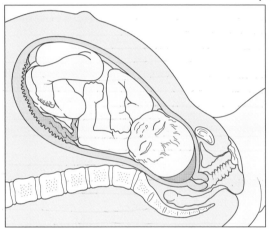

Fig 10.7 Late pregnancy. The fetal head has engaged in the transverse diameter of the pelvic brim, and some flexion of the head on the chest has occurred. The cervix is soft but is not yet effaced and the amniotic membranes are intact.

During the active part of the first stage of labour, the fetal head descends more deeply into the maternal pelvis and flexes (*Fig. 10.7*, *Fig. 10.8* and *10.9*).

The management of the first stage of labour

The patient should be made as comfortable as possible and should choose whether she prefers to remain in bed, walk about, sit on a chair and so on. If there is a common room on the delivery floor she may prefer to go there to be with other women. If the presenting part has not descended into the pelvis, she should remain in bed, but should be propped up on pillows with a back rest so that the full weight of her uterus does not press on the descending aorta and inferior vena cava, impeding blood flow to the uterus and its return to the heart.

It is customary to withhold solid food during labour as the contents remain in the stomach, and if a general anaesthetic is required for a forceps or a caesarean delivery, the acid stomach contents may be regurgitated and inhaled causing Mendelson's syndrome. Today few inhalational anaesthetics are given during childbirth and it is known that fasting does not reduce the acidity of the stomach contents. There seems no good reason why a woman at low risk of an operative procedure requiring general anaesthesia should not be permitted, if she wishes, to eat a low-residue, low-fat diet (such as tea, fruit juice, toast, lightly cooked eggs or biscuits). Food eaten during labour may reduce the chance of maternal acidoketosis.

Obstetricians who believe that oral feeding should be withheld once labour has been established usually set up an intravenous infusion. It is now generally agreed that I.V. infusions are not required in the first 12 hours of labour, regardless of the presence of ketosis. The patient's lips can be kept moist and she may suck ice. If intravenous fluids are deemed necessary the amount should not exceed

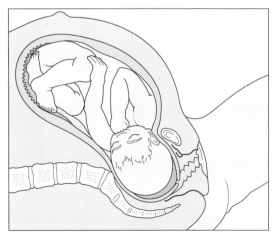

Fig 10.8 Early labour. There has been further flexion of the fetal head, and it has moved more deeply into the true pelvis, causing pressure on the bladder and rectum. The cervix has become effaced but has not yet begun to dilate and the membranes are intact.

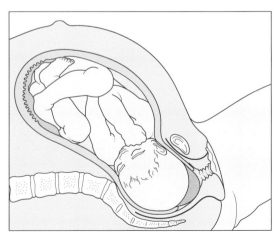

Fig 10.9 Late first stage of labour. The cervix is now 7cm dilated and further flexion of the fetal head has occurred. The membranes are still intact.

1500ml in 12 hours) and normal saline 500ml should alternate with Hartmann's solution 500ml. Glucose infusions providing more than 25g of glucose during labour should be avoided as they may cause fetal hyperinsulinaemia and neonatal hypoglycaemia.

Specific care in the first stage

The following steps should be followed:

- Support and comfort the patient and inform her about the progress of labour.
- Complete the partogram.
  i.   Check pulse, temperature and blood pressure every 2 hours.
  ii. Monitor the frequency, strength and intensity of the uterine contractions.
  iii. Monitor the fetal heart rate once active labour has started, every 15 minutes in the first stage and every 5 minutes in the second stage of labour. The normal variation is 120–160 beats per minute. If the rate mains below 100bpm between contractions and particularly if meconium is passed, fetal distress may be imminent and the situation should be assessed (see Chapter 24). Although the fetal heart is usually monitored between contractions, a more informative way is to auscultate the heart immediately after a contraction. In some hospitals continuous fetal heart monitoring is practised using a transabdominal transducer.
  iv. When labour has been established, perform a vaginal examination every 2 hours to determine the dilatation of the cervix and the descent of the fetal head (or breech).
  v.   Discuss with the patient her need for analgesics or epidural anaesthesia (see pages 82–84).

Determine the position of the fetal presenting part, usually the head, in relation to the maternal pelvis, dividing the pelvis into 45° segments. Right refers to the right side of the woman, left to her left side. If the vertex presents the occiput is the point of reference; if the breech presents the sacrum is the point of reference; if the face presents the chin is the point of reference. In *Fig. 10.5* (page 71) the positions and frequency of vertex presentations are shown.

THE SECOND STAGE OF LABOUR

The second stage of labour begins when the cervix is fully dilated, to complete the formation of the curved birth canal, and ends with the birth of the baby. The second stage of labour is the expulsive stage during which the fetus is forced through the birth canal. The uterine contractions become more frequent, recurring at 2–5 minute intervals and are stronger, lasting 60–90 seconds. The fetal head descends deeply into the pelvis, and reaching the gutter shaped pelvic floor, rotates anteriorly (internal rotation) so that the occiput lies behind the symphysis pubis *(Fig. 10.10)*. Anterior rotation occurs in 98 per cent of

cases. In 2 per cent of cases the head rotates posteriorly so that the occiput lies in front of the sacrum.

The uterine contractions are now supplemented by voluntary muscle contractions. Simultaneously with the uterine contraction, the patient holds her breath, closes her glottis, braces her feet, and taking a breath, holds it, grunts and contracts her diaphragm and her abdominal muscles, to force the fetus lower in her pelvis. The energy expended causes her pulse to rise, and she sweats. As the uterine contraction diminishes and ceases, she relaxes and often dozes.

As the fetal head is pushed deeper into the pelvis the patient may complain of intense pressure on her rectum or pains radiating down her legs, due to pressure on the sacral nerve plexus or obturator nerve *(Fig. 10.11)*. Some 15 minutes later the anus begins

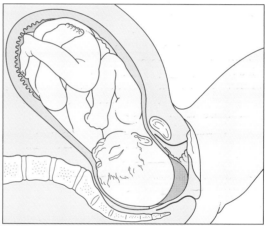

Fig 10.10 Early second stage. The cervix is fully dilated and the head is beginning to rotate at the level of the ischial spines. Rotation is through 90°, so that the occiput lies in the anterior segment of the pelvis and the sagittal suture of the fetal head in the antero-posterior diameter of the pelvis. The membranes are intact and bulge in front of the head.

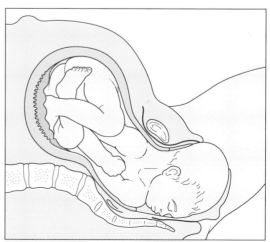

Fig 10.11 Late second stage. The head is broaching the vulval ring ('crowning'). The membranes have ruptured. The perineum is stretched over the head.

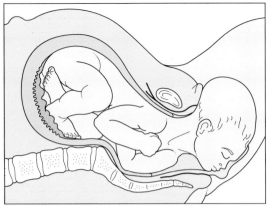

Fig 10.12 Birth of the head. As the fetal head is pushed through the vulval ring it extends on the neck, and the perineum is swept over the face. The direction of movement of the head is now upwards. The uterus has retracted to fit closely over the fetal body. The shoulders are still in the transverse diameter of the mid pelvis.

to open, exposing its anterior wall, and the head can be seen inside the vagina. With each contraction the fetal head becomes a little more visible, retreating a little between contractions but advancing slightly all the time (Fig 10.11).

The head now presses on the posterior wall of the lower vagina and the perineum becomes thinner, stretched, its skin tense and shining (Fig. 10.12). The woman complains of a 'bursting' feeling and a desire to push even without a uterine contraction. Soon a large part of the head can be seen between the stretched labia, and the parietal bosses become visible. The further sequence of the birth is shown in Fig. 10.13 and is now described. With an extra effort the baby's head is born, extending at its neck, so that the forehead, the nose, the mouth and the chin appear in sequence. Mucus streams from the baby's mouth and nose. After a short pause, the head rotates into a transverse diameter (external

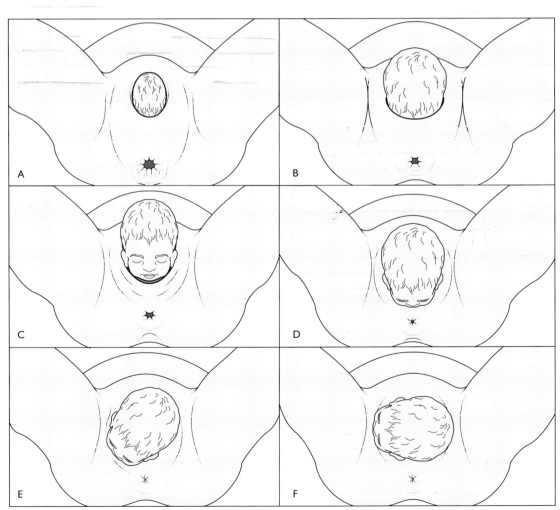

Fig 10.13 Birth of the head. A sequence showing the progressive distension of the perineum by the head, which extends as it is born. The perineum sweeps over the forehead, face and chin. Once the head is born it drops slightly and then restitution (external rotation) occurs.

rotation). This brings the shoulders into the anterior posterior diameter of the lower pelvis. The shoulders are born next, the anterior shoulder stemming from behind the symphysis and the posterior shoulder rolling over the perineum, followed by the baby's trunk and legs. The baby gasps once or twice and cries vigorously. The uterus contracts to a size found at a 20-week pregnancy.

The management of the second stage of labour

In the second stage of labour the active cooperation of the expectant mother is needed, to add the voluntary muscle contractions of her diaphragm and abdominal muscles to the involuntary uterine contractions, which together increase the downward pressure on the fetus. As the contractions are very painful, the woman may need more analgesics, or if she has had an epidural anaesthetic it may need 'topping up'. Some women find relief by back massage or by moving into another position, including sitting up.

Throughout the second stage of labour a medical attendant (and/or the woman's husband or partner) should be present helping and encouraging the woman to bear down with each uterine contraction and to relax in between. As there is much energy expenditure, sweating is usual and the patient will feel more comfortable if she can have cool face cloths to wipe away the sweat.

During the second stage of labour most women prefer to recline on a bed at 45° to the horizontal, supported, if the woman wishes, by her partner. Some women choose to sit up, squat or kneel until the baby's head is visible at the vulva.

The actual birth of the baby is easier to manage if the woman is reclining on a bed, but there is no justification for putting her legs in stirrups.

The mother's contractions are recorded and the fetal heart is auscultated every 15 minutes. If the fetal heart falls below 100 beats per minute, and the bradycardia persists for more than 2 minutes, action should be taken to determine the cause. This will include a vaginal examination to make sure that the umbilical cord has not prolapsed. The position of the patient should be changed as this may affect the fetal heart rate.

THE BIRTH OF THE BABY

The head

As the fetal head (for this is the usual presenting part) becomes visible between the labia, the woman should be prepared for the birth. With each contraction the patient pushes and the fetal head becomes more visible, retracting slightly between contractions. When the area of the visible head has increased to 5cm, and the perineum is thin and distended, the vulva should be swabbed with chlorhexidine (1:1000). The medical attendant who will deliver the baby now scrubs up and put on gloves and gown. With each contraction, the fetal head is flexed by the index finger of one of the attendant's hands, whilst the perineum is 'protected' by a pad which covers the perineum and the distended anus and is held in the attendant's other hand. In some cases the perineum tears in spite of the protection; in others a deliberate incision (an episiotomy) is made to avoid the perineum tearing. This is discussed later.

The manoeuvres described permit the head to be born slowly, until the parietal bosses are visible (when the head is said to be 'crowned'). The mother now ceases to push with a contraction unless asked to do so by the medical attendant. Instead she is asked to pant during each painful contraction.

To be born the fetal head now has to extend, and this is aided by the attendant's left hand keeping the head flexed and the right hand holding the perineal pad pushing the chin upwards. The forehead, nose, mouth and chin emerge and the head is born, the perineum being pressed back behind the chin. The baby's eyes are swabbed with sterile water and the baby's head is rotated (or rotates itself) through 90. The attendant now puts a finger inside the woman's vagina to feel if the umbilical cord is around the baby's neck. If it is, a loop of the cord is brought down.

The shoulders

As the baby's head rotates, mucus streams from its mouth and nose. With the next contraction, the rotated head is grasped gently between the attendant's two hands, which are placed over the side of the head, and the head is drawn posteriorly so that the anterior shoulder is released from behind the pubic bones (Fig. 10.14).

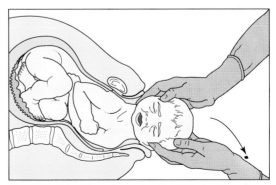

Fig 10.14 Birth of the anterior shoulder. With the birth of the head the shoulders reach the pelvic floor and, directed by the levator 'gutter', rotate to lie in the antero-posterior diameter of the pelvic outlet. The head therefore rotates 'externally', or undergoes 'restitution', to its position at the onset of labour. The anterior shoulder (in this case the right one) is appearing from behind the symphysis. The birth of the shoulder is aided by downward and backward traction of the head by the obstetrician.

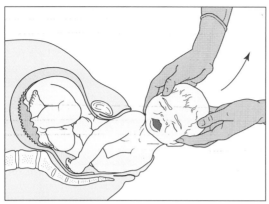

Fig 10.15 The birth of the posterior shoulder. The obstetrician aids the birth by lifting the head gently upwards whilst maintaining traction. This prevents damage to the perineum.

Following the birth of the anterior shoulder, the baby is swept upwards in an arc to release the posterior shoulder, followed by the body and the legs (*Fig. 10.15*).

The mother should now be able to see and touch her baby. The baby is then laid between the mother's legs and its mouth and fauces are sucked clear using a suction apparatus or a soft tube and bulb. The reason for placing the baby between the mother's legs is that as it is below the level of the placenta its circulation will receive an additional 60ml of blood as it drains from the placenta. One-third of this amount is received in the first 30 seconds after the birth and the remainder in the next 2–3 minutes. In normal cases (where the baby is not hypoxic) the attendant should not clamp, divide and tie the umbilical cord for about 2–3 minutes.

THE NEWBORN BABY

The neonate lies between its mother's legs, usually taking its first breath within seconds and starting to cry, and to move its arms and legs. It is checked for good respiratory effort and its colour and its alertness. Either an Apgar score is taken (*Table 10.2*) or the Basic Resuscitation Programme suggested in the UK is adopted (*Fig. 10.16*). Most babies establish respirations easily and quickly, but a few are born in a mild or severe hypoxic state. This problem is discussed further in Chapter 23. The baby is checked for gross malformations. It is then given to the mother for cuddling and suckling. This early mother-baby contact encourages (but is not essential for) bonding, and if the baby is put to the breast this helps to 'bring in' the milk.

Two other issues need discussion. These are the use of prophylactic eye drops to prevent gonococcal ophthalmic infection and the routine use of vitamin K.

Prophylactic eye drops

There is no indication for the routine use of prophylactic eye drops or ointment as gonorrhoea is uncommon. In selected cases, tetracycline 1 per cent eye ointment is the treatment of choice.

Vitamin K

Most neonates develop vitamin K deficiency by the third day of life. This predisposes the baby to a bleeding diathesis (haemorrhagic disease of the newborn) caused by the depression of clotting factors II, VII, IX, and X. The baby may bleed from the gastrointestinal tract, the umbilical cord or from skin punctures. A late onset variety of vitamin K deficiency may affect breast fed babies between 4–6 weeks after birth. It manifests as gastrointestinal bleeding or intracranial haemorrhage. To prevent these possible problems it is currently recommended that all newborn babies should be given phytomenadione (vitamin K_1) either 1.0mg intramuscularly at birth or 1.0mg orally at birth, at 3–4 days and at 6 weeks of age. The further care of the newborn infant is described Chapter 11.

Apgar Scoring Method for Evaluating the Infant			
Sign	0	1	2
Colour	Blue; pale	Body pink; extremities blue	Completely pink
Respiratory effort	Absent	Weak cry; hypoventilation	Good; strong cry
Muscle tone	Limp	Some flexion of extremities	Active motion; extremities well flexed
Reflex irritability (response to stimulation of sole of foot)	No response	Grimace	Cry
Heart rate	Absent	Slow (below 100)	Fast (over 100)

Table 10.2 Apgar scoring method for evaluating the infant (from Apgar and associates).

THE THIRD STAGE OF LABOUR

The third stage of labour extends from the birth of the baby to the expulsion of the placenta and membranes.

Separation of the placenta takes place through the spongy layer of the decidua basalis, as the result of uterine contractions being added to the retraction of the uterus which follows the birth of the child. The retraction of the uterus reduces the size of the placental bed to one quarter of its size in pregnancy, with the result that the placenta buckles inwards, tearing the blood vessels of the intervillous space,

and causing a retroplacental haemorrhage, which further separates the placenta. The process starts as the baby is born and placental separation is usually complete within 5 minutes, but the placenta may be held in the uterus for longer because the membranes take longer to strip from the underlying decidua. Following the separation of the placenta, the lattice arrangements of the myometrial fibres effectively strangle the blood vessels supplying the placental bed, reducing further blood loss and encouraging formation fibrin plugs in their torn ends *(see Fig. 10.17)*.

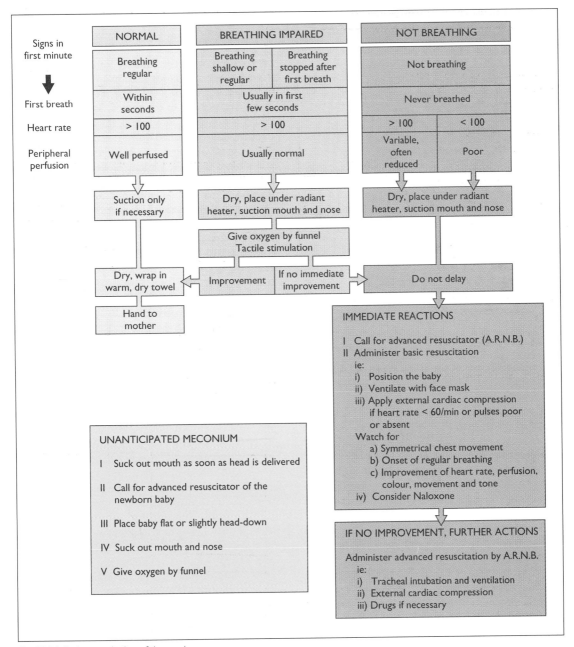

Fig 10.16 Basic resuscitation of the newborn.

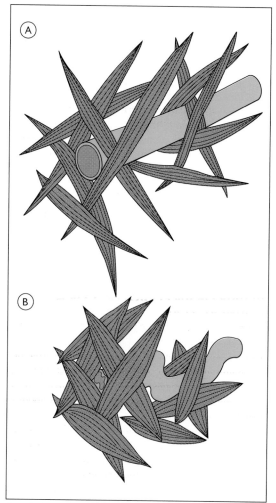

Fig 10.17 Diagram showing how the uterine muscle forms a 'living ligature' to occlude blood vessels.

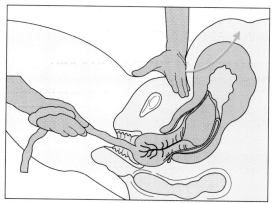

Fig 10.18 Controlled cord traction.

by 'fiddling' with the fundus, for example, unless haemorrhage demands action. Once the signs indicate that the placenta has been expelled from the uterus and is lying in the vagina, a uterine contraction is obtained by 'rubbing up' the uterus. The contracted uterus is pushed down towards the pelvis, so that it acts as a piston to expel the placenta and membranes from the vagina. The expelled placenta is grasped and twisted around with continuing traction to make the membranes into a twisted cord and so that they are expelled intact.

Active management

As the fetal head is being born, an intramuscular injection of Syntometrine 0.5ml or of Syntocinon 10U is given. If the woman is hypertensive, Syntometrine is avoided as the ergometrine content may increase the hypertension. In this case an intravenous injection of Syntocinon 10U is given with the birth of the anterior shoulder of the baby.

The delivery of the baby following the injection is conducted slowly over 60 seconds. The umbilical cord is divided and clamped 2 minutes after the birth. The slowness is because the oxytocic effect takes about 2 minutes to produce a strong uterine contraction. The attendant's left hand is placed on the uterus to detect the contraction. When it occurs, the hand is placed suprapubically and pushes the uterus upwards, whilst the right hand grasps the umbilical cord and pulls the placenta out of the vagina in a controlled manner *(Fig. 10.18)*. The membranes are drawn out of the vagina intact by twisting them into a rope and pulling them out with a sponge forceps or the hand. In 1–2 per cent of cases the placenta is retained, but no blood loss occurs. After a 10-minute delay another attempt is made to pull the placenta out by controlled cord traction. If this fails, manual removal of the placenta is necessary (see page 180). This is a disadvantage of the active management of the third stage of labour. The advantages of active management are that post-

The management of the third stage of labour

There are two methods of managing the third stage of labour:

- The traditional management.
- Active management.

The traditional management. The placenta and membranes are allowed to separate without interference. The ulnar border of one hand is placed on the uterine fundus, and the signs of placental separation are awaited. These are:

- A gush of blood.
- The fundus rises in the abdomen and becomes spherical.
- That part of the umbilical cord which can be seen at the vulva, lengthens.
- If the fundus is lifted upwards the umbilical cord does not shorten.

Ten to twenty minutes pass before these signs appear. No attempt is made to hasten the separation,

partum haemorrhage (a loss of >500 ml of blood) is reduced from 4 per cent to 2 per cent of all deliveries and the third stage of labour is shortened.

INSPECTION OF THE PLACENTA AND MEMBRANES

The placenta and membranes are held up by the umbilical cord and the fetal surface is examined, attention being paid to the blood vessels to see if there is any run to the edge of the membranes, indicating a possible succenturiate lobe. The membranes are examined to make sure that no part remains in the uterus. The maternal surface of the placenta is next examined, any clots being washed away, so that the cotyledons can be inspected. The maternal surface is held in both hands and fitted together to make sure that no cotyledon has been left in the uterus. If any cotyledon is missing or if most of the membranes have been left in the uterus or vagina, a doctor should explore the vagina and the uterine cavity under sterile conditions.

RETAINED PLACENTA

A retained placenta is one which has remained in the uterus for more than 1 hour. As retained placenta may be associated with haemorrhage, action should be taken to remove it. The causes of retained placenta are:

- Incarceration of a separated or partially separated placenta when, following the injection of an oxytocic drug the closing cervix traps it.
- Uterine atony, which is accompanied by bleeding.
- A morbidly adherent placenta. In this relatively uncommon condition (> 1:1500 births), the trophoblast has invaded the decidua and myometrium to varying degrees (placenta accreta) or has penetrated to the serosal coat (placenta percreta).

Management

If postpartum bleeding is marked, attempts should be made at once to find if the placenta has separated as described earlier, and attempts should be made to deliver it. If these measures fail it should be removed manually (see page 180).

Should the placenta be retained for one hour with little bleeding the above procedures should be undertaken.

A placenta accreta or percreta may resist attempts at manual removal and hysterectomy should be performed.

INSPECTION OF THE GENITAL TRACT FOR DAMAGE

Following the expulsion of the placenta and membranes, bleeding usually ceases. If the perineum has been torn or an episiotomy made, the tear or incision is now repaired after inspecting the vagina for damage. If a difficult forceps delivery has been made, the cervix should be inspected to exclude a lateral tear.

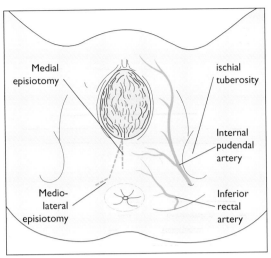

Fig 10.19 Types of episiotomy.

REPAIR OF AN EPISIOTOMY OR A PERINEAL TEAR

Episiotomy

Episiotomy, a deliberate incision in the stretched perineum and vagina, was first suggested 200 years ago, to prevent a ragged perineal tear occurring. If the attending doctor thinks that the perineum is about to tear because of its distension by the fetal head, the perineum is infiltrated with local anaesthetic, unless the woman has already had an epidural anaesthetic. The episiotomy incision may be midline or mediolateral (Fig. 10.19). The midline incision has the advantage that no large blood vessels are encountered and it is easier to repair. Its disadvantage is that it may extend into the rectum. If a large episiotomy is needed, for example when a difficult midforceps delivery is anticipated, a mediolateral episiotomy is preferred.

One method of repairing an episiotomy is shown in Fig. 10.20. This repair is the least painful postoperatively, particularly when 2/0 polyglycolic suture material is used.

Another method is to use continuous suture to repair the vagina and interrupted sutures for the perineal muscles and skin. The standard repair of an episiotomy is shown in Fig 10.21.

Perineal tears

Four degrees of perineal tears are recognized:

- *First degree.* Damage to the fourchette and the underlying muscles is exposed.
- *Second degree.* The posterior vaginal wall and the perineal muscles are torn but the anal sphincter is intact.
- *Third degree.* The anal sphincter is torn, but the rectal mucosa is intact.
- *Fourth degree.* The anal canal is opened, and the tear may spread to the rectum.

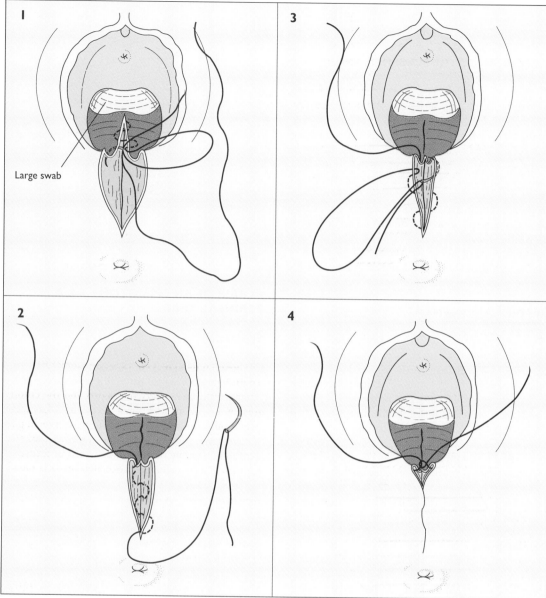

Fig 10.20 (1) Suture of the vaginal wall. (2) The suture of the vaginal wall has been completed and the perineal muscles are being sutured. (3) The subcuticular suture of the perineal skin starting posteriorly and finishing deep to the hymen. (4) The two strands of catgut are tied, and cut short. The knot disappears beneath the vaginal mucosa.

First degree tears are easy to repair; one or two sutures is all that is needed. Second and third degree tears need more care and their repair is shown in *Fig. 10.21*. Repair of fourth degree tears requires considerable skill, and it is essential to secure the apex of the tear or a rectovaginal fistula may result. The anal sphincter retracts when torn and its exposed ends must be identified and rejoined by sutures *(Fig. 10.22)*.

Postoperative care
The degree of postoperative pain and oedema depends on the method of delivery (forceps deliveries are followed by more oedema) and the quality of suturing. Most women need analgesics for a few days. A woman who has had the traditional interrupted sutures experiences more pain, but most patients can walk and have showers. Perineal swabbing is not usually necessary unless there is marked perineal oedema.

Episiotomies and perineal tears are not without longer-term discomfort. Twelve weeks after giving birth, 5 per cent of women still experience some degree of pain and 15 per cent have perineal discomfort. Sexual intercourse may be painful or uncomfortable for up to 20 weeks.

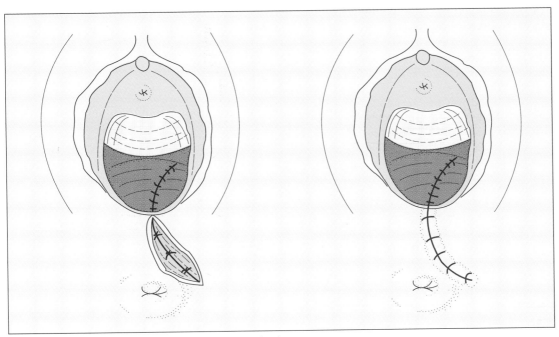

Fig 10.21 Standard method of repair of an episiotomy or perineal tear.

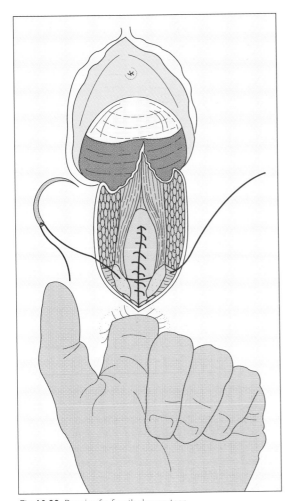

Fig 10.22 Repair of a fourth degree tear.

LACERATIONS OF THE LOWER GENITAL TRACT

After a difficult delivery the vagina and the clitoral area should be inspected for lacerations. Any large laceration should be sutured. Continued bleeding in spite of a firmly contracted uterus suggests an internal laceration. The vagina and cervix should be inspected with good illumination. If a lacerated cervix is found, the tear is sutured, care being taken to include the apex of the tear *(Fig. 10.23)*.

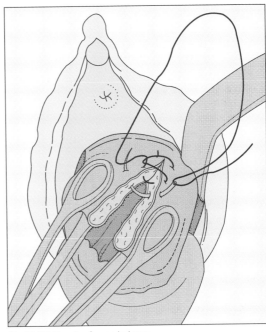

Fig 10.23 Repair of a cervical tear.

MANAGEMENT OF THE IMMEDIATE POST-DELIVERY PERIOD

The woman should remain in the delivery room for one hour. The medical attendants will check regularly that the uterus is contracted, that there is no excessive blood loss and that the vital signs are normal. During this time the baby will be checked thoroughly for abnormalities (see page 87), cleansed and returned to the mother to enable the parents to celebrate the birth.

Before the woman leaves the delivery room, the attendant must be sure that:

- The mother is in good general condition.
- The uterus is well contracted and contains no clots.
- The perineum has been properly repaired.
- The woman is not in pain from the repair.
- She does not have a full bladder.

PAIN RELIEF DURING CHILDBIRTH

The pain of childbirth varies considerably between women. Because of this a woman has the right to know that analgesics and anaesthetics are available for her, and she can decide when she needs pain relief. If the medical attendants decide when a woman needs pain relief, it reduces the autonomy of the woman and is not always effective. For example, surveys of women made some time after birth in Britain, Norway and Australia showed that between 15 and 20 per cent were disappointed by a lack of effective pain relief during their labour.

The ideal obstetric method of pain relief should:

- Do no harm to the mother or her baby.
- Not prevent the patient cooperating, particularly in the second stage of labour.
- Not interfere with normal uterine activity.

PAIN RELIEF IN LABOUR

In early labour (the latent phase) when uterine contractions are not particularly painful most women do not require pain relief. If the woman is very apprehensive a short acting benzodiazipine drug may be given, but not many women request it.

Most women seek pain relief once the active phase of the first stage begins. There are several methods: non pharmacological and using drugs.

NON PHARMACOLOGICAL METHODS

The *non pharmacological methods* need to be taught during the pregnancy by a trained person, so that by the time labour begins the woman understands what she has to do. They include; massage and touch; relaxation techniques; rhythmical movements; hot and cold (e.g. showers or baths); transcutaneous electrical nerve stimulation (TENS). The effectiveness of these techniques is not clear, but some women find them very helpful in relieving pain.

Later in the active phase when the contractions become stronger, a woman may choose to continue with nonpharmacological methods, but must be made aware that if they do not provide adequate pain relief she may obtain a *pharmacological method*. She must not be made to feel that she has failed if she seeks *narcotics or epidural anaesthesia*. Of the narcotics, pethidine in a dose of 100–150mg intramuscularly at intervals is chosen by many women (the opioid is effective in about 15 minutes and the effect lasts for 2-3 hours). There is some concern that if pethidine is given within 2 hours of birth, the baby may have a delayed onset in breathing after birth. If this occurs it is easily and effectively treated by injecting an opioid antagonist, for example, naloxone into the umbilical vein, or intramuscularly.

An alternative method of giving pethidine, which is available in some hospitals, is Patient Controlled Analgesia. Using PCA the woman controls the dose she is receiving (within limits) The method is attractive to some women, particularly after a caesarean section, but is not widely used.

NITROUS OXIDE AND OXYGEN

In most cases a fifty-fifty mixture of nitrous oxide and oxygen is given in an Entotox machine. The patient breathes the mixture during a contraction in the active phase of the first stage and during the second stage of labour. It can be used to supplement the pain relief provided by pethidine. To be effective it has to be used properly. Even if used properly, rather less than 50 per cent of women obtain satisfactory pain relief; 20 per cent obtain some relief and 30 per cent find the method ineffective.

EPIDURAL ANALGESIA.

Epidural anaesthesia has become increasingly popular in recent years and would be chosen by more women if the service were more readily available. In Britain, for example, the Social Services Committee has recommended strongly that the Health Authorities should provide an anaesthetic service in all major obstetric units that is available within a few minutes of receiving a call. The Committee also recommends that only trained doctors should give an epidural anaesthetic.

Epidural anaesthesia is the most effective way of relieving the pain of childbirth, and provides complete relief of contraction pain in 95 per cent of labouring women. It provides great flexibility in pain management. For example, should the delivery require forceps, vacuum extraction or be by caesarean section, epidural anaesthesia avoids possible adverse biochemical effects associated with a general anaesthetic, and can provide postoperative pain relief. The disadvantages of epidural anaesthesia are that a few women complain of dizzyness or shivering; that it may increase the duration of the second stage and lead to an increase in operative vaginal delivery.

Serious side effects are uncommon. The most worrying are transient hypotension, which occurs in 20 per cent of patients, and dural tap (in 1 per cent), which is followed by severe headache in half of the women. Rather more women complain of backache in the puerperium (15 per cent v. 10 per cent who did not have an epidural)

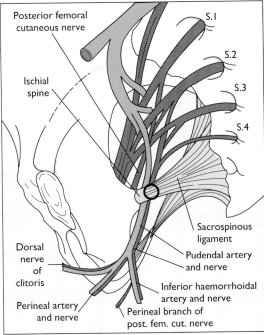

Fig 10.24 The course of the pudendal nerve. The area in the circle which lies just medial to and below the tip of the ischial spine is the area into which the local anaesthetic is infiltrated.

LOCAL ANALGESIA

Local analgesia is a choice in the relief of pain during childbirth for women who have not had an epidural anaesthetic and who require a forceps or vacuum extraction delivery, the repair of an episiotomy or a perineal tear and in some cases of breech delivery. Two techniques are available. These are pudendal nerve block and perineal nerve infiltration. To understand the techniques, knowledge of the nerve supply of the vulva and lower vagina is needed.

The nerve supply of the vulva

The female vulva is innervated mainly by branches of the pudendal nerve. The pudendal nerve, derived from S2, S3 and S4 leaves the pelvis medial to the sciatic nerve through the greater sciatic foramen. It then crosses the external surface of the ischial spine and re-enters the pelvis through the lesser sciatic notch and, passing along the lateral wall of the ischio-rectal fossa, divides into branches which supply most of the perineum (*Fig. 10.24*). Further sensory branches to the skin of the perineum are derived from the ilio-inguinal nerve, the pudendal branch of the posterior femoral cutaneous nerve and the genital branch of the genito-femoral nerve (*Fig. 10.25*).

The technique of pudendal nerve block

A 10cm, 20 gauge needle and, if available, a needle director are required. Two fingers are introduced into the vagina to palpate the ischial spine, the guide containing the needle being introduced in the groove between the index and middle finger to impinge on the spine. The guide is then directed to lie just medial to, and below, the ischial spine and the

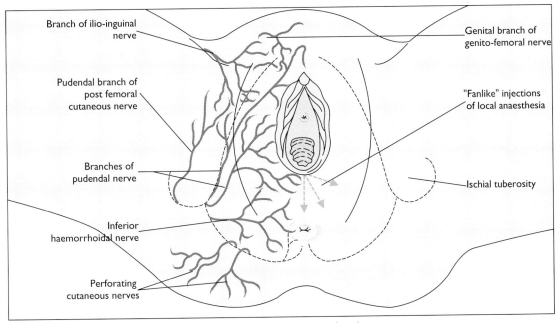

Fig 10.25 Innervation of the perineum. On one side the nerves are shown, on the other, 'fanlike' local anaesthesia.

needle is advanced 1cm beyond the guide (if no guide is available the needle is introduced between the fingers to the same site) and pushed through the sacrospinous ligament (*Fig. 10.26*); 10ml of 0.5% lignocaine is injected behind each ischial spine, and a further 10ml is used to make a perineal infiltration. Anaesthesia should be effective within 5 minutes and it should be tested. The lower vagina and perineum become insensitive to pain. The use of pudendal nerve block is not without problems. For example, the needle may be difficult to introduce accurately in a relatively mobile patient, particularly when the fetal head is deeply engaged.

The technique of perineal nerve infiltration
Using a 7.5cm, 22 gauge needle, and 20ml of 0.5–1 % lignocaine, the perineum is infiltrated in a fan-like manner, the base being the posterior fourchette at the midline. Three lines of infiltration are required, one medially as far as the anal sphincter and midway between the skin and the vaginal mucosa, and two others at 45° to block the nerves as they reach the perineum (*Fig. 10.25*). The analgesia is effective in about 3 minutes and lasts between 45 and 90 minutes. It should be tested by pricking the skin with a sharp needle before any procedure is begun.

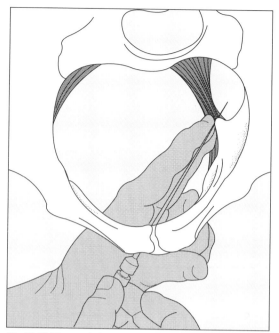

Fig 10.26 Transvaginal pudendal nerve block shown diagrammatically.

11

THE PUERPERIUM

By convention the puerperium lasts for six weeks from the day of the birth of the child. During this time the physiological and morphological changes which occurred during pregnancy revert to the non-pregnant state. It is also a time when the woman takes on the responsibility of caring for a dependent, demanding infant. This may cause problems, particularly if she finds it difficult to adjust to being a mother.

THE PHYSIOLOGICAL AND ANATOMICAL CHANGES

The *endocrinological changes* which occurred during pregnancy rapidly revert. Within hours of the expulsion of the placenta the levels of the placental hormones, human placental lactogen (hPL) and chorionic gonadotrophin (hCG), fall rapidly. Within 2 days hPL is undetectable in serum and by the 10th day after birth, hCG can no longer be detected. The serum levels of oestrogen and progesterone fall rapidly in the first 3 puerperal days reaching non-pregnant levels by the 7th day after birth. They remain at this level if the woman chooses to breast-feed; if she does not, oestradiol begins to rise, indicating follicular growth. Among breast-feeding women human pro-lactin (hPr) levels rise following suckling.

The *cardiovascular system* reverts to the non-pregnant state during the first 2 puerperal weeks. In the first 24 hours the additional burden on the heart caused by the hypervolaemic state persists, after which time the blood and plasma volume return to the non-pregnant state. This occurs by the second puerperal week. In the first 10 days after birth the raised coagulation factors occurring during pregnancy persist but are balanced by a rise in fibrinolytic activity.

MORPHOLOGICAL CHANGES IN THE GENITAL TRACT

The perineum and vagina. Following the birth the perineum is either damaged or intact. The damage will have been repaired, but oedema of the tissues may have occurred and will persist for some days. The vaginal wall is swollen, bluish and pouting. It rapidly regains its tonicity, although it is fragile for one or two weeks.

The *uterus* undergoes the most marked changes. At the end of the third stage of labour, the uterus is the size of a 20-week pregnancy and weighs about 1000g. It rapidly becomes smaller and by the end of the first puerperal week it weighs about 500g. Its involution can be demonstrated by the fact that its size is reduced on abdominal examination by one finger-breadth a day, to the extent that on the 12th day after the birth it cannot be palpated abdominally. Its involution continues after this time more slowly, but by the end of the 6th puerperal week it is only slightly larger than it was before the pregnancy.

Concurrently with the involution of the uterus, the *placental site* becomes smaller. It is rapidly covered after the birth with a fibrin mesh, and thrombosis occurs in the vessels supplying it. Beneath the placental site, macrophages, lympho-cytes and polymorphs form a 'barrier' which also extends throughout the endometrial cavity. Within 10 days the placental site has shrunk to a diameter of 2.5cm, and a new growth of covering epithelium has occurred, which also covers the remainder of the uterine cavity. The superficial tissues of the uterine lining and placental site continue to be shed for 6 weeks, and form part of the lochia.

The *lochia* is the term used for the discharge from the genital tract which follows childbirth. For the first 3–4 days it consists of blood and remnants of trophoblastic tissue, mainly from the placental site. As the thrombosed vessels of the site become organized the character of the lochia changes. From the 3rd to the 12th day after the birth its colour is reddish-brown, but after this time, when most of the endometrial cavity has been covered with epithelium, it changes to a yellow colour. Occasionally some of the thrombi at the end of the vessels break, releasing blood and the lochia becomes red once more for a few days.

THE CONDUCT OF THE PUERPERIUM

In contrast with 25 years ago, a recently delivered woman is no longer confined to bed. For instance, she may start walking about as soon as she wishes, go to the toilet when required and rest when she feels tired. Often an afternoon nap is all that she needs. Some women prefer to remain in bed for the first 24 hours after the birth, and women who have had an extensive repair of a torn perineum or a large episiotomy may choose to remain in bed for longer. Visitors are no longer restricted, but common sense must prevail and if the new mother is tired, they should be asked to leave.

A function of the medical attendants is to make sure that the tissues are healing properly, and that the uterus is involuting normally. But this function is less important than helping a woman to breast-feed if she chooses to do so, and providing information about the care of the infant when the mother goes home.

There is no longer a fixed time for remaining in hospital after the birth. A woman may choose to go home after 1 or 2 days or may prefer to remain in hospital for 5 days. An advantage of the longer stay is that lactation and breast feeding is established during this time.

CARE OF THE PUERPERAL WOMAN

With early ambulation the care of the puerperal woman has becomes more simple. Regular checks are made of the temperature and pulse. The perineum is inspected each day to observe the degree of oedema (if any) and the sutures. Many women who have a damaged and repaired perineum experience considerable pain. The woman may need analgesics, and may find it more comfortable to sit on a rubber ring. This matter is discussed further on page 80.

The character and amount of the lochia is observed and recorded and the height of the uterine fundus above the symphysis is checked daily.

Uterine contractions continue after the childbirth. They are usually painless, but some women experience painful uterine contractions (afterpains) especially when breast-feeding. The woman may ask for analgesics.

URINARY TRACT PROBLEMS

Micturition may be difficult in the 24 hours after childbirth because of a reflex suppression of detrusor activity caused by the pressure on the bladder base during the birth. As a diuresis occurs following the birth, the woman may be uncomfortable. If she is unable to pass urine, catheterization may be required. After catheterization, 60ml of chlorhexidine solution should be instilled into the bladder, to reduce the risk of urinary tract infection. This is more likely to occur in the puerperium than later because the pregnancy induced dilatation of the renal pelvis and ureters and the relaxation of the bladder muscle take about 3 weeks to disappear.

About 10 per cent of puerperal women experience urinary incontinence (usually 'stress incontinence'). This incontinence persists for a few weeks and then ceases in all but a few women. Pelvic floor exercises (see page 293) may speed up the resolution of problem more quickly.

BOWEL PROBLEMS

A few women become *constipated* in the puerperium. in most cases spontaneous relief is obtained; if not, stool softeners such as biscodyl rectal suppositories may be prescribed.

Women who have *haemorrhoids* during pregnancy often complain that they are more painful in the postpartum period. One woman in 20 develops haemorrhoids for the first time during the birth, but in most cases these settle in two or three weeks.

BACKACHE

Backache often occurs in the last quarter of pregnancy and persists after birth, or it may occur for the first time in the puerperium. Backache affects about 25 per cent of puerperal woman, but over half of them had complained of backache before becoming pregnant. The pain can be considerable, particularly if the woman has no help in caring for her baby. It may persist for months but eventually settles.

CARE OF THE NEONATE

Today in most hospitals facilities exist for rooming in, the baby lying in a cot close to the mother's bed, mother and baby being treated as a dyad. This has made the care of a healthy newborn infant much easier.

CHECKING FOR CONGENITAL ABNORMALITIES

A check for major abnormalities is made immediately after birth before the baby is given to the mother to celebrate her or his birth. A full check is made during the baby's first day of life. The procedure is described in *Table 11.1*.

THE CARE OF THE UMBILICAL CORD

The umbilical cord is inspected, the clamp removed, and the cord is tied and cut close to the umbilicus 24 hours after birth. The area is smeared with chlorhexidine cream, but no cord dressing or binder is used.

WEIGHT LOSS

A newborn infant may be expected to lose between 5 and 10 per cent of its birth-weight during the first 4 days of life. This causes no problems for a healthy mature baby. From the 4th day the infant will be obtaining sufficient breast milk (or breast milk substitute) to start gaining weight. No fluids other than those obtained from the breast or bottle need be given. Extra fluids should be avoided in breast-fed babies as they interfere with the smooth establishment of lactation. The only reason for extra fluids is if the baby develops 'dehydration fever' .

DEHYDRATION FEVER

Because a neonate's temperature control is not very efficient, dehydration fever may affect a few infants in first days of life in hot, humid weather. The infant develops a high fever, looks dehydrated, and has a dry mouth and a depressed anterior fontanelle. It is vigorous and thirsty, unlike an infected infant, which is languid and febrile. Dehydration fever rarely occurs in infants who room-in and breast-feed on demand. The treatment is to replace the fluid and salt lost by giving oral feeds of 200ml 1/5 normal saline per kg body-weight per 24 hours.

Examination of a Newborn Baby
Examine baby one hour after a feed when he/she is likely to be calm, quiet and with open eyes. Get mother to undress the baby.
1. Observe posture movements, check for skin abnormalities.
2. Palpate neck for goitre or sternomastoid tumour.
3. Look at eyes, see if he/she will follow side-to-side movement of examiner's face.
4. Measure occipito-frontal circumference, feel skull and fontanelles.
5. Get baby to open mouth; examine for cleft palate.
6. Examine the chest for signs of respiratory distress (note the respiratory rate should be less than 60).
7. Examine the pericardium for cardiac murmurs.
8. Palpate abdomen.
9. Examine external genitalia, feel for femoral pulses.
10. Check Moro and traction manoeuvres: *Moro*: When picked up, the baby extends and abducts arms and fingers and opens eyes; he/she then flexes and abducts arms. *Traction*: When lifted by grasping hands, the baby flexes arms and keeps head in the plane of trunk.
11. Pick up baby in prone position; check muscle tone, examine spine (scoliosis), anus.
12. Examine hips To examine the left hip, the doctor steadies the infant's pelvis between the thumb of the left hand on the symphysis pubis and the fingers behind the sacrum. The examiner grasps the child's left thigh in the right hand and attempts to move the femoral head gently forwards and then backwards out of the acetabulum. If the head of the femur is felt to move, with or without an audible 'clunk', dislocation, or dislocability is diagnosed. If there is any doubt after the examination, real-time ultrasound is used to detect a displaced hip. In about 10 per cent of the cases the babies' hips produce a soft 'click' rather than a 'clunk', and there is no evidence of abnormal movement of the femoral head. These babies must be examined again before discharge from hospital. If one month later the click has changed into a clunk, and abnormal movement between the femoral head and the acetabulum is found, the ultrasound examination is repeated.

Table 11.1 Examination of a newborn baby.

THE STOOLS

In the first two days of life the infant's faeces are sticky and greenish-black in colour. As microorganisms invade the gut the colour of the faeces changes to yellow with the occasional passage of greenish faeces. Breast-fed babies usually defaecate a soft stool which has little smell. Bottle-fed infants do not defaecate as regularly and the stool when expelled is firmer in consistency, dark yellow in colour and occasionally has an offensive smell.

JAUNDICE

Most babies develop transient jaundice which is benign and self-limiting. A few infants develop more marked jaundice. If this occurs within 24 hours of birth, persists, and the jaundice extends onto the infant's trunk or thighs, serum bilirubin measurements are made. A serum bilirubin reading of >250mmol/L is of concern as kernicterus may occur. Advice from a paediatrician should be obtained. Treatment is phototherapy or, in severe cases, exchange transfusion.

INFANT FEEDING

The establishment of maternal lactation and breast-feeding, or, if the mother chooses not to breast-feed, the establishment of feeding with breast milk substitutes, is one of the most important tasks of those caring for the infant.

LACTATION AND BREAST-FEEDING

During pregnancy the breasts develop considerably. Fat is deposited around the glandular parts of the breasts. Oestrogen leads to an increase in the size and number of the ducts, and progesterone increases the number of alveoli. Human placental lactogen (hPL) also stimulates alveolar development and may be involved in the synthesis of casein, lactalbumin and lactoglobulin by the alveolar cells.

In spite of this activity, lactation is inhibited during pregnancy, although levels of human prolactin (hPr) rise throughout the pregnancy. The reason for this is that the high levels of oestrogen occupy binding sites on the alveoli which prevent them from responding to the lactogenic properties of hPr. In late pregnancy the breasts secrete a thickish, yellowish fluid, colostrum, which is rich in immune antibodies. The production of colostrum increases after the birth until it is replaced by breast milk.

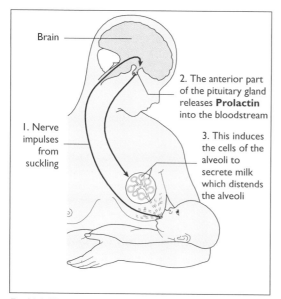

Fig 11.1 The prolactin reflex.

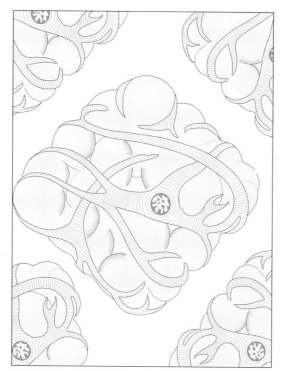

Fig 11.2 Myoepithelial cells surrounding a partially filled villus

As mentioned earlier, the level of oestrogen falls rapidly in the 48 hours following childbirth. This permits circulating hPr to act on the alveolar cells to initiate and maintain lactation.

Lactation is encouraged by early and frequent suckling, as this reflexly causes the pituitary gland to secrete hPr (*Fig. 11.1*). On the other hand, negative emotions, including the fear of failing to breast-feed, may reduce the secretion of prolactin, by promoting the release of prolactin-inhibiting factor (dopamine) from the hypothalamus.

By the 2nd or 3rd day after the birth, hPr has induced the alveolar cells to secrete milk, which is thin and bluish in colour. Initially the milk distends the alveoli and the small ducts, causing the breasts to become full, engorged and tender. Turgid veins can be seen beneath the skin and the milk ducts can be felt as tender strings in the breast tissue. The engorgement is due to the absence of ejection of milk through the large ducts to the nipple.

THE MILK EJECTION REFLEX

The milk filling and distending the alveoli is unavailable to the infant until myoepithelial cells (*Fig. 11.2*) which surround the alveoli and smaller ducts contract in response to the milk ejection (or 'let-down') reflex. The reflex is initiated by suckling, and is mediated via the hypothalamus and pituitary gland which releases oxytocin into the bloodstream (*Fig. 11.3*).

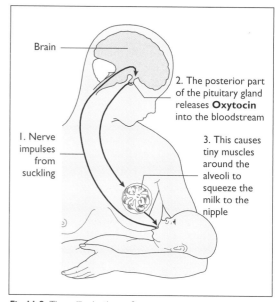

Fig 11.3 The milk ejection reflex.

The oxytocin causes contractions of the myoepithelial cells and milk is ejected from the alveoli and small ducts to flow to the large ducts and the sub areolar reservoirs. Oxytocin may also inhibit the release of dopamine from the hypothalamus, further encouraging the secretion of milk.

Negative emotional and physical factors can reduce the let-down reflex so that for lactation to be established the mother must be confident that she can breast-feed. The medical attendants should encourage her to be confident.

A joint statement by WHO and UNICEF was published in 1989 which showed how the support needed for successful lactation could be obtained (*Table 11.2*).

THE MAINTENANCE OF LACTATION

The most effective way of maintaining lactation is regular suckling, so that both the prolactin and the milk ejection reflexes are initiated frequently, and abnormal distension of the alveoli by milk is prevented. If distension occurs, the alveoli are unable to secrete milk efficiently and at the same time suckling is avoided because of pain in the breasts. A consequence of this is that the inhibition of the reflex which prevents the release of dopamine from the hypothalamus is lost and alveolar activity diminishes, with a further reduction of milk secretion.

THE ESTABLISHMENT OF BREAST-FEEDING

The establishment of successful breast feeding requires:
- That milk secretion occurs in the alveoli.
- That the milk ejection reflex is efficient.
- That the mother is motivated to breast-feed (she may need support to keep motivated).

As mentioned in *Table 11.2*, breast-feeding is more readily established if:
- The baby is given to the mother to caress and suckle soon after birth.
- The baby rooms-in with the mother and the staff treat them as a dyad.
- The baby is allowed to suckle frequently from birth for a short period each time to help 'bring the milk in'.
- Once the milk is flowing the baby is fed on demand, including at night.
- No feeds of water or of glucose water are given to the infant by the nursing staff without the express agreement of the mother and her doctor.
- The nursing staff help the establishment of lactation by adopting a positive approach to the mother and are unhurried and supportive during the time she establishes breast-feeding.

THE TECHNIQUE OF BREAST-FEEDING

The mother should be shown how to stroke the infant's mouth with her nipple, to induce the 'rooting' reflex in which the baby opens her or his mouth and searches for the nipple.

Ten Steps to Successful Breast-feeding
A joint WHO/UNICEF statement (1989) Every facility providing maternity services and care for newborn infants should:
1. Have a written breast-feeding policy that is routinely communicated to all health-care staff.
2. Train all health-care staff in the skills necessary to implement this policy.
3. Inform all pregnant women about the benefits and management of breast-feeding.
4. Help mothers initiate breast-feeding within a half-hour of birth.
5. Show mothers how to breast-feed and how to maintain lactation even if they are separated from their infants.
6. Give new-born infants no food or drink other than breast milk unless medically indicated.
7. Practise rooming-in. Allow mothers and infants to stay together 24 hours a day.
8. Encourage breast-feeding on demand.
9. Give no artificial teats or pacifiers (also called dummies and soothers) to breast-feeding infants.
10. Foster the establishment of breast-feeding support groups and refer mothers to them on discharge from hospital or clinic.

Handwritten margin notes:

maybe me de- orally

(Hand) written policy
Training health care staff
Inform mothers. benefits
Help initiate br. feeding
Maintain be. feeding
° Food drink to new born
Rooming in 24/24
Demand B/F
no dummies
B/F Support groups.
on discharge.

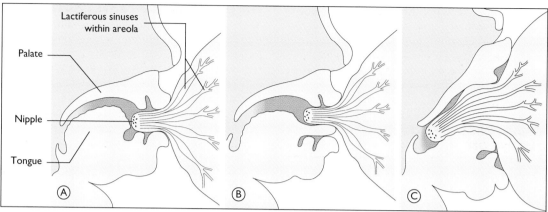

Fig 11.4 Ideal position of nipple in infant's mouth. In A and B the nipple is being chewed; in C the nipple is well within the baby's mouth.

She then holds her breast with the nipple between her forefinger and middle finger, so that the nipple becomes more prominent and the infant is able to put its gums on the areola and not on the tender nipple (*Fig. 11.4*). This technique enables the baby to breathe when suckling (*Fig. 11.5*).

The mother is shown how to detach the infant's mouth from the nipple without causing her pain. This is done by putting her little finger into the corner of the baby's mouth to break the suction before detaching the baby from her nipple (*Fig. 11.6*).

As mentioned earlier, very few babies managed in this way require additional fluids in the first 4 days of life. However, if the baby becomes clinically dehydrated, water may be given by a spoon or dropper after a feed. A feeding bottle should be avoided as it may stop the baby learning properly how to suck at the breast.

BREAST ENGORGEMENT

It takes a few days to adjust the supply of milk to the demand, mainly because the milk ejection reflex is not yet operating properly. During this time the breasts of some women become engorged as described earlier. Treatment depends on the severity of the engorgement. Many nurses claim success if hot and cold towels are applied alternately to the breasts. They claim that the towels stimulate increased blood flow through the engorged areas of the breasts. Another method is to

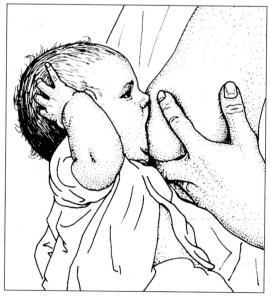

Fig 11.5 The technique of breast-feeding.

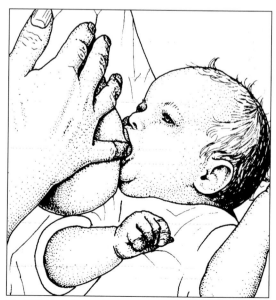

Fig 11.6 How the mother releases her nipple from the baby's mouth.

stimulate the milk ejection reflex using an electric breast pump (the Egnell pump). Severe and painful engorgement may be reduced by prescribing small doses of bromocriptine (a dopamine) for 24–48 hours.

If possible the mother should continue to breast-feed in spite of the engorgement of her breasts, to stimulate the milk ejection reflex.

BREAST PROBLEMS DURING LACTATION

Cracked nipples

Aggressive suckling by the baby may lead to cracked nipples, particularly if the nipple is not well within the infant's mouth. The nipple should be treated with chlorhexidine cream and a nipple shield used to protect the abraded area during feeding. If the cracking is severe, the baby should not be fed from the affected breast, which should be emptied manually or by using a breast pump.

Milk stasis

This may occur early in lactation and be associated with, or follow, breast engorgement. It is due to pressure on the main duct of a lobule by the engorged alveoli. It usually settles without treatment but may lead to non-infectious inflammation of the breast. It is thought the pressure in some of the alveoli permits seepage of milk into the surrounding breast tissues, which causes the non infectious breast inflammation. Treatment of both forms, if needed, is to try to help the mother feed her baby more often and to empty the breasts manually after each feed.

Acute mastitis

Most cases of acute mastitis in the mother are caused by organisms acquired from the infant's nasopharyngeal or umbilical areas which harbour colonies of staphylococci or streptococci that develop within a few days of birth.

Acute mastitis occurs at the end of the first week following birth. The mother develops a fever and a tender, red, firm-to-hard area is felt in one of the breasts. Treatment is to prescribe analgesics and antibiotics. As most infections are caused by staphylococci, currently flucloxacillin is preferred. If it is not too painful, the mother should continue suckling the baby. If pus develops in the infected area of the breast, causing a breast abscess, incision of the abscess and drainage for 24 hours may be required.

Proper attention to breast feeding reduces the chance of acute mastitis developing. The breasts should be emptied after a feed, as incomplete emptying of the breasts leaves stagnant milk in the system which may become infected. Cracked nipples should be treated, as microorganisms may invade through the cracks. Rooming-in reduces the chance of cross-infection between babies and of mastitis in the mother.

THE SUPPRESSION OF LACTATION

Women who choose not to breast-feed or who stop breast-feeding may require to have lactation suppressed. Lactation will diminish and cease if the baby no longer suckles. At first the breasts become engorged, but if supported by an appropriately sized bra, will become less engorged in a few days and lactation will cease. An alternative is for the woman to be prescribed a prolactin inhibitor (dopamine receptor agonist), such as bromocriptine, pergolide or cyclofenil. Bromocriptine is given by mouth in a dose of 2.5mg twice daily for 14 days; alternatively, a single 40mg injection may be used.

BREAST-MILK SUBSTITUTES

More than 95 per cent of women can breast-feed if they want to. Although most women choose to breast-feed immediately after childbirth, by the 6th week of the puerperium, fewer than 60 per cent of women are still breast-feeding.

Women who do not breast-feed choose one of the breast-milk substitutes (formula milks) available. They are based on cow's milk, modified as far as possible to have the same proportions of protein, fat, carbohydrates, minerals and vitamins as human milk.

Provided that the formula milk is prepared according to the manufacturer's directions the baby will thrive, although she or he is not as well protected against infection as a breast-fed infant. This is of importance in the developing countries and among poor women in all countries.

PSYCHOLOGICAL PROBLEMS IN THE PUERPERIUM

The birth of a baby places considerable 'stress' on the mother. She has the responsibility of caring for a demanding infant, she has to continue to care for her husband or partner, her nights are usually disturbed and she may not feel competent or confident about her ability as a mother.

It is not surprising that it takes time for her to adjust to being a mother and that she may suffer psychological disturbances.

A large number of women become temporarily sad and emotional between the 3rd and 5th day after the birth (Third Day Blues), and about 10 per cent of women become more severely depressed. Postpartum depression is mentioned here and discussed more fully on page 182.

THIRD DAY BLUES

Why so many women develop third day blues is not known. Speculation about its aetiology includes hormonal imbalance (although none has been identified), reaction to the excitement of childbirth, and uncertainty by the mother about her ability to care for her dependent child. Another factor in Western culture may be the expectation that a mother immediately loves her baby, when in reality, mother love is a learned behaviour. The condition leads to bursts of crying, to irritability and in some cases to general depression. Successful management of this malaise consists of one of the medical or nursing staff talking with the woman, explaining what is occurring, and if the woman wishes, restricting visitors. There is some evidence that 'third day blues' are less likely to occur if maternal-infant bonding has occurred and if rooming-in is practised. 'Third day blues' is a misnomer as the inability to adjust to parenthood, with feelings of inadequacy, tiredness, reduced sexuality, emotional lability and, in a small proportion of women, severe depression, may persist for weeks or months.

ADJUSTMENT TO PARENTHOOD AND PUERPERAL DEPRESSION

Few doctors understand that adjustment to parenthood is difficult for most women. Women have been brought up to believe that they should be good housekeepers, excellent lovers and experienced mothers all at the same time. Yet on return home after childbirth, the persistent demands of the newborn baby on the energy, the time and the emotions of a woman may cause considerable stress. This stress is aggravated by the nuclear family and the tendency for young people to live at some distance from their close relatives, who, in other cultures, are readily available to offer help and consolation. The stress becomes intensified as the mother realizes that she has the sole responsibility for a small, unpredictable infant who needs attention day and night. She had not realized that the baby would cry so much, for so little apparent cause. Her sleep is constantly broken and fatigue is added to her feelings of maternal inadequacy. Her relationship with her husband requires adjustment; and this can be emotionally disturbing, particularly if he does not do his share of parenting. As the baby occupies so much of her time, the mother finds that she cannot keep the house as clean as she would wish, and feels guilty that she is not the efficient housewife she believed she was.

The fatigue induced by the demands of the baby, the emotional readjustment in marital relations, the guilt experienced over an untidy house and lack of a helpful counsellor, often induces depression. In about 5 per cent of women the depression becomes so severe that medical help is sought, usually between the 2nd and 7th week of the puerperium. The presenting symptoms are mainly changes in mood: tearfulness, feelings of inadequacy and inability to cope predominate. These changes are labile, and tend to become worse towards evening, when associated psychosomatic complaints of fatigue, anorexia and nausea may occur. Doctors all too frequently offer sedation or psychotropic drugs, when explanation, reassurance and advice would be even more useful. It is also important to tell parents of community-based help organizations

such as the La Lèche League in Britain and the USA, and the Nursing Mothers Association and Play Groups in Australia. These organizations provide 24-hour home counselling and home visiting when needed. Their activities in helping women adjust to parenthood can be of great value in reducing the incidence of puerperal depression.

SEXUALITY AFTER BIRTH

After childbirth the demands of the new baby occupy a good deal of a mother's time. Moreover, if the mother has had a perineal tear or an episiotomy repaired, her perineum and vagina may be tender for several weeks. It is not unexpected that her desire for sexual intercourse is reduced. Sexual intercourse is not the only way of obtaining sexual pleasure and she may welcome touching, cuddling and stimulating her husband or partner to orgasm if he wishes. When she is ready the couple can resume sexual intercourse. Women may consult a doctor about their lack of sexual feeling after the birth and supportive advice is helpful.

PERINATAL BEREAVEMENT

About 12 babies in every 1000 are either stillborn or die in the first 28 days of life. They constitute perinatal deaths. Many of these babies are born preterm, are of low birth-weight and about 25 per cent have severe congenital malformations. Parents whose baby dies in the perinatal period have grief reactions similar to those which follow the loss of any loved person. At first the mother (and often the father) feels numb and 'shocked'. After a few days the reaction changes to a desire to understand why the baby died, or to expressions of anger or guilt about events in pregnancy or during labour. Over the next 2 or 3 months many parents are likely to review the events surrounding the baby's death, often repeatedly. More than 50 per cent of mothers suffer from depression and anxiety which may last for months, but in time, the couple adjust, often embarking on a new pregnancy.

The severity and duration of the bereavement reaction may be reduced if the parents are given the opportunity to talk with the attending medical and nursing staff soon after the baby's death. The talk should take place in a quiet private area, not in an open ward. Most parents want to understand what has gone wrong explained in clear, simple language. A few become angry, blaming the staff for the child's death. The doctor or nurse should listen to the parents with sympathy and understanding and explain as clearly as possible the events surrounding the death.

In addition, the staff member should give information to the parents about the grief reaction which may be expected and should provide reassurance that nothing the mother did, or failed to do, caused the death of the child.

Parents who wish to see their dead child (even if malformed) should be given the opportunity, so that they may mourn their loss. If they do not wish to see the child at that time, a photograph, a footprint and perhaps a lock of the child's hair should be kept with the mother's records, as later the parents may regret their decision not to have seen their child.

Before the parents see the baby they should be told how the infant will look. If deformities are present, they should be described (perhaps with the aid of a photograph). The baby is presented to the parents clothed and wrapped, and when they become accustomed to him or her, the baby is undressed by them. This procedure is often emotional, and support from a health professional may be invaluable. The parents should be told that they can spend as much time as they wish with the baby, and should be encouraged to name the child. Many parents wish to have a photograph of their dead baby. When the mother leaves hospital it is important to suggest that she makes contact with her family doctor (or health visitor) and should be told about community-based helping organizations in her area.

One woman in every five whose baby is stillborn or who dies in the neonatal period will suffer severe symptoms of bereavement (sleeplessness, depression and withdrawal). Women who have little or no support from husband, partner or family, who are cared for by insensitive health professionals, and who lack a caring environment are more likely to be affected severely. These women, particularly, need help from sympathetic health professionals who listen, communicate and counsel.

There is some evidence that parents cope better, psychologically, with the next pregnancy if conception is delayed for a few months, but the decision has to be made by the couple, rather than imposed by a doctor. During the pregnancy, continuity of care is important, and supportive, communicating, sympathetic health professionals help to reduce possible mothering difficulties and puerperal problems.

CHILD ABUSE

Women who find difficulty in coping with their baby, or who have strange, disturbed behaviour whilst in hospital, are more likely to abuse their baby after discharge. The prevalence of child abuse before the age of 3 is not known exactly, but it is probable that at least 6 per 1000 live-born children are abused. Mothers who have social problems, who have no supportive partner or relative, or who have marital problems are more likely to abuse their child. It is possible, by simple observation in the puerperium, to identify some 'vulnerable' women, and this is part of postnatal care. Preventive intervention by family doctors, paediatricans and social workers has been shown to reduce the prevalence of child neglect and abuse.

THE POSTNATAL CHECK

It is usual for the mother (and her baby) to be asked to return for a postnatal check 6–8 weeks after the birth. The purpose of this visit is for the woman to discuss her adjustment to parenthood, her need for information about child care, her sexual relationships and contraception. The doctor will refer to the records to recall if any complications arose in pregnancy or during childbirth which need follow-up. The doctor also examines the woman (and her baby if he or she is not being seen by a paediatrician).

The examination includes inspection of the perineum and vagina to ascertain that any damage has healed and to determine the muscle tone. A vaginal speculum is used to visualize the cervix and a pap smear is made if indicated. A bimanual examination is made to check that the uterus has involuted completely.

Most of the visit is spent in discussing the woman's problems if she has any. Contraception is also an important area for discussion and advice (see Chapter 33).

It should be noted, however, that if the woman has decided not to breast feed, contraception should be discussed with her in the last quarter of pregnancy and started 21 days after the birth.

Perinatal mortality - 12/1000

12

'MINOR' COMPLICATIONS OF PREGNANCY

The physiological and anatomical changes which occur during pregnancy may lead to complications which although minor in medical terms may cause considerable distress and discomfort to many pregnant women. They are listed in alphabetical order.

BACKACHE

Backache is common in late pregnancy and is felt over the sacroiliac joints. It is due to relaxation of the ligaments and muscles supporting the joints, and is probably also caused by progesterone and, possibly, relaxin. It is usually worse at night and may prevent the woman from sleeping.

It is thought that if women avoid wearing high heels (whenever practicable) and have a good posture the incidence of backache decreases. However, this has not been shown in any well designed study.

CERVICAL EVERSION AND DISCHARGE

The high levels of oestrogen in pregnancy may increase the eversion of the endocervical columnar cells so that they appear as a red ring around the external cervical os. Exposed to the vagina, the cells may secrete mucus – causing a non infective vaginal discharge. The condition has erroneously been called a cervical 'erosion'.

CONSTIPATION

The reduced gut motility aggravated in late pregnancy by the pressure of the enlarged uterus, makes constipation common in pregnancy. Treatment is to increase dietary fibre (for example by eating wholemeal instead of white bread) and attempting to defaecate after a meal. If the constipation is causing discomfort the woman may be prescribed purified senna (Senokot) or the contact laxative, bisacodyl.

'DISPLACEMENTS' OF THE UTERUS IN PREGNANCY

RETROVERSION
In 10 per cent of women the uterus is normally retroverted; moreover, retroversion of the uterus does not hinder conception, and so when examined vaginally in the early weeks of pregnancy some women will be found to have a retroverted uterus. In nearly all cases the uterus becomes anteverted spontaneously, usually between the 9th and 11th week of pregnancy. Very rarely the uterus remains retroverted

until after the 14th gestational week and becomes incarcerated in the cul-de-sac. If this occurs the woman complains of frequency of micturition and dysuria. If the position of the uterus is not corrected, the symptoms increase in severity and eventually there is retention of urine and an enormously distended bladder. Finally, retention of urine with overflow occurs. Examination shows a smooth, soft cystic tumour arising in the pelvis and palpable abdominally in the midline. Treatment is to insert a catheter and to decompress the bladder slowly. When this is done the uterus usually becomes anteverted but may need to be anteverted using the fingers by pushing up in the posterior fornix and manipulating the uterus to one side of the sacral promontory.

Incarceration of a uterus in pregnancy can be prevented if a woman who is seen before the 10th week of pregnancy and is found to have a retroverted uterus is examined again at the 12th week. If the uterus is still retroverted, the doctor manipulates it to become anteverted.

PENDULOUS ABDOMEN
Women who have had several children and who have a wide separation of the recti abdominis muscles, may find in late pregnancy that the uterus becomes pathologically anteverted – the pendulous abdomen.*(Fig 12.1)*. In late pregnancy it can cause considerable discomfort and in labour may delay the birth because the fetal head does not enter the pelvis easily. Treatment is to wear a firm binder in pregnancy. In labour a binder should be applied and the woman should pull her uterus up.

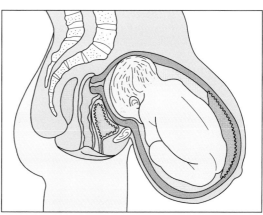

Fig 12.1 Pendulous abdomen. The patient was Indian, aged 36, gravida 4.

UTEROVAGINAL PROLAPSE

In multiparous women, particularly in the developing countries, uterovaginal prolapse may complicate pregnancy. In the early weeks of pregnancy the prolapse may become more prominent. As the uterus becomes an abdominal organ the pressure on the vagina is relieved to some extent and the prolapse becomes less obvious, but occasionally a swollen, infected cervix may protrude through the vulva. The prolapse causes few problems during labour and cervical dilatation is usually rapid.

PREGNANCY AFTER A VAGINAL REPAIR FOR PROLAPSE

This is considered on page 290.

DYSPNOEA

By the 15th week of pregnancy 1 woman in 4 complains of dyspnoea on exertion. The proportion increases as pregnancy advances so that by the fourth quarter of pregnancy three quarters of pregnant women are dyspnoeic. The condition is probably due to a lack of adaptation to progesterone-induced hyperventilation. There is no specific treatment and the patient should be reassured that the breathlessness will not harm her or her fetus.

HEARTBURN

Relaxation of the lower oesophageal sphincter permits the regurgitation of some of the stomach contents causing irritation of the lower oesophagus. It is also possible that a similar relaxation of the pyloric sphincter permits a reflux of bile into the stomach, which may then be regurgitated into the lower oesophagus. The woman complains of heartburn, which increases as the pregnancy advances. Treatment is difficult. Frequent small meals, avoidance of spicy food and cigarettes and the use of antacids may relieve the discomfort. If antacids fail, 'floating' antacids such as sodium alginate – sodium bicarbonate mixture (Gaviscon) or metoclopramine may give relief. If the heartburn occurs predominantly at night, the use of extra pillows to prop up the expectant mother may help.

HAEMORRHOIDS AND VARICOSE VEINS

Haemorrhoids and varicose veins of the legs and occasionally the vulva become increasingly common as pregnancy advances. Haemorrhoids often become larger or may appear for the first time during childbirth. They may persist for several months after the birth and cause pain. Varicose veins increase in size in late pregnancy. Treatment is for the woman to lie or sit with her feet up as much as possible, and, if the veins are painful or disfiguring, to wear elastic stockings. The latter should be put on before the woman gets out of bed in the morning. Surgical treatment for either condition is generally contraindicated in pregnancy.

INSOMNIA

Many pregnant women find that their sleep pattern is altered. In early pregnancy they may sleep for longer than usual. In late pregnancy, because of the discomfort of the enlarged uterus, leg cramps and backache, sleep may be disturbed. The short term use of hypnotics may help.

LEG CRAMPS

The cause of leg cramps is not known. They tend to occur more frequently in the second half of pregnancy, usually at night. Various treatments, including calcium tablets have been tried, but have no value except as a placebo. Some women obtain relief if the foot of the bed is raised about 25cm.

MICTURITION

Frequency of micturition

Increased frequency of micturition is common in early pregnancy, when it is due to a supra-normal excretion of urine by the kidney, and in the last weeks when the pressure of the fetal head causes direct irritation of the trigone.

Urinary incontinence

Urinary incontinence affects over 50 per cent of pregnant women to some extent. Usually only a small leakage of urine occurs occasionally. There is no treatment and it resolves in the puerperium.

NAUSEA AND VOMITING

Nausea due to pregnancy affects over 75 per cent of women and vomiting occurs in half of them. The symptoms usually begin at the 6th gestational week and cease by the 12th, although they may continue throughout the pregnancy. The symptoms are more common in women who have a history of unsuccessful pregnancies, or who are carrying a multiple pregnancy. One-quarter of women who have the symptoms will experience them again in a subsequent pregnancy.

The cause appears to be due either to the effect of the rising levels of oestrogen, or to the high levels of human chorionic gonadotrophin acting on the chemoreceptor trigger zone in the midbrain. Once the body has become habituated to the new hormonal environment, the nausea and vomiting cease in most women. In addition, psychological factors may act on the emetic centre in the cerebral cortex.

Nausea and vomiting may be graded as:

- **Mild.** Mild nausea (and occasional vomiting) affects 45 per cent of pregnant women, and is the most common form. The nausea usually occurs in the morning ('**morning sickness**') but may be provoked by travel or emotional stress at any time of the day.
- *Treatment.* The patient should be advised to eat frequent small meals during the day; to take fluid between (not with) meals, and to avoid fatty or spicy foods. If she wishes, a centrally acting sedative such as meclozine (25–50mg, three times a day) may be prescribed.
- **Moderate.** Moderate nausea and vomiting affects 5 per cent of all pregnant women, or 10 per cent of all women suffering from nausea. The symptoms may occur at any time of the day or night. The patient feels miserable and may become mildly dehydrated.
- *Treatment.* The treatment suggested for the mild form applies to the moderate form, but most of the women choose to take a sedative. If the mild sedative used for the mild form does not relieve the symptoms, promethazine (25mg morning and evening) may be needed. The drug produces marked sleepiness, which reduces its value.
- **Severe.** This form is uncommon affecting 1 in 1000 pregnant women. The nausea is continuous and the vomiting frequent. This is the reason for its name – **hyperemesis gravidarum**. The woman rapidly becomes dehydrated and acidoketotic.
- *Treatment.* The patient should be admitted to hospital and treatment started urgently to avoid the possibility of liver damage. An intravenous line is established and dehydration and ketosis corrected by infusing 1 litre of 5% dextrose followed by 1 litre of Hartmann's solution if electrolyte disturbance is detected. The infusion should provide 3–4 litres a day and is continued until hydration and electrolyte balance have been corrected. The fluid intake and output is recorded. The urine is checked twice daily for acetone, bile, sugar and specific gravity. Plasma electrolytes are measured daily. If vomiting persists, the patient should be given metoclopramide (10mg IM) as needed. During the time that the infusion is running, the patient may have dry ice to suck, and oral feeding should be withheld. Once the vomiting has ceased the patient is treated in the same way as for the moderate form of nausea. She should remain in hospital for 2 days after the vomiting has ceased and has begun to gain weight.

OEDEMA

Oedema, particularly of the legs is, in the absence of hypertension, a normal physiological adaptation to the pregnant state. The cause is water stored in the ground substance of connective tissue. In pregnancy the increased secretion of oestrogen alters the ground substance from a colloid-rich, water-poor matrix to a colloid-poor, water-rich matrix. In addition, in late pregnancy, increased mechanical obstruction to the venous return from the legs adds to leg oedema. Oedema around the ankles and lower legs is more common towards evening, in hot humid climates and in obese women. Treatment is for the woman to sit or lie with her legs elevated. There is no place for diuretics.

Oedema, associated with a rise in blood pressure, requires further investigation, particularly when the hands or face become oedematous (see Chapter 16).

PALPITATIONS, FAINTING AND HEADACHES

These symptoms are common in pregnancy and are caused by altered cardiovascular dynamics. The patient should be examined and reassured that she has no organic lesion. Auscultation of the heart may reveal a soft systolic murmur, which is due to the hypervolaemic circulation occurring during pregnancy. Murmur of this kind is not a sign of cardiac damage. Some women feel faint when lying on their back in late pregnancy, because the pressure of the uterus reduces venous return to the heart (supine hypertension). Pregnant women should avoid lying flat on their backs. Headaches also appear to be due to the altered vascular dynamics.

PLACIDITY AND DROWSINESS

These are common symptoms in pregnancy. They are due to the increase in circulating progesterone. There is no treatment.

PUBIC SYMPHYSIS DIASTASIS (PELVIC OSTEOARTHROPATHY)

In a few women abnormal relaxation of the ligaments surrounding the pubic joint permits the pubic bones to move on each other, when the woman walks or exerts herself. This movement may put strain on the sacroiliac joints. Pubic symphysis diastasis may occur during pregnancy or start in the puerperium. The pain may persist for the remainder of the pregnancy or for several weeks after the birth, which makes care of the neonate difficult. The patient complains of severe pubic pain, backache and sacral pain. Examination shows that the pubic joint is very tender when pressed. The diastasis can be confirmed by ultrasound or x-ray examination *(see Fig 12.2)*. Treatment is bed rest on a firm mattress, with the patient nursed as far as is possible on one or other side. A firm binder may relieve some of the pain.

SWEATING

Because of the vasodilatation and increased peripheral circulation, pregnant women 'feel the heat' and often sweat profusely, particularly in hot, humid climates. No treatment is available apart from frequent cool showers.

VAGINAL DISCHARGES

In pregnancy the quantity of normal vaginal secretions increases and many women complain of a non-irritant vaginal discharge. Vaginal infections, particularly candidosis, are more frequent among pregnant women than non-pregnant women. Vaginal discharges are discussed on p 248.

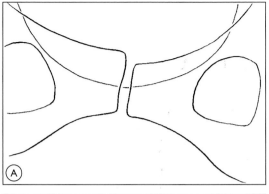

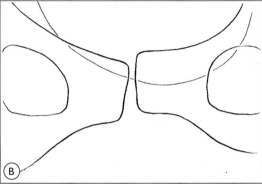

Fig 12.2 Pelvic symphysis diastasis. The patient was 39 weeks pregnant. The sliding movement of the symphysis is shown when (A) the patient stands on her right leg; (B) the patient stands on her left leg (redrawn from radiographs).

13

ABORTION

Abortion is defined as the expulsion of a fetus before it reaches viability. Because of different definitions of viability in different countries, the World Health Organization (WHO) has recommended that a fetus is viable when the gestation period has reached 22 or more weeks, or when the fetus weighs 500g or more. As the term 'abortion' does not differentiate between spontaneous and induced abortion, many obstetricians refer to the former as 'miscarriage'. Most abortions occur naturally (or are induced) between the 6th and 10th week of pregnancy.

Data from several countries estimate that between 10 and 15 per cent of clinically diagnosed pregnancies end as an abortion. Abortion is more frequent among women over the age of 30 and increases further among women over the age of 35. Abortion increases in frequency with increasing gravidity: 6 per cent of first or second pregnancies terminate as an abortion; with 3rd and subsequent pregnancies the rate increases to 16 per cent.

THE AETIOLOGY OF SPONTANEOUS ABORTION

The causes of abortion are:
- Ovofetal.
- Maternal.

In the early weeks of pregnancy (0–10 weeks) ovofetal factors account for most abortions; in the later weeks (11–22 weeks) maternal factors become more common. *(Table 13.1).*

OVOFETAL FACTORS

Ultrasonic examination of the fetus and subsequent histological examination show that in 70 per cent of cases, the fertilized ovum has failed to develop properly or the fetus is malformed. In 40 per cent of these cases chromosomal abnormalities are the underlying cause of the abortion. In 20 per cent of abortions, the trophoblast has failed to implant adequately.

MATERNAL FACTORS

Systemic maternal disease, particularly maternal infections, account for 2 per cent of abortions. A further 8 per cent are associated with uterine abnormalities, such as congenital defects, uterine myomata, particularly submucous tumours, or cervical incompetence (see page 104). Psychosomatic causes have been suggested as leading to an abortion but the evidence is difficult to evaluate.

THE MECHANISMS OF ABORTION

The immediate cause of abortion is the partial or complete detachment of the embryo by minute haemorrhages in the decidua. As the placental function fails, uterine contractions begin, and the process of abortion is initiated. If this occurs before the 8th week, the defective embryo, covered with villi and some decidua, tends to be expelled en masse (the so-called 'blighted ovum'), although some of the products of conception may be retained either in the cavity of the uterus or in the cervix. Uterine bleeding occurs during the expulsion process.

Between the 8th and the 14th week, the above mechanism may occur or the membranes may rupture expelling the defective fetus but failing to expel the placenta, which may protrude through the external cervical os, or remain attached to the uterine wall. This type of abortion may be attended by considerable haemorrhage.

Between the 14th and the 22nd week, the fetus is usually expelled followed by the placenta after an interval. Less commonly the placenta is retained. Usually bleeding is not severe, but pain may be considerable, resembling a 'miniature labour'.

It is clear from this description that abortion is attended by uterine bleeding and pain, both of varying intensity. Although abortion is the cause of bleeding per vaginam in early pregnancy in over 95 per cent of cases, less common causes such as ectopic gestation, cervical bleeding from the everted epithelium or from an endocervical polyp; hydatidiform mole; and, rarely, cervical carcinoma, must be excluded.

VARIETIES OF SPONTANEOUS ABORTION

For descriptive purposes the abortion is classified according to the findings when the woman is first

Aetiological Factors in 5000 Abortions	
Fetal or ovular	**Percentage**
Defective ovofetus	60
Defective implantation or activity of trophoblast	15
Maternal	
General disease	2
Uterine abnormalities	8
Psychosomatic	?15

Table 13.1 Aetiological factors in 5000 abortions.

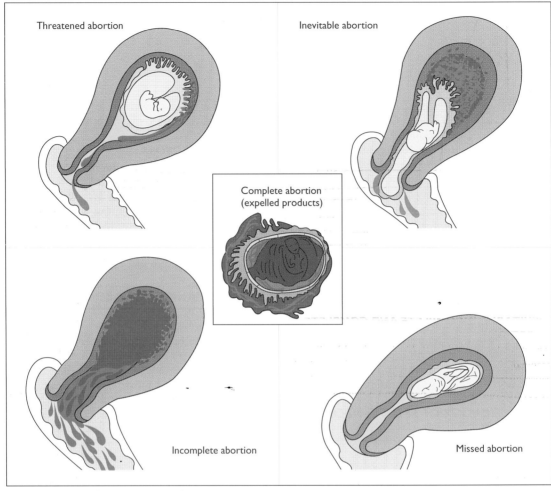

Fig 13.1 The types of abortion which may be seen.

examined, but one kind may change into another if the aborting process continues. If infection complicates the abortion, the term *septic abortion* is used. The various types of abortion are shown in *Fig 13.1* and each will be considered separately later.

Four other varieties of abortion are defined. *Recurrent abortion* is diagnosed if the woman has had three or more diagnosed abortions. *Missed abortion* occurs when the dead fetus is retained in the uterus for a period of time. *Induced (therapeutic) abortion* occurs when the pregnancy is terminated for medical reasons under rigid guidelines. *Illegal (criminal) abortion* is diagnosed when the pregnancy is terminated outside those guidelines.

THREATENED ABORTION

Threatened abortion is diagnosed when a pregnant woman develops uterine bleeding with or without painful uterine contractions; other causes of bleeding in early pregnancy should be excluded. Vaginal examination (or vaginal speculum examination) shows that the cervix is not dilated.

A real-time pelvic ultrasound examination will clarify the diagnosis. This may show:
• A normally sized amniotic sac and a fetus whose heart is beating.
• An empty amniotic sac.
• A missed or incomplete abortion.
Only if the first finding is obtained is the diagnosis confirmed. The ultrasound finding also provides the information that the pregnancy will continue (in 98 per cent of cases), and the patient can be reassured. She should also be informed that in about 5 per cent of cases the pregnancy will be curtailed and a preterm baby born.

The use of ultrasound examination has meant that the treatment of threatened abortion has changed in recent years. It is no longer normal practice to insist that the woman remains in bed until the bleeding has ceased. However, if the woman feels more comfortable there, she may do so. It is now known that drugs, hormones (progesterone) and sedatives have no effect except as a placebo, and should be avoided.

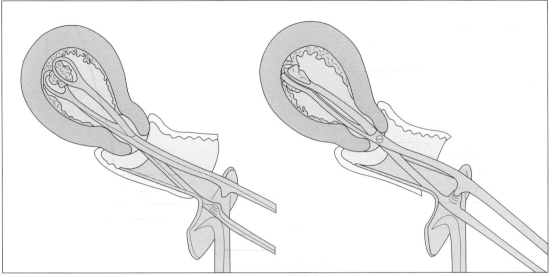

Fig 13.2 The use of sponge forceps for clearing placental tissue from the uterus.

INEVITABLE, INCOMPLETE AND COMPLETE ABORTION

Abortion becomes *inevitable* if uterine bleeding is associated with strong uterine contractions which cause dilatation of the cervix. The woman complains of severe colicky uterine pains and a vaginal examination shows a dilated cervical os with part of the conception sac bulging through. Inevitable abortion may follow signs of threatened abortion, or more commonly, starts without warning.

Soon after the onset of symptoms of inevitable abortion, the abortion occurs either *completely*, when all the products of conception are expelled, or *incompletely* when either the pregnancy sac or the placenta remains, distending the cervical canal. In most cases the abortion is incomplete. Unless the doctor has been able to inspect all the material expelled from the uterus, or has had an ultrasound picture made which shows an empty uterus, the abortion should be considered incomplete.

Treatment

A woman who is diagnosed as having an inevitable or an incomplete abortion and who is not in hospital should be transferred to one without delay. Before effecting the transfer, the examining doctor should give an analgesic to the patient (if required) and should make a vaginal examination. Any products of conception found protruding from the cervix should be removed by finger or sponge forceps, as to leave them may lead to shock. If the woman is bleeding heavily an intramuscular injection of ergometrine 0.5 mg should be given.

In hospital, intervention is required unless the abortion is proceeding quickly and with minimal blood loss. On admission of the patient a vaginal examination is made and any products of conception in the cervix are removed by finger or sponge forceps.

Should there be any doubt about the completeness of the abortion, the patient is taken to the operating theatre and the uterus evacuated using a sponge forceps *(Fig 13.2)*, followed by a careful, gentle curettage. Towards the end of the curettage, an injection of ergometrine 0.25mg is given intravenously and intramuscularly.

Follow-up

Following a complete abortion, or one which has been completed surgically, bleeding usually ceases within 10 days. If placental remnants have been left in the uterus, the bleeding may persist beyond this time, varying in severity, and may be accompanied by uterine cramps. Examination will show a bulky uterus with a patulous os. Treatment is to give further injections of ergometrine or ergometrine tablets or to recurette the uterus carefully. Tissue removed should be sent for histopathology, as very rarely a choriocarcinoma is present.

A women who is Rhesus negative should be given a prophylactic injection of anti-D gammaglobulin, and a Kleihauer test should be performed to determine the amount of fetal blood cells in her circulation.

SEPTIC ABORTION

Although less common than formerly, because of better care in hospital and fewer 'backyard abortions', infection may complicate some spontaneous and induced abortions. In 80 per cent of cases the infection is mild and is localized to the decidua. The organisms involved are usually endogenous and are most commonly *anaerobic streptococci, staphylococci or E. coli.* In 15 per cent of cases the infection is severe, involving the myometrium and may spread to involve the Fallopian tubes. If the infection spreads from the cervix it may involve the parametrium or the pelvic cellular tissues. In 5 per cent of cases there is generalized peritonitis or vascular collapse, which is due to the release of endotoxins by *E. coli* or *Cl. welchii* and is termed endotoxin shock.

Clinical features

In infections limited to the decidua, a malodorous, pink vaginal discharge is usual and the patient may develop pyrexia. In more severe spreading infections, pyrexia occurs, but its extent may not be related to the severity of the infection. Tachycardia is usual: a pulse rate of >120 per minute indicates that spread has occurred beyond the uterus. Examination may show a tender lower abdomen; vaginal examination shows a boggy, tender uterus with evidence of extra-uterine spread.

Investigations

A high vaginal or cervical swab is made and if the temperature is >38.4°C a blood culture should be taken. In severe infections serum electrolytes and coagulation studies should be undertaken.

Treatment

Antibiotics are administered at once, the precise one chosen depending on local conditions, but in general a broad-acting antibiotic and one effective against anaerobes is selected. Twelve hours after starting antibiotics, or sooner if haemorrhaging is severe and the uterus is not empty, its contents are evacuated by careful curettage. If the infection is not controlled in spite of these measures hysterectomy may be indicated.

ENDOTOXIN SHOCK

As mentioned already this life-threatening condition follows 5 per cent of septic abortions. Endotoxins released by *E coli* and *Cl welchii* are neutralized initially by phagocytes but if this protection fails, vaso-constriction of the postcapillary vessels occurs with resulting pooling of blood, a failure of venous blood to reach the heart and a reduced cardiac output. As well, the gram-negative endotoxins may act directly on the blood vessels and heart, releasing substances which profoundly affect the cardiovascular system.

Clinical signs include pyrexia, rigors, hypotension, tachycardia and hypoventilation. A patient with these signs is acutely ill and should be transferred to an intensive care unit with the least delay.

MISSED ABORTION

In a few cases of abortion, the dead embryo or fetus and placenta are not expelled spontaneously. If the embryo dies in the early weeks, it is likely to be anembryonic or 'blighted'. In other cases a fetus forms but dies. Multiple haemorrhages may occur in the choriodecidual space, which bulge into the empty amniotic sac. This condition is called *carneous mole (Fig 13.3)*. It is thought that although the fetus has died, progesterone continues to be secreted by surviving placental tissue, which delays the expulsion of the products of conception.

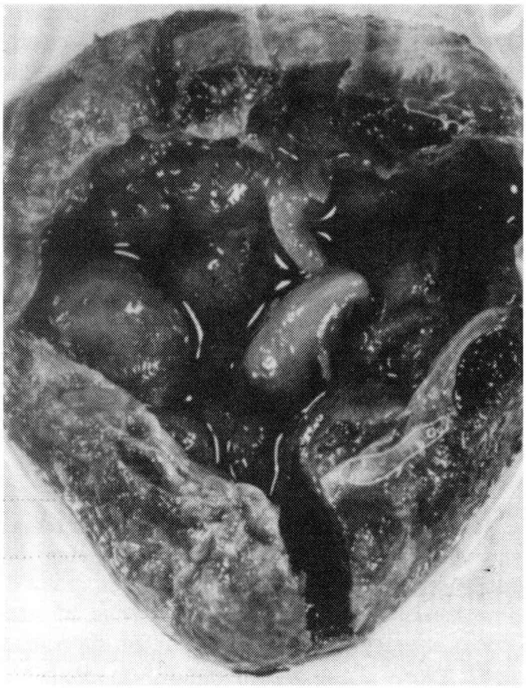

Fig 13.3 Carneous mole - a small fetus can also be seen in the centre.

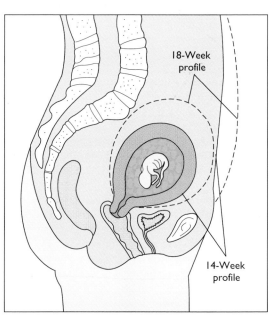

Fig 13.4 Missed abortion. The duration of the pregnancy is 18 weeks but the uterus has failed to enlarge beyond the size of a 14-week gestation. Note that the abdomen is flat.

When the fetus dies at a later stage of the pregnancy, but before the 22nd gestational week, and is not expelled, it is either absorbed or mummified. The liquor amnii is absorbed and the placenta degenerates. Fetal death after the 22nd week is discussed on page 106.

Clinical aspects

The patient usually has a history of threatened abortion, which settles down, but she complains of a dirty, brown discharge which persists. Examination, at intervals, shows that the uterus fails to grow (*Fig 13.4*) and symptoms indicating early pregnancy disappear.

The diagnosis can not usually be made for about 21 days, but can be established earlier by ultrasound examination.

Treatment

There is no medical need to treat missed abortion urgently as most cases end in a spontaneous abortion. Information and support must be given to the parents once they become aware that the fetus has died in utero, as this can be a very traumatic experience. The reason for delaying evacuation of the uterus must also be explained. Some women remain anxious after an explanation has been given and request that the abortion is completed. This is best effected using mifepristone and misoprostol or prostaglandins as described on page 105.

If a spontaneous abortion has not occurred within 28 days, the pregnancy should be terminated, as coagulation defects may result.

The termination procedure depends on the size of the uterus. If it is <12 weeks gestational size, the uterus can be evacuated by sponge forceps and curette after cervical dilatation. If the uterus is > 12 weeks gestational size, either mifepristone 600mg followed 36 hours later by misoprostol (300mg repeated in 2 hours) or prostaglandin E$_2$ vaginal pessaries (20mg) every 3 to 6 hours are effective.

RECURRENT (HABITUAL) ABORTION

A few women have the misfortune to miscarry successively. It has been estimated that after one abortion the risk of another is 20 per cent; after 2 abortions it is 25 per cent and after 3 abortions, 30 per cent. A woman who has three or more successive abortions is termed a recurrent aborter. As well as having a 30 per cent chance of aborting again, if she avoids this outcome she is at greater risk than a non-aborter of delivering a preterm baby, but has at least a 75 per cent chance of delivering a healthy infant at term.

The aetiological factors in recurrent abortion vary depending on the population studied, but two large series of over 100 subjects in each offer some idea of the aetiology (*Table 13.2*). In *Table 13.2* the causes marked with a query are speculative.

Investigation and treatment of a recurrent aborter

A careful medical and obstetrical history may reveal systemic disease or suggest cervical incompetence. A vaginal examination may show uterine myomata or cervical incompetence, and the diagnosis can be clarified if a transvaginal ultrasound image is made. Ultrasound will also detect uterine malformations. **Submucous myomata** or **uterine septa** may be removed by abdominal surgery or under hysteroscopic vision. **Cervical incompetence** is discussed later.

If **endometrial infection** is considered a causative factor, (as some specialists do) endometrial tissue cultures may be made to detect *T. gondii* and urealyticum. Treatment is to prescribe appropriate antibiotics.

Endocrine dysfunctions, for example, polycystic ovarian disease (see page 212) may be excluded by transvaginal ultrasound scanning. Other endocrine disorders, such as thyroid disease and diabetes, are no longer believed to be causes of recurrent abortion.

Although it is usual to investigate both parents for **chromosome abnormalities**, they account for only 5 per cent of recurrent abortions at the most, and no treatment is available.

Immunological causes for recurrent abortion have been investigated for the past 10 years. The theory is that if the two parents share several HLA sites, the fetus may not be able to provide a sufficient stimulus to enable the mother to produce blocking antibodies to the allogenic fetus, with the result that the fetus is aborted. A clinical study which supports

Recurrent Aborters		
	% of abortions occurring	
Possible aetiology	**<12 week**	**>12 week**
Not known	62	35
Uterine malformations or abnormality	3	10
Cervical incompetence	3	30
Chromosome abnormality	<5	<4
?Endometrial infection	15	15
Endocrine dysfunction	3	3
Systemic disease	1	1
?Sperm factors	3	1
?Immune factors	?	1

Table 13.2 The aetiology of recurrent abortion.

this theory had the finding that if a woman who has had recurrent abortions changes her partner, her chance of aborting falls to that normally experienced by women in the community. Treatment suggested is to immunize the woman between pregnancies with paternal leukocytes, pooled donor cells or trophoblast membrane preparations to enhance her immune system. Four of five clinical trials using this approach have failed to show any statistical benefit from immunotherapy.

A few women, with an **autoimmune disease,** especially the **antiphospholipid syndrome, and systemic lupus erythematosus,** have a strong blocking antibody reaction, which, it is believed, may lead to recurrent abortion. SLE must be excluded before immunotherapy is used as SLE may be aggravated. If SLE is identified by laboratory tests, aspirin (75mg daily), corticosteroids or low-dose heparin may permit the pregnancy to continue to fetal viability, although the published results are not impressive.

General measures

Women who are recurrent aborters need considerable support and care. They should be advised to stop smoking, to avoid sexual intercourse and not to travel. The results from this regimen are as good as those following the use of multivitamins, hormones (including human chorionic gonadotrophin), metallic chemicals , thyroid extract, and acupuncture, all of which are advocated from time to time.

Cervical incompetence

About 20 per cent of women who have recurrent abortions in the second quarter of pregnancy will be found to have cervical incompetence. The diagnosis is based on:

- A history of recurrent abortions occurring after the 12th week of gestation, usually starting with painless leaking of amniotic fluid.
- The easy passage of a size 9 cervical dilator through the internal os of the cervix when the woman is not pregnant, and the absence of a 'snap' on its withdrawal.
- The gradual dilatation of the internal cervical os to >3cm during pregnancy as detected by ultrasound or repeated vaginal examinations.

If cervical incompetence is diagnosed, treatment is to place a soft unabsorbable suture (such as Mersilk 4) around the cervix at the level of the internal cervical os *(Fig 13.5)*. The patient may return home the same night or stay in hospital for a day depending on circumstances. There is no place postoperatively for the use of progesterone, uterine relaxants or narcotics.

Following cervical circlage 10 per cent of women abort; 10 per cent give birth prematurely and the remainder give birth after the 36th week of pregnancy. Cervical circlage should not be made if the membranes have ruptured. If abortion becomes inevitable following circlage, the suture must be cut. In all other cases it is left until about 7 days prior to term, when it is cut and the women may then be expected to give birth vaginally.

THE PSYCHOLOGICAL EFFECTS OF SPONTANEOUS ABORTION

For most women a spontaneous abortion is a distressing occurrence: over 90 per cent express a grief reaction which persists for a month in 20 per cent of cases. During the period when the abortion threatens or is occurring, many women are distressed by not knowing what the outcome will be; others are distressed by being told to rest in bed without any further explanation.

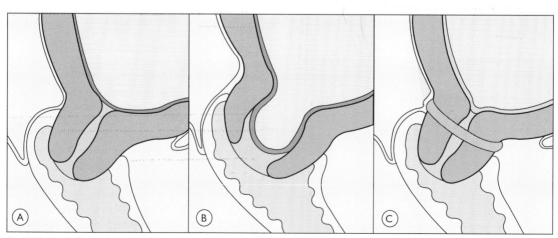

Fig 13.5 Cervical incompetence. (A) Normal cervix at 16 weeks; (B) Incompetent cervix at 16 weeks; (C) 'Cerclage' with an unabsorbable suture.

Too little information is given by many doctors after an abortion has occurred, both in general and in hospital practice, about the reason for the abortion and the outcome of a future pregnancy. Women need counselling on these matters and need to have an opportunity to express their feelings. There are three main questions to which most women require answers: the first is, Why did the abortion occur?; the second, Is there anything that I did or did not do which caused the abortion? and the third, Is my next pregnancy likely to end in a miscarriage? Some women are too embarrassed to ask these questions, even so the doctor should provide answers sensibly and sympathetically even if the questions are not asked. This will reduce the period of grief and distress that usually follows a spontaneous abortion.

INDUCED ABORTION

In many countries, induced (therapeutic) abortion is now legal. The exact conditions vary but the purposes of legalizing abortion are:

- To enable all women, irrespective of social or economic status, after counselling to obtain an abortion performed by a trained health professional in hygienic surroundings.
- To reduce the frequency of 'illegal' abortions performed in unhygienic surroundings, which are often associated with high morbidity and mortality.

The main reasons for the abortion are shown in *Table 13.3*. In most developed countries where abortion is legal over 95 per cent are performed for social or psychiatric reasons. It should be stressed that women rarely seek an abortion without considerable thought, and are receptive to and welcome counselling during this difficult time. It is also

---

Indications for Therapeutic Abortion
Social
Psychiatric: Severe neuroses, psychoses
Medical Severe cardiac disease, heart failure Severe chronic renal disease, renal failure Malignant disease, especially breast or uterine cervix
Fetal Viral infections Haemolytic disease Genetic defects Congenital defects incompatible with normal life (e.g. anencephaly, spina bifida)

Table 13.3 Indications for therapeutic abortion.

---

evident that in many cases the pregnancy could have been prevented if effective contraceptive precautions had been taken.

TECHNIQUE OF INDUCED ABORTION

Abortion is safest when it is performed between the 6th and the 12th gestational week. Termination of the pregnancy may be surgical or medical.

The surgical approach is to evacuate the uterus using a suction curette, under local or general anaesthesia. Following curettage, uterine bleeding persists for about 6 days, often being light in the first 2 days after the termination. Most gynaecologists give the woman a course of doxycycline to prevent infection.

Medical methods of termination are available if the pregnancy is less than 9 weeks' gestation. They include the administration of a single dose of the progesterone antagonist, mifepristone 200mg, in countries where this medication is available. The mifepristone tablet is followed 36–48 hours later by a prostaglandin E_1 vaginal pessary (gemeprost) 1mg every 6 hours for 4 doses. If the abortion has not started within 24 hours, gemeprost 1mg is given 3 hourly for up to 4 more doses. (An alternative is oral misoprostol 200µg repeated after 2 hours). Bleeding usually starts during the interval between the mifepristone and the gemeprost vaginal pessary or oral misoprostol, and uterine contractions start within 4 hours of the administration of either drug. The pain may be severe and most women require narcotics. Nausea and/or vomiting affects one-third of patients. Bleeding persists for about 9 days, with a mean loss of 75ml (20–400ml). Over 98 per cent of women abort using this regimen, but 10 per cent require curettage for persistent heavy bleeding.

After the 12th gestational week the uterus may be evacuated by dilating the cervix and by removing the fetus and placenta by sponge forceps and curettage. This is a fairly bloody and prolonged procedure. An alternative is to use the mifepristone/gemeprost regimen. Over 80 per cent of women require narcotics for pain, and nausea or vomiting occurs in 30 per cent. Following the abortion, one-third of women require evacuation of the uterus for retained products of conception.

THE SEQUELAE OF INDUCED ABORTION

An induced abortion performed before the 12th gestational week in a well-equipped and -staffed clinic is followed by few complications. Less than 1 per cent of women develop infection, and the mortality rate is less than 1 per 100 000 abortions. After the 12th gestational week the rate of complications rises to 3–5 per cent and the mortality increases to 9–12 per 100 000. There is no reduction of the woman's fertility or any increase in the risk of spontaneous abortion, preterm birth or fetal loss in a subsequent pregnancy.

THE PSYCHOLOGICAL EFFECTS OF INDUCED ABORTION

An expert panel in the USA in 1990 reported that 'legal abortion of an unwanted pregnancy does not pose a psychological hazard for most women'. Most women feel grief and guilt after a termination but less than 10 per cent show evidence of anxiety or depression persisting for more than a month. Most of the women adversely affected were ambivalent about having the abortion or were pressured by parents or partner into terminating the pregnancy. This finding emphasizes that a woman seeking an abortion should be counselled before the procedure takes place and should continue to receive support (if she chooses) during and after the operation.

FETAL INTRA-UTERINE DEATH

The World Health Organization has recommended that a fetus should be considered viable if the gestation period has reached 22 or more completed weeks or when the fetus weighs 500g or more. A fetus born after this time must be registered as a birth, either alive or stillborn. Not all countries have accepted the WHO recommendation. For example Britain categorizes a pregnancy ending before the 24th week of pregnancy as an abortion, and registration of a stillbirth is not required, although a live birth has to be registered.

Fetal intra-uterine death may follow pregnancy-induced hypertension, maternal diabetes mellitus, and other complications of pregnancy. In most cases labour begins soon after the death and the baby is stillborn. In a few cases the dead fetus is retained in the uterus.

CLINICAL ASPECTS

The mother notices that fetal movements have ceased and Doppler examination fails to detect any fetal heart sounds. Apart from the psychological upset to the expectant mother when she realizes that her baby has died in the uterus and her concern that the dead fetus will decay and will infect her, medical problems are unlikely, at least in the first 3 weeks after the fetal death has been diagnosed. After this time, disseminated intravascular coagulation and hypofibrinogenaemia may arise with potential serious consequences to the woman.

DIAGNOSIS

The history provides evidence that the fetus has died. This is confirmed by Doppler examination. In addition an ultrasound examination may show overlapping of the bones of the fetal skull (Spalding's sign).

MANAGEMENT

The parents should be offered bereavement counselling and support. They should be made aware that the dead fetus will not cause any harm to the woman in the first 3 weeks after the death, and that in most cases labour will start before this time. The management of the labour should be discussed with the patient and she should be assured that she will be given analgesics to reduce or eliminate the pain of childbirth. In the event that she wishes to view and hold her fetus she should be made aware that it will be macerated.

The woman may choose to await spontaneous labour or to have labour induced. If spontaneous labour has not started by 3 weeks after the diagnosis, or if she chooses immediate treatment, labour is induced by prostaglandin E_2 vaginal pessaries or gel as described on page 185. Alternatives are to prescribe mifepristone 600mg a day for 3 days or the prostaglandin analogue, sulprostone, 1µg /minIV until the fetus is expelled. It is claimed that there are fewer gastrointestinal side effects if sulprostone is used. Using any of the methods, 50 per cent of women will expel the fetus in 12 hours and 90 per cent in 24 hours.

If the woman chooses to await the spontaneous onset of labour, frequent blood checks should be made by observing the clotting time of the blood or by estimating fibrinogen levels.

14

EXTRA-UTERINE PREGNANCY – ECTOPIC GESTATION

Most extra-uterine pregnancies occur in the Fallopian tubes (ectopic gestation), but rarely the fertilized ovum may implant on to the ovarian surface or the uterine cervix. Extremely rarely the fertilized ovum implants on to the omentum (abdominal pregnancy).

The incidence of ectopic gestation is rising in the developed countries and is currently running at a rate of 1 in 80–150 pregnancies. The reason for the increase is not clear but the rise seen may be associated with increased sexual activity and an increased incidence of pelvic inflammatory disease, or to earlier diagnosis using ultrasound.

AETIOLOGY

The aetiology of ectopic gestation is not known. Implantation of the fertilized ovum can only take place when the zona pellucida has partially or completely disappeared. This could occur if the passage of the fertilized ovum along the Fallopian tube is delayed because of tubal damage following infection. Implantation may occur in:

- the fimbriated end of the Fallopian tube (in 17 per cent of cases).
- in the ampulla (in 55 per cent of cases).
- in the isthmus (in 25 per cent of cases).
- in the interstitial portion of the tube (in 2 per cent of cases) (Fig 14.1).

OUTCOME FOR THE PREGNANCY

In most cases the pregnancy terminates between the 6th and 10th week in one of several ways.

TUBAL ABORTION

This occurs in 65 per cent of cases and is the usual termination in fimbrial and ampullary implantation (Fig. 14.2). Repeated small haemorrhages from the invaded area of the tubal wall separate the ovum which dies, and is either:

- Absorbed completely.
- Aborted completely through the tubal ostium into the peritoneal cavity.
- Aborted incompletely, so that the clot-covered conceptus distends the ostium.
- Forms a tubal blood mole.

TUBAL RUPTURE

This occurs in 35 per cent of cases, and is more common when the implantation is in the isthmus. Whilst the rupture of the ampulla usually occurs between the 6th and 10th week, rupture of the isthmus occurs earlier, frequently at the time of the first missed period. The trophoblast burrows deeply and eventually erodes the serosal coat of the tube, the final break being sudden or gradual. Usually the ovum is extruded through the rent and bleeding continues.

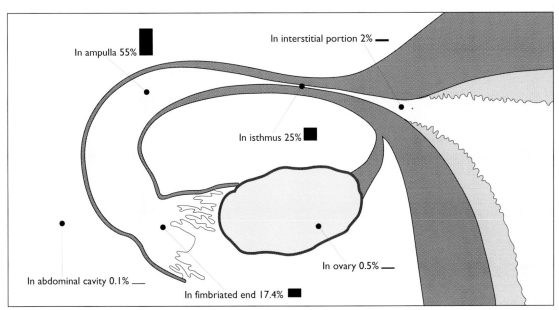

Fig 14.1 Sites of ectopic gestation implantation, with the relative frequency of occurrence.

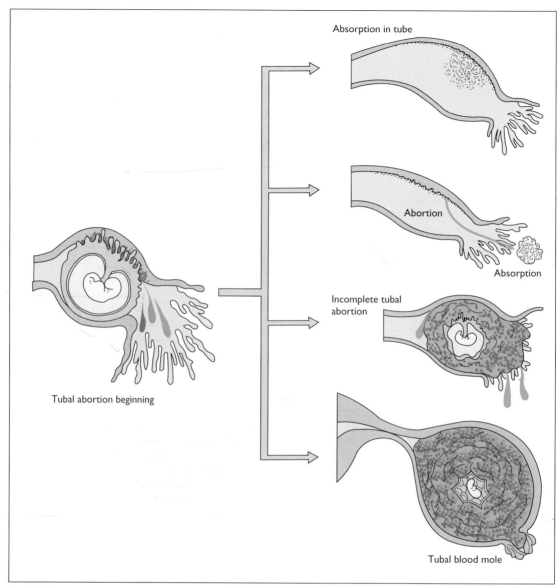

Fig 14.2 The sequelae of tubal abortion shown diagrammatically.

If the rupture is on the mesenteric side of the tube, a broad ligament haematoma will form *(Fig. 14.3)*.

SECONDARY ABDOMINAL PREGNANCY

Very rarely the extruded ovum continues to grow, as sufficient trophoblast maintains its connection with the tubal epithelium, and later the trophoblast covering the ovisac attaches to abdominal organs. A few of these pregnancies advance to term, and in a very few the fetus dies early and is converted into a lithopaedion.

CLINICAL ASPECTS

The possibility of an ectopic gestation should always be considered in a woman of childbearing age espe-

cially if there is a history of acute salpingitis. The history is of greater importance than the physical signs, as these can be equivocal. Usually there is a short period of *amenorrhoea*, although in 20 per cent of cases this may not be present. The *pain* is lower abdominal in site, but not distinguishable from that of abortion. However, in ruptured ectopic gestation *fainting* is usual, although this may only be momentary. *Vaginal bleeding* follows the pain, and may be mistaken for bleeding due to a delayed menstrual period or an abortion. The bleeding is slight, brownish in colour and continuous, and clots are rarely present *(Table 14.1)*.

Two clinical patterns occur, and are due to the extent of the damage to the tube wall by the invading trophoblast. The first is subacute, the second acute.

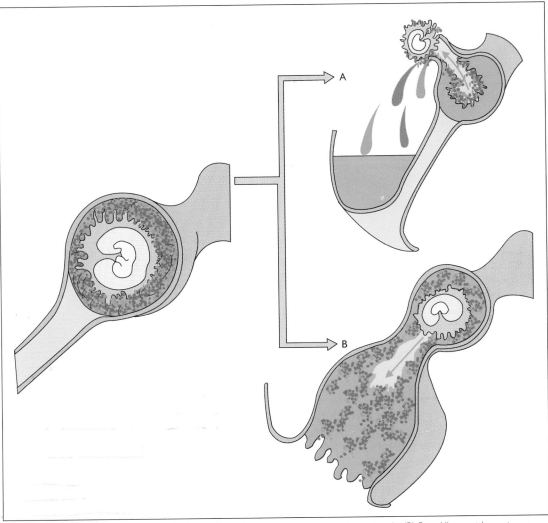

Fig 14.3 The sequelae of tubal rupture. (A) Intraperitoneal haemorrhage and pelvic haematocele; (B) Broad ligament haematoma.

SUBACUTE

After a short period of amenorrhoea, the patient complains of some lower abdominal discomfort, which may be so mild that she considers it normal for pregnancy. Occasionally there is an attack of sharp pain and faintness, due to an episode of intraperitoneal bleeding, and if these symptoms are marked she will seek advice, particularly if the episode is followed by slight vaginal bleeding. Examination may reveal tenderness in the lower abdomen, and vaginal examination may show a tender fornix, or a vague mass, but the signs may be insufficient to make a diagnosis. If the patient is observed, further episodes of pain are likely, and the blood loss per vaginam persists, until acute collapse supervenes (indicating tubal rupture or incomplete tubal abortion), or the symptoms cease (indicating complete abortion with or without a pelvic haematocele).

ACUTE–DRAMATIC

Sudden collapse with little or no warning is more common when the implantation is isthmal, but is not the most frequent type of the acute clinical pattern. It is more usual for the acute rupture to

Symptoms and Signs in Ectopic Gestation	
	percentage
Abdominal pain	90
Amenorrhoea	80
Vaginal bleeding	70
Adnexal tenderness	80
Abdominal tenderness	80
Adnexal mass	50

Table 14.1 Symptoms and signs in ectopic gestation.

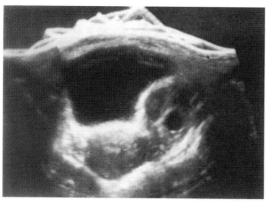
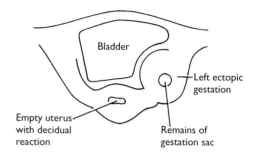

Fig 14.4 Ectopic gestation (ultrasound – transverse scan). Line drawing showing the identification of relevant points.

supervene upon the subacute, but the mild symptoms of the latter may have been thought to be normal occurrences in pregnancy and ignored.

As the tube ruptures, the patient is seized with a sudden acute lower abdominal pain, sufficiently severe to cause fainting. The associated internal haemorrhage leads to collapse, pallor, a weak, rapid pulse, and a falling blood pressure. Usually the condition improves after a short time, as the haemorrhage diminishes or ceases, but abdominal discomfort persists, and pain is felt in the epigastrium or is referred to the shoulder. A further episode of haemorrhage and collapse is likely, and continued bleeding can be suspected from increasing pallor and a falling haemoglobin level.

On examination the patient is shocked, the lower abdomen is tender with some fullness and muscle guarding. Vaginal examination, which should only be carried out in hospital, shows extreme tenderness on movement of the cervix from side to side.

DIAGNOSIS

Although in acute cases the presence of internal bleeding is obvious and the diagnosis not in doubt, in subacute cases it can be extraordinarily difficult. Laboratory tests may help, but in most instances are not particularly informative. A radio-immuno-assay for serum levels of βhCG, should be made. A negative result (< 1ng/ml) indicates that the woman is not pregnant, and ectopic gestation can be excluded. If the βhCG test is positive, a pelvic ultrasound examination should be made, preferably using a transvaginal probe. If this shows an empty uterus (Fig. 14.4), and particularly if it shows a sac and fetus in the Fallopian tube the diagnosis is certain and a laparoscopy or a laparotomy should be made. On the other hand if ultrasound shows an intra-uterine pregnancy, a concurrent ectopic pregnancy is extremely unlikely. If the diagnosis remains in doubt a laparoscopy will clear the matter up.

If ultrasound is not available, or is equivocal, the presumptive diagnosis should be confirmed by laparoscopy.

The diagnosis of suspected ectopic gestation is summarized in *Fig. 14.5*.

TREATMENT

If the patient is seen in her home and ectopic gestation is suspected, she should be transferred to hospital without making a vaginal examination. If she is in shock an intravenous line should be set up and transfer quickly arranged. Morphine may be given if the woman is in pain.

As mentioned, if there is any doubt about the diagnosis a pelvic ultrasound examination should be made to establish if the pregnancy is intra- or extra-uterine.

Once the ectopic gestation has been diagnosed, the treatment is surgical. Several approaches are possible. The gynaecologist may:

- Perform a laparotomy and either excise the Fallopian tube containing the ectopic gestation, or incise the tube over the ectopic gestation and 'milk' it out.
- Insert a laparoscope to inspect the Fallopian tube and if possible, under laparoscopic vision, incise along the superior border and suck the ectopic gestation out of the tube.
- If the tube has not ruptured, inject methotrexate into the ectopic gestation so that the viable trophoblast and embryo are absorbed; or give an intramuscular injection of methotrexate 50mg/m².

PROGNOSIS

Fewer than 60 per cent of women who have had an ectopic gestation become pregnant again. Three-quarters of the women voluntarily avoid pregnancy, and one-quarter are involuntarily infertile. In a subsequent pregnancy the risk of a second ectopic gestation is 10 per cent compared with a risk of <1 per cent in other women.

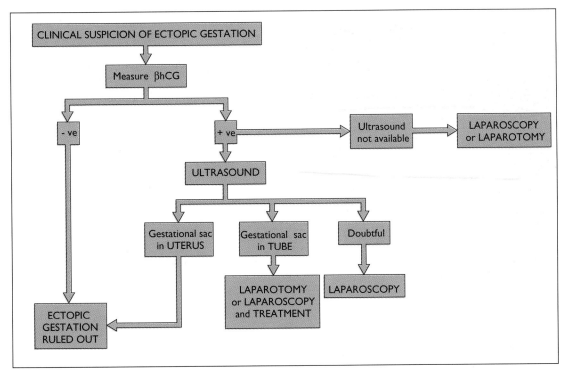

Fig 14.5 Algorithm for diagnosis of suspected ectopic gestation.

Serial βHCG's

15

ANTEPARTUM HAEMORRHAGE

Antepartum haemorrhage is defined as significant bleeding from the birth canal which occurs after the 20th week of pregnancy. The causes and proportions of cases of antepartum haemorrhage are shown in *Table 15.1*. In fewer than 0.05 per cent of cases the bleeding is due to a cervical lesion, such as a cervical polyp, or rarely, a cervical carcinoma. As a vaginal examination is usually made early in pregnancy, the local cervical conditions which may cause bleeding in the second half of pregnancy are usually diagnosed before the 20th week.

PLACENTA PRAEVIA

In this condition the placenta is implanted, either partially or wholly, in the lower uterine segment and lies below (praevia) the fetal presenting part. The extent of implantation may be minor, in which case vaginal birth is possible, or major when it is not *(Fig 15.1)*.

Placenta praevia occurs in 0.5 per cent of all pregnancies, and accounts for 20 per cent of all cases of antepartum haemorrhage. It is three times as common in multiparous women as in primiparous women, and no other aetiological factor has been detected.

The bleeding occurs when the lower uterine segment is increasing in length and shearing forces between the trophoblast and the maternal blood sinuses occur. The first episode of bleeding occurs after the 36th gestational week in 60 per cent of cases; between the 32 and 36th week in 30 per cent; and before the 32nd week in 10 per cent.

The Incidence of the Causes and Proportions of Antepartum Haemorrhage	
	Incidence %
Placenta praevia	0.5
Accidental haemorrhage	
Unknown origin	3.0
Abruptio placentae	
Moderate grade	0.8
Severe grade	0.2
Cervical bleeding	0.05

Table 15.1 The incidence of the causes and proportions of antepartum haemorrhage (derived from hospital reports).

SYMPTOMS AND DIAGNOSIS

The bleeding is painless, causeless and recurrent. The presenting part is usually high and often not central to the pelvic brim. The diagnosis is made should an ultrasound image show that the placenta is praevia *(see Fig 15.2)*.

If a routine ultrasound examination is made late in the second quarter of pregnancy, the report may show that there is a low-lying placenta. This does not mean that the placenta will be praevia later in pregnancy and a further ultrasound examination should be made at about the 30th week.

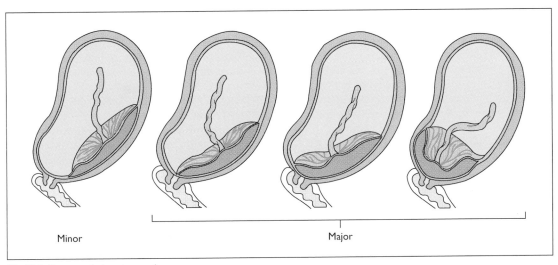

Minor   Major

Fig 15.1 Degrees of placenta praevia.

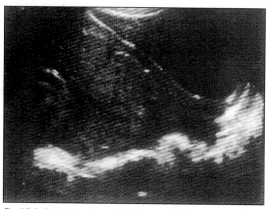
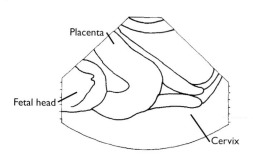

Fig 15.2 Sagittal section, major degree of placenta, praevia in fourth quarter. Cervix and vagina on right.

MANAGEMENT OF PLACENTA PRAEVIA

The first episode of significant bleeding usually occurs in the patient's home, and usually is not heavy. The patient should be admitted to hospital and no vaginal examination made, as this may start torrential bleeding. In hospital the patient's vital signs are checked, the amount of blood loss assessed, and blood cross-matched. Heavy blood loss may require transfusion. The abdomen is palpated gently to determine the gestational age of the fetus, its presentation and its position. An ultrasound examination is made soon after admission, to confirm the diagnosis.

Further management depends on the severity of the bleeding and the gestational age of the fetus.

In cases of severe bleeding urgent treatment to deliver the baby (and the placenta) is required irrespective of the gestational age of the fetus. If the bleeding is less severe, expectant treatment is appropriate if the fetal gestational age is <36 weeks. As the bleeding tends to recur the woman should remain in hospital. An episode of severe bleeding may lead to urgent delivery but in most cases the pregnancy can continue until the 36 week when the choice of delivery depends on whether the placenta praevia is of minor or major degree. Women who have a minor degree of placenta praevia may choose to await birth at term or may wish to have labour induced, provided that the conditions are suitable (see page 185). Placenta praevia of major degree is treated by caesarean section at a time determined by patient and doctor, although usually it is performed at an early date, as a severe bleed may occur at any time.

COMPLICATIONS OF PLACENTA PRAEVIA

Episodes of heavy bleeding may occur at any time, during which the fetus may die from hypoxia. Following the birth, postpartum haemorrhage may occur because the trophoblast has invaded the poorly supported veins of the lower uterine segment. In most cases the haemorrhage ceases after administration of oxytocics, but occasionally the bleeding cannot be staunched and caesarean hysterectomy is required.

The perinatal mortality is less than 50 per 1000. The maternal mortality is low, provided the case is managed by an experienced obstetrician and no vaginal examination is performed before admission to hospital.

ACCIDENTAL HAEMORRHAGE

The term 'accidental haemorrhage' derives from an observation made in 1775 that in placenta praevia haemorrhage is inevitable, whilst in the other group of antepartum haemorrhage it is due to some 'accidental' circumstance. About 4.0 per cent of pregnant women develop accidental haemorrhage, which can be subdivided into three groups. In the first, the bleeding is slight, and when the placenta is examined after the birth, no retroplacental bleeding can be observed. This group is classified as **antepartum haemorrhage of unknown aetiology.** It accounts for 75 per cent of cases of accidental haemorrhage.

In the second and third group of cases, there is evidence of retroplacental bleeding. The amount of blood lost to the circulation may be moderate or severe. These two groups are classified as **abruptio placentae.** Abruptio placentae accounts for 25 per cent of cases of accidental haemorrhage. In four-fifths of cases of abruptio placentae the amount of blood lost to the circulation is moderate (<1500ml) and in one-fifth the blood loss is severe (>1500ml).

AETIOLOGY AND PATHOLOGY OF ABRUPTIO PLACENTAE

The aetiology is obscure, the only relevant association being multiparity. Hypertensive diseases in pregnancy are associated with abruptio placentae in about 15 per cent of cases, but it is not clear whether the hypertension is an aetiological factor.

The cause of the retroplacental bleeding is damage to the walls of the maternal venous sinuses supplying the placental bed. The bleeding spreads and separates the placenta to varying degrees. The blood then trickles down between the uterine

Comparison of the Clinical Picture in the Various Grades of Accidental Haemorrhage			
	Severity of bleeding		
	Mild	Moderate	Severe
Pulse	No change	Raised	Raised
Blood pressure	No change	Lowered	Lowered
Shock	None	Often	Always
Oliguria	Rare	Occasionally	Common
Hypofibrinogenaemia	Rare	Occasionally	Common
Uterus	Normal	Tender	Tender and tense
Fetus	Alive	Usually dead	Dead
Blood loss in litres	Less than one	1–3	3–6

Table 15.2 Comparison of the clinical picture in the various grades of accidental haemorrhage.

decidua and the amniotic sac to appear in the vagina and vulva (revealed haemorrhage) or is retained behind the placenta (concealed haemorrhage). In a few cases of severe bleeding the blood is forced by intra-uterine pressure between the myometrial fibres towards the serosal layer of the uterus. If the amount of blood is large, the uterus has the appearance of a bruised, oedematous organ, described as **apoplexie uteroplacentaire**. This is a rare occurrence in today's obstetric practice.

In severe cases of abruptio placentae shock may result from the distraction and separation of the myometrial fibres. Another complication is the release into the circulation of thromboplastins, from the damaged vessels, which cause widespread intravascular coagulation. The microthrombi are dissolved by fibrinogens, mainly plasmin, with the release of fibrin degradation products and the possible development of consumption coagulopathy. In severe cases some microthrombi escape lysis and are deposited in the endothelium of the vessels supplying the glomeruli of the kidneys. This may lead to tubular necrosis and oliguria or anuria.

SIGNS, SYMPTOMS AND TREATMENT OF ANTEPARTUM HAEMORRHAGE

The symptomatology is related to the degree of bleeding and the extent of placental separation *(Table 15.2)*.

SLIGHT HAEMORRHAGE

The amount of blood lost is less than 500ml. There is no disturbance of the maternal or fetal condition. An ultrasound examination shows that the placenta is not lying in the lower uterine segment and no retroplacental clots can be seen. If the patient has been admitted to hospital she may go home once the bleeding ceases, or if the pregnancy has advanced to 37 weeks she may choose to have labour induced by amniotomy, provided that the condition of the cervix is suitable.

ABRUPTIO PLACENTAE: MODERATE PLACENTAL SEPARATION AND HAEMORRHAGE

Usually at least one-quarter of the placenta has separated and >1000ml of blood has been lost to the circulation. The woman complains of abdominal pain and the uterus is tender because blood has infiltrated between the muscles fibres of the uterus. The patient may be shocked, with a high pulse rate, but paradoxically in 5 per cent of cases the pulse rate is within the normal range until delivery, when it rises precipitously. The fetus is hypoxic and may show abnormal heart rate patterns on a cardiotocogram.

ABRUPTIO PLACENTAE: SEVERE PLACENTAL SEPARATION AND HAEMORRHAGE

In cases of severe placental separation, at least 1500ml of blood has been lost to the circulation. The woman is usually in shock. Her uterus is firm to hard, and very tender. The fetus is almost always dead. As pregnancy-induced hypertension is associated with about one-third of cases, the blood pressure may be in the normal range in spite of the shock. Most coagulopathies occur in this group.

The management of abruptio placentae

The management is to restore the blood lost, to prevent coagulopathy and to monitor urinary output:
- At least 1500ml of blood should be transfused in cases of moderate separation, and 2500ml in cases classified as severe separation. The first 500ml of blood is transfused rapidly. Rapid blood transfusion prevents renal 'shut down' and anuria. The central venous pressure is monitored and the remainder of the transfusion adjusted accordingly. The blood loss and the height of the fundus are monitored.
- Venous blood is examined 2-hourly for evidence of coagulopathy and if present this is treated. Adequate rapid transfusion and amniotomy or caesarean section usually prevent it from occurring.

- Urine output is measured 2 hourly. Oliguria may occur but diuresis follows the birth provided that sufficient blood has been transfused.
- If the fetus is alive the decision has to be made whether to perform a caesarean section or to artificially rupture the amniotic membranes (ARM). If the latter procedure is chosen it should be performed even in the presence of shock and a hard uterus. The uterus is not inert and release of intra-uterine pressure will reduce the shock. An infusion of oxytocin may be started after the ARM. The fetal heart is monitored and if the fetus develops distress, a caesarean section is performed.

MATERNAL AND FETAL LOSS

Maternal mortality depends on the speed and adequacy of treatment. Today few women should die from abruptio placentae. Fetal mortality depends on the degree of placental separation.

HYPERTENSIVE DISEASES IN PREGNANCY

Between 5 and 8 per cent of pregnancies are complicated by hypertensive diseases. These are pregnancy-induced hypertension, essential hypertension, and hypertension due to chronic renal disease. All of the hypertensive states may lead to eclampsia (fits).

PREGNANCY-INDUCED HYPERTENSION

Pregnancy-induced hypertension (PIH) was previously called `toxaemia of pregnancy' or pre-eclampsia. PIH accounts for 80 per cent of all cases of hypertension in pregnancy and affects between 3 and 8 per cent of patients, mainly primigravidae, in the second half of pregnancy.

CLASSIFICATION
There is no generally accepted classification of PIH. In each case the patient's blood pressure is measured at the level of the heart, with the woman propped up or lying on her side, after a rest of 10 minutes if she is an outpatient.

Potential PIH
The patient's blood pressure measured as described has risen by >30 points systolic or >15 points diastolic over her basal diastolic blood pressure. This should be taken as a warning that the woman may develop PIH, and she should be seen more frequently by a health professional.

Mild PIH (also known as gestational ✓ hypertension)
The patient's diastolic blood pressure is 90–99 torr, and the elevation is detected on at least two occasions separated by 6 hours. The urine does not show significant protein (<30mg/dl). Mild PIH poses little risk to the woman or to the fetus.

Moderate PIH ✓
The patient's blood pressure lies in the range 140–170/100–110, confirmed on two occasions after resting. If significant urinary protein is found (>30 and <300 mg/dl) the category is changed to severe PIH.

Severe PIH (also known as pre-eclampsia or gestational proteinuric hypertension)
The patient's blood pressure exceeds 170/110 and/or marked proteinuria is present. Severe PIH affects about 1 per cent of primigravidae.

Imminent eclampsia
In addition to the signs of severe PIH, the patient complains of severe headache, blurring of vision or epigastric pain and her reflexes are exaggerated.

Oedema
Oedema may occur in all grades of PIH but is of little diagnostic significance unless it is generalized, as oedema occurs as frequently in women who have no antenatal disorder.

THE PATHOGENESIS OF PIH
The aetiology of PIH is not known but there is increasing evidence that the disorder is due to an immunological disturbance in which the production of blocking antibody is reduced (see page 24). This may prevent the invasion of maternal spiral arteries by trophoblasts to any significant extent leading to impairment of placental function. As pregnancy advances, placental hypoxic changes induce proliferation of cytotrophoblasts and thickening of the trophoblastic basement membrane which may affect the metabolic function of the placenta. The endothelial cells of the placenta secrete less vasodilator prostacyclin and the platelets more thromboxane, leading to generalized vasoconstriction and decreased aldosterone secretion. The results of these changes are a reduction by 50 per cent in placental perfusion, maternal hypertension and a reduced maternal plasma volume. If the vasospasm persists, trophoblastic epithelial cell injury may occur, and trophoblast fragments are carried to the lungs where they are destroyed, releasing thromboplastins. In turn, thromboplastins cause intravascular coagulation and deposition of fibrin in the glomeruli of the kidneys (glomerular endotheliosis) which reduces the glomerular filtration rate and indirectly increases vasoconstriction. In advanced, severe cases fibrin deposits occur in vessels of the central nervous system, leading to convulsions.

→ liver cell injury

PREVENTION OF PIH
Knowledge of the physiopathology of PIH, although rudimentary, has suggested ways of preventing the disorder. None has been successful, with the possible exception of aspirin which has been shown to reduce the platelet production of proaggregatory vasoconstrictor thromboxane A_2. Alas, the daily administration of aspirin (75mg) to women who have a higher risk of developing PIH has proved ineffective.

THE MANAGEMENT OF PIH

The management of PIH is shown in *Table 16.1*. The table shows that there is no concensus about treatment, and few double-blind studies have been made.

The aim of treatment is to permit the continued growth of the fetus until it is sufficiently mature to survive outside the uterus, or it is estimated that the risk of intrauterine death is greater than extrauterine existence. The duration of treatment depends on:

- The severity of PIH.
- The duration of the pregnancy.
- The patient's response to treatment.

PIH diagnosed before week 32 of pregnancy

Before the 32nd week of pregnancy the objective is to keep the fetus in utero until the 35th week or longer. Fetal well-being is monitored by daily fetal movement counts, or thrice-weekly cardiotocograph examinations (see page 149). A sinister sign is slow fetal growth, which can be detected by serial ultrasound examinations or perhaps by Doppler uteroplacental blood flow measurements. In cases of severe PIH,

serum urate measurements may give an indirect index of fetal well-being. A level of >0.35 mmol/l on three successive readings is taken by some obstetricians to indicate that delivery should be effected rapidly.

Platelet counts are made at intervals in cases of severe PIH. In most cases a reduced platelet count returns to normal after the birth, but a few patients who have severe PIH complain of upper abdominal pain, nausea or vomiting. If the platelet count is <100 000 the woman may have the HELLP syndrome (thrombolysis, elevated liver enzymes, low platelets). Treatment is to correct the thrombocytopaenia and deliver the fetus.

If the PIH worsens, pregnancy must be terminated, usually by caesarean section.

PIH diagnosed between the 32nd and 35th week of pregnancy

PIH diagnosed between the 32nd and the 35th week is managed in the same way as before the 32nd week, but should delivery of the fetus be indicated the choice is caesarean section or induction of labour.

Summary of the Management of Pregnancy-induced Hypertension		
Classification	**Nursing responsibilities**	**Obstetrician's treatment**
1. Potential PIH	Report significant rise in blood pressure, or excessive weight gain, to obstetrician	Usually no treatment required. See patient in 7 days
2. Mild PIH	Report rise in blood pressure or excessive weight gain to obstetrician	Possible admission to hospital, depending on socio-economic conditions. If not admitted, see patient in 3 days. ?Atenolol 100mg each evening
3. Moderate PIH	In hospital: 1. Four-hourly recording of the blood pressure 2. Twice-daily urine testing for protein 3. Regular observation of the patient's condition, including fluid intake and output 4. Bed rest but toilet privileges allowed	1. Probably admit to hospital 2. Sedation (if indicated) 3. Labetalol (starting) 100mg b.d. or atenolol (starting) 100mg in evening or oxprenolol (starting) 20mg t.d.s. or methyldopa, (starting) 250mg t.d.s.

4. Severe PIH	1. Two-hourly blood pressure recording for 6 hours, then 4-hourly
	2. Urine testing for protein and acetone twice daily
	3. Fluid intake and output recorded
	4. Careful observation of the patient for the signs of imminent eclampsia
	5. Complete bed rest for 24 hours, thereafter possible toilet privileges
		1. Admit to hospital
		2. Depending on the severity of the illness:
		  (a) labetalol intravenously or orally
		  (b) diazoxide 30mg intravenously every 60 seconds until diastolic BP <90, then diazepam 10–20mg parenterally or orally
		3. ?Intravenous frusemide 20mg or stable plasma protein substitute (SPPS), if gross oedema present
		4. ?Caesarean section

5. Imminent eclampsia	The patient requires careful systematic observation and accurate recording of the findings as eclampsia is a possible outcome. The blood pressure requires frequent estimation at intervals determined by the obstetrician. Fluid intake and urinary output must be measured meticulously, and the urine tested quantitatively for protein	1. Diazoxide 30mg intravenously every 60 seconds until diastolic BP <90, then diazepam 10–20mg parenterally or orally 2. Labetalol intravenously 3. ?Caesarean section

Table 16.1 Summary of the management of pregnancy-induced hypertension.

PIH diagnosed after the 35th week of pregnancy

PIH diagnosed after the 35th week of pregnancy should be controlled rapidly and labour induced or a caesarean section performed depending on the condition of the fetus and the state of the cervix (see page 185).

Women with PIH should not become postdates as the risk of intrauterine death increases after term.

Care after birth

The woman needs to have 4-hourly blood pressure readings taken for 7 days after birth, and if the blood pressure remains high, antihypertensive agents should be continued. Proteinuria often persists for longer and is of little consequence. One-third of the women will have non-proteinuric hypertension in a subsequent pregnancy but the rate of recurrence of severe PIH is less than 5 per cent.

ECLAMPSIA

The purpose of the treatment of hypertensive disorders in pregnancy is to prevent eclampsia. The word arises from the Greek 'like a flash of lightning' and this is how the disease may occur.

Eclampsia is characterized by convulsions and coma, which usually occur in patients who have severe PIH or imminent eclampsia and in patients in whom gestational proteinuria has been superimposed on chronic hypertension. With better antenatal care and early recognition and treatment of PIH and chronic hypertension, the incidence of eclampsia has fallen. In developed countries eclampsia occurs in 1:2000 pregnant women but in the developing countries the incidence is higher.

PHYSIOPATHOLOGY

The changes which occur in severe PIH are more marked in eclampsia: vasospasm is intense, with tissue hypoxia; the glomerular filtration rate is further reduced and urinary output falls; intracellular water retention impedes cellular metabolism and cerebral oedema may occur; blood viscosity increases, platelet levels fall and coagulation defects arise.

CLINICAL PICTURE

The convulsion is preceded by a disorientation stage during which the woman becomes restless, twitches and develops spasmodic respiration. Within a minute she passes into the tonic stage of the convulsion: her back arches, her hands clench, she grimaces; her breathing ceases and she becomes cyanosed. In this stage she may bite her tongue. She then passes into the clonic stage of the convulsion, when her body jerks uncontrollably, frothy saliva may fill her mouth, and her breathing becomes stentorous. Finally she becomes comatose *(Fig. 16.1)*. The coma may persist for an hour or longer or recurrent convulsions may occur.

The convulsions occur in late pregnancy in 40 per cent of cases; intrapartum in 30 per cent; and a few hours after the birth in 30 per cent.

MANAGEMENT OF ECLAMPSIA

The aims of treatment are:
- To control the fits by relieving the generalized vascular spasm and decreasing the sensitivity of the brain to stimuli.
- To reduce the blood pressure.
- To deliver the fetus.

Nursing care

The quality of the nursing care of an eclamptic patient is crucial. The patient is nursed on her side with her head and shoulders raised and a catheter is inserted into her bladder. The attending nurses must:
- Detect any changes presaging a second convulsion.
- Prevent the woman injuring herself during a convulsion.
- Provide continuous oxygen.
- Keep the mouth and fauces clear of any saliva by suction.
- Monitor vital signs and urinary output.

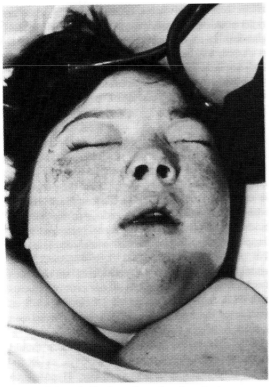

Fig 16.1 Eclampsia. The face of an eclamptic patient.

The Drug Treatment of Eclampsia		
Drug	**Dose regimen**	**Comments**
Diazoxide	30mg i.v. every 60 secs until diastolic BP <100	May reduce uterine contractions
Diazepam	40mg in 500ml Hartmann's solution. Adjust rate to maintain diastolic BP <100	
Labetolol	200mg in 500ml Hartmann's. Initial dose 0.5mg/kg/hr. Increase by 0.5mg/kg/hr every 20min to maintain diastolic BP <100. Max dose 3mg/kg/hr	
Magnesium sulphate	1gm i.v. and 10gm i.m. initially. 2g i.m. if fits recur	Blurred vision with i.v. $MgSO_4$; painful lumps at i.m. injection site.
Phenytoin	15mg/kg i.v. over 30min then oral phenytoin for 5 days	Chosen by some obstetricians to control fits
Hydralazine	Only use if other drugs fail to control convulsions. Dose: 10mg i.v. over 15min; i.v. infusion 25mg in 500ml Hartmann's to maintain diastolic BP <100	Severe headache, tachycardia hyperreflexia ?later: lupus syndrome

Table 16.2 The drug treatment of eclampsia.

Medical care

The attending doctor should prescribe antibiotics and choose one of the available treatments to reduce the blood pressure and control the fits. There is no 'best' treatment, as the numbers of cases of eclampsia are too few to warrant comparable studies. Currently used treatments are shown in *Table 16.2*. If cardiac failure occurs, frusemide 20mg may be given intravenously, but because of the hypovolaemia it should be used with care.

Once good control of the blood pressure and the convulsions has been gained, the pregnancy should be terminated. Depending on the period of the gestation, the health (alive or dead) of the fetus and its presentation, and on the condition of the cervix, delivery may be effected by caesarean section or labour may be induced using prostaglandins or by amniotomy. In most cases of eclampsia, induction of labour is followed rapidly by the birth of the infant. As postpartum haemorrhage may occur, prophylactic intravenous syntocinon should be given with the birth of the infant. The patient should continue to be monitored for the first 4 days of the puerperium at least.

PROGNOSIS IN PIH AND ECLAMPSIA

Today few women in the developed countries should die from severe PIH or from eclampsia. The situation in the developing countries is not so good: the maternal mortality after eclampsia varies between 3 and 20 per cent depending on the speed of starting treatment. Most deaths are from cerebral haemorrhage or cardiac failure.

CHRONIC (ESSENTIAL) HYPERTENSION

Most women with chronic hypertension have been diagnosed before the pregnancy; a few women are found to be hypertensive at the first antenatal visit. In the absence of a secondary cause for hypertension (for example, renal artery stenosis or phaeochromacytoma), a raised blood pressure (>140/90) which persists and is present before pregnancy or detected before the 20th gestational week is diagnostic of essential hypertension. It is important to remember that the small physiological fall in blood pressure in the first half of pregnancy may be exaggerated in women who have chronic hypertension, and some cases may be missed.

Essential hypertension complicates 1–3 per cent of pregnancies, and is more frequent among women over the age of 35.

PHYSIOPATHOLOGY

The generalized vasospasm of essential hypertension, is counterbalanced by an increased stroke volume and heart rate, which maintains an adequate blood flow to most organs with the exception of the uterus. Although uterine blood flow is increased in normal pregnancy, the increase is less in women who have essential hypertension and the higher the blood pressure the less the increase. This may reduce fetal growth and increase perinatal loss.

Pregnancy affects the course of essential hypertension. In 60 per cent of affected women, a rise in blood pressure occurs, and in 30 per cent significant proteinuria (>300mg/l) is detected. The changes usually occur after the 30th week of pregnancy.

Essential hypertension with superimposed protein-uria is indistinguishable from severe PIH.

TREATMENT

The aims of treatment are:
- To obtain and to maintain as good a blood supply to the uterus as possible.
- To control the level of the blood pressure and prevent the superimposition of proteinuria.
- To terminate the pregnancy if the patient's condition deteriorates markedly, or if the fetus fails to grow adequately in the last quarter of pregnancy.

Maintenance of uterine blood supply

Usually the woman is instructed to rest more to improve the uterine blood supply, particularly in the first quarter of pregnancy, but the benefits of this have not been confirmed.

Control of the hypertension

Most patients will be taking an antihypertensive drug. Consultation should be made with a physician to confirm that the drug is required and that it is safe to be given during pregnancy. Diuretics should be avoided as these agents reduce plasma volume and uteroplacental blood flow. Most experience has been obtained using methyl dopa, but it appears that beta-blockers such as atenolol, labetolol and calcium-channel blocker inhibitors are safe. ACE inhibitors should be avoided.

Avoidance of problems

The woman should be seen more frequently during the antenatal period, the frequency depending on the severity of the hypertension. Her lifestyle should be checked, and if she is obese, a reduction diet should be prescribed. Her salt intake should be regulated.

If the fetus shows signs of growth retardation, biophysical tests for fetal well-being should be started (Chapter 22), and if conditions deteriorate induction of labour should be discussed with the patient. It is safer for the fetus to be born earlier rather than later, and the patient should not become postdates as the perinatal loss increases.

RENAL DISEASE IN PREGNANCY

Less than 0.2 per cent of pregnant women and <5 per cent of women with hypertension in pregnancy have renal disease. In most cases the diagnosis is known before pregnancy, but routine examination of a midstream urine specimen (which is made to detect symptomless bacteriuria) may occasionally detect an affected woman. Most affected women have no impairment of renal function. Renal function is tracked by periodic serum creatinine measurements. If the level rises to >0.18mmol/l and there is evidence of poor fetal growth, either renal dialysis or induction of labour should be performed after consultation with a renal physician.

Indications for Aspirin.

Immediate Mx in rooms/surgery. Pregnant ♀ 170/110.
Sublingual nifedipine → drazepam - (Phenytoin)
site IV drip ⟶ ambulance → labour ward.

17

CARDIOVASCULAR, RESPIRATORY AND HAEMATOLOGICAL DISORDERS

CARDIOVASCULAR COMPLICATIONS IN PREGNANCY

It will be recalled that pregnancy places an increased strain on the heart because of the increased rate and stroke volume. The burden on the heart reaches its maximum at about the 28th week of pregnancy and continues into the puerperium. If a pregnant woman has heart disease, the increased strain may affect her well-being.

At present in the developed countries, between 0.2 and 0.5 per cent of pregnant women have heart disease. In 30 per cent of the cases, a woman has mitral valve disease; in 20 per cent, ventricular septal defect; in 15 per cent, atrial septal defect; in 15 per cent, aortic stenosis; and in the remainder, other defects.

DIAGNOSIS

In most cases the diagnosis has been established before the pregnancy, but the doctor should auscultate the woman's heart at the first antenatal visit. Any suspicious signs, particularly a diastolic or a loud systolic murmur, should lead to a referral to a cardiologist.

MANAGEMENT IN PREGNANCY

The initial assessment of the pregnant woman should be made in conjunction with a cardiologist, after which the medical management of the pregnancy can be carried out by the attending doctor, the patient being referred to a cardiologist at intervals. The aims of management are:

- To avoid those factors which predispose the woman to heart failure.
- Should failure occur, to treat it vigorously.

Factors which predispose to heart failure include anaemia; infections, particularly urinary tract infections; and the development of hypertension. If any of these are found, treatment should be started.

The woman's cooperation and that of her family should be obtained. Her daily activities should be evaluated and changes suggested if this is appropriate.

The patient should be seen at intervals of no more than 2 weeks up to the 28th week of pregnancy and thereafter weekly by a doctor (if it causes less stress on the woman, it could be her GP in collaboration with the obstetrician and the cardiologist). At each visit cardiac function is assessed by inquiring about breathlessness on exertion, or if she has a cough or orthopnea. Her lungs are auscultated to detect rales.

Many cardiologists place the woman in categories suggested by the New York Heart Association and plan the management on this. Initially most pregnant women are in Class 1 or 2, but during pregnancy some degree of cardiac decompensation may occur.

Class 1

The patient has no symptoms, although signs of cardiac damage are present. She can undertake all physical activities.

In this class, no additional treatment is needed.

Class 2

The woman is comfortable at rest but ordinary physical exertion usually causes fatigue, palpitations and occasionally dyspnoea. Most patients in this class do not require treatment but if the woman's social conditions are unfavourable or if signs of a deterioration in cardiac reserve occur, she should be admitted to hospital.

Class 3

Less than ordinary physical exertion causes dyspnoea and fatigue, although the patient is comfortable when resting. Most women in this class should be admitted to hospital for rest, but home conditions and responsibilities have to be assessed and help provided if needed.

Class 4

Women in this class are seriously ill. The patient is breathless even when resting. Hospital admission is mandatory.

Heart failure

Should the woman develop heart failure the principles of treatment are no different from those of non-pregnant women. Digoxin is given to control the heart rate and increase the time for blood flow into the left ventricle. Diuretics (such as frusemide) are given if pulmonary oedema is present. There is no consensus if women who are not in cardiac failure should be given prophylactic digoxin; but most experts agree that if the woman is at risk of atrial fibrillation or has mitral heart disease and an enlarged left atrium, digoxin is indicated.

MANAGEMENT DURING CHILDBIRTH

Most women who have heart disease have an easy spontaneous labour and there is no indication for inducing labour owing on account of the cardiac condition. During labour the patient should be nursed either on her side or well propped up, as compression of the aorta in the supine position may cause marked hypotension. The woman's fluid balance and her pulse rate should be checked at intervals. If her pulse rate is >110bpm between contractions and she has not been receiving digoxin, she should be 'digitalized'. The place of prophylactic antibiotics is not clear, but many cardiologists recommend that they are given from the onset of labour and for the first 5 puerperal days.

Delay in the second stage of labour should be treated by forceps, but there is no place for a prophylactic forceps delivery. The third stage is conducted in the same way as in non-cardiac patients, and active management using syntometrine is safe, unless the woman is in heart failure.

THE PUERPERIUM

The burden on the heart continues into the puerperium. For the first 24–48 hours the patient must receive constant observation for signs of decompensation. The woman should be nursed propped up and remain in bed for the first 2 days of the puerperium and in hospital for 7 days.

PROGNOSIS FOR MOTHER AND BABY AND FOR FUTURE PREGNANCIES

With good antenatal care the risk to the mother or fetus is not increased during the current pregnancy. Only women in classes 3 and 4 should be dissuaded from having a further pregnancy, until the condition of the heart has been assessed and further treatment including surgery discussed.

THROMBOEMBOLISM IN PREGNANCY

One third of the 0.5 per cent of women who develop thromboembolism during pregnancy and the puerperium do so during the pregnancy period. Treatment in pregnancy is to prescribe heparin, initially intravenously (40 000 units/day by continuous infusion in normal saline) to obtain a concentration of 0.6–1.0u/ml. Once full heparinization has been obtained for 3–7 days, the infusion may be replaced by calcium heparin given subcutaneously.

RESPIRATORY CONDITIONS

ASTHMA

The effect of pregnancy on asthma is variable, but most asthmatic women experience fewer attacks. Asthma has no effect on the course of pregnancy, labour or the birth weight of the infant. Treatment is in no way different from that of a non-pregnant asthmatic woman.

PULMONARY TUBERCULOSIS

Although the prevalence of pulmonary tuberculosis is low in most developed countries, it appears to be increasing with increased movement of populations.

A patient diagnosed as having active tuberculosis in the first half of pregnancy should be treated with isoniazid and ethambutol. After the 20th week of pregnancy, rifampicin may be used.

The management of labour does not differ from that for a non-infected woman. If the mother's sputum shows acid-fast bacilli, the baby should be separated from her, vaccinated with BCG and remain separate for about 6 weeks. If the mother's sputum has no acid-fast bacilli, the baby should be vaccinated with BCG but may remain with her and be breast-fed if the mother wishes to breast-feed.

ANAEMIA IN PREGNANCY

In the developing countries, anaemia poses a considerable danger to pregnant women. In the developed countries anaemia in pregnancy is less common, but some women, particularly of the lower socioeconomic groups become anaemic in pregnancy.

A healthy adult woman has a total body iron content of 3500–4500mg. Of this 75 per cent is held in the erythrocytes as haemoglobin; 20 per cent is held in body stores, mainly the bone marrow and reticuloendothelial system as a ferritin complex, and the remaining 5 per cent is held in muscles and enzyme systems, mainly as myohaemoglobin.

The life of an erythrocyte is 100–120 days; each day erythrocytes die and release iron, and new erythrocytes are formed which use this released iron. However, each day a loss of 1mg of iron occurs through the death of epithelial cells. In women, iron is also lost each month in menstrual discharge. This averages about 1mg a day. Thus a non-pregnant woman needs 2mg of iron a day to maintain her iron balance. The average 'mixed' diet of a woman in the developed countries provides 12–15mg of iron of which 14–20 per cent is absorbed. For most women this provides sufficient iron to maintain iron balance. In the developing countries where the diet consists mostly of complex carbohydrates and vegetables, more dietary iron is needed daily as the cereals contain phytates which prevent iron absorption. In addition, many women living in these countries are infested with hookworm which may cause a considerable loss of blood in the stools. These reasons (and malabsorption of iron in some women) provide the explanation of the higher prevalence of anaemia in pregnant women in the non-industrialized countries.

Pregnancy imposes an increased demand for iron to meet the needs of the woman's larger red cell mass and additional muscle formation, particularly that of the uterus. This amounts to 425mg spread out over the 40 weeks of pregnancy. The fetus requires about 300mg of iron, mostly in the last quarter of pregnancy, and the placenta, 25mg. Thus pregnancy places a demand for 750mg of iron, less the 250mg saved from the cessation of menstruation. The demand is not constant throughout the pregnancy, but increases as pregnancy advances *(Table 17.1)*.

Iron Requirements in Pregnancy				
	Over period		Daily needs	
Week	Net maternal needs[1]	Fetoplacental needs	Total daily need	Daily intake required[2]
	mg	mg	mg	mg
1–9	90	40	2.3	10–12
10–19	112	65	2.5	10–12
20–29	112	120	3.3	14–16
30–39	112	200	4.5	18–22

Notes

1. The net maternal needs are calculated from:

Replacement of iron lost from epithelial cells	1mg/day
Increase in red cell mass and muscle development	1.6mg/day
Less Savings due to amenorrhoea	1mg/day
Net daily needs	1.6mg/day

2. Assumes a daily utilization rate of 20 to 25 per cent of dietary elemental iron.

Table 17.1 Iron requirements in pregnancy.

THE DIAGNOSIS OF ANAEMIA IN PREGNANCY

Most cases of anaemia in pregnancy are due to iron deficiency, but in areas where people from southeast Asia, southern Europe and Africa live, or to where they have migrated, thalassaemia and sickle cell anaemia occur. In a few cases of severe anaemia (<65g/l), megaloblastic anaemia may be present.

For these reasons all pregnant women should have a sample of blood tested for the presence of anaemia at the first antenatal visit. The test is repeated at the 30th and 36th week of pregnancy. The number of tests varies, depending on local circumstances *(Table 17.2)* but a haemoglobin or a haematocrit estimation is always made.

If clinical anaemia is detected (Hb <105g/l), the MCV and serum ferritin should be measured, as a reduced Hb may merely indicate that the patient has a large blood volume.

TREATMENT

Treatment depends on the severity of the iron deficiency and the length of time available between diagnosis and the expected date of the birth. If the anaemia is detected before the 36th week of pregnancy and the haemoglobin level is >65g/l, oral iron may be given. The dose should not exceed 200mg of elemental iron a day because of gastrointestinal upset, and the more severe the anaemia the greater the amount absorbed. Treatment should be started with one-third of the dose required and gradually built up. The iron tablets should be taken 8-hourly so that absorption may occur throughout the 24 hours. A daily increase of about 1.5g/l may be expected, and if this response has not occurred over a 2-week period, the case should be reviewed and

megaloblastic anaemia suspected. If the woman is unable to take oral iron, or if the time to delivery is short, or the haemoglobin level <65g/l, parenteral iron should be substituted for oral iron. The regimen and dosage is provided in the manufacturer's product information sheet. Blood transfusions should be avoided if possible, for obvious reasons.

Women who have severe anaemia should also be given folate 5mg a day, as the severe anaemia may mask megaloblastic (folate-deficient) anaemia. The lower the haemoglobin level the greater the chance that the woman has megaloblastic anaemia. Megaloblastic anaemia may be suspected if >7% of neutrophils have five or more lobes, and confirmed by examining a bone marrow film for megaloblasts. Treatment is to prescribe folate 5–10mg daily by mouth unless the woman has tropical sprue or coeliac disease, when folate should be given parenterally. In addition, iron tablets should be prescribed.

SHOULD PROPHYLACTIC IRON BE GIVEN?

It is important to diagnose anaemia in pregnancy, as anaemic women have a higher mortality ($\times$3–5 that for non-anaemic women) and the stillbirth rate is increased 6-fold. This raises the question: 'Should all pregnant women receive prophylactic iron tablets?' Tradition decrees that all women should be prescribed iron tablets, but the evidence is that most women fail to take them regularly because of nausea or constipation (which may or may not be due to the iron tablets). A healthy woman, whose haemoglobin is within the normal range and who eats a mixed diet, probably does not need to take additional iron, at least in the first half of pregnancy. A women whose diet is less balanced or who lives in a developing country needs iron. The daily amount needed for a woman in the

The Diagnosis of Anaemia in Pregnancy	
Haemoglobin	< 10.5g/dl
Haematocrit	<0.30
MCV	An MCV of <70fl indicates possible beta-thalassaemia. If found, an estimation of haemoglobin A_2 and haemoglobin electrophoresis should be made.
MCH	<28pg
MCHC	<32g/dl
Serum ferritin	A level of <50µg indicates a strong possibility that anaemia will develop, whilst a level <10µg/l indicates severe depletion of iron stores. In this case iron tablets should be prescribed, irrespective of the haemoglobin level. Some authorities estimate serum ferritin at 24, 30 and 36 weeks to ensure that iron deficiency does not occur.

Table 17.2 The diagnosis of anaemia in pregnancy.

industrialized countries is 85mg of elemental iron, which can be obtained from any of the available iron preparations (none is better than any other); a woman in the non-industrialized countries needs 120–140mg a day, because of the increased severity of anaemia and the phytate in her diet which hinders absorption of iron. She should also take vitamin A (2.4mg) and 500µg of folate.

THE THALASSAEMIAS

The thalassaemias are a genetically determined group of blood disorders, characterized by a reduced production of one or more of the α- or β- chains of globin which make up haemoglobin. All forms of thalassaemia are inherited as an autosomal recessive trait. In α-thalassaemias the α-chains accumulate and eventually precipitate causing severe anaemia (thalassaemia major or Cooley's anaemia). The β-thalassaemias may be either heterozygous, when they are symptomless or homozygous when they produce severe anaemia.

Thalassaemia in a woman who is anaemic in pregnancy can be excluded if the MCV is >80fl. An MCV of <80fl indicates that haemoglobin electrophoresis should be performed; an HbA_2 greater than 3.5 indicates a β-thalassaemia trait.

If either α- or β-thalassaemia is diagnosed, the father of the child should have a full blood count and electrophoresis. If he is a carrier of the trait, genetic counselling should be obtained.

A pregnant woman carrying the thalassaemia trait has a 30 per cent chance of becoming anaemic and a similar chance of developing urinary tract infection. Thalassaemia in the fetus can be detected in the first quarter of pregnancy by chorionic villus sampling and in the second quarter by sampling fetal cord blood under ultrasonic guidance or by fetoscopy. If the tests are positive, termination of the pregnancy may be offered to the parents.

OTHER HAEMOGLOBINOPATHIES – SICKLE CELL ANAEMIA

In these cases a defective gene on the chromosome responsible for haemoglobin synthesis leads to the production of abnormal haemoglobin and an erythrocyte life of less than 15 days. The episodes of erthryocyte destruction may cause severe haemolytic anaemia and bone pains, because of infarction of the vessels supplying the bones.

The most common abnormal haemoglobin is haemoglobin S or C which causes sickle cell disease. The condition mainly affects Africans from east and west Africa.

All pregnant women suspected of carrying an abnormal haemoglobin should be given folate 15mg daily routinely, and frequent haemoglobin estimations made. If the haemoglobin level falls below 60g/l a direct or an exchange transfusion should be made. Infections, especially urinary tract infection, should be treated, and prophylactic antibiotics given during childbirth and the puerperium. If a bone pain crisis occurs, heparin should be given and the haemoglobin measured every 2 hours, a fall of >2g indicating the need for an exchange transfusion.

ISO-IMMUNIZATION IN PREGNANCY

Abnormal haemoglobinopathies affect Africans and southeast Asians predominantly; in contrast, Rhesus iso-immunization mainly affects Caucasians and south Asians.

Rhesus iso-immunization is caused by a complex antigen, consisting of three pairs of alleles, occupying a locus on a chromosome. The antigen was discovered more than 50 years ago on erythrocytes of the rhesus monkey. Only one of these pairs, D, is likely to cause iso-immunization in humans. Eighty-five per cent of

Caucasians have the D antigen, and are termed Rhesus positive, whilst 15 per cent are Rhesus negative. If a woman who is Rhesus negative conceives by a man who is Rhesus positive, the fetus may be Rhesus negative or positive depending on whether the man is heterozygous or homozygous for the Rhesus antigen. In the case of a Rhesus positive fetus, its blood cells may cross the placenta during pregnancy or, more commonly, during labour, in sufficient numbers to stimulate antibody production against the Rhesus antigen in the mother. In the next pregnancy if the fetus is again Rhesus positive, the anti-D antibodies may cross the placenta from mother to fetus and attach to antigen sites on the surface of the fetal erythrocytes. In the presence of complement the antigen–antibody complex causes lysis of the fetal erythrocytes, which shows as haemolytic disease.

THE RHESUS PROBLEM

As Rhesus iso-immunization occurs only if a Rhesus negative mother is impregnated by a Rhesus positive man (or has received a transfusion of Rhesus positive blood which only occurs exceptionally rarely today). All pregnant women should be tested to determine their Rhesus group at the initial antenatal visit. If the woman is found to be Rhesus negative, the father of the fetus should be asked to be tested. If he is found to be Rhesus negative there is no Rhesus problem. If he is Rhesus positive, iso-immunization may occur. This is unlikely in a first pregnancy, but increases in likelihood with subsequent pregnancies, unless preventive measures are taken. These will be discussed later in the section.

A Rhesus negative woman whose partner is Rhesus positive has her serum tested again for iso-agglutinins every 4 weeks from the 24th week of pregnancy. If the level of Rhesus iso-agglutinins is found to be positive in a titre of 1:8 or greater, further assessment is made by amniocentesis and testing a sample of amniotic fluid for the level of bilirubin, as this correlates fairly well with the degree of destruction of the fetal erythrocytes. In the absence of bilirubin, the absorption spectrum of amniotic fluid over the range of 360 to 630nmol is expressed as a straight line. The presence of albumin-bound bilirubin produces a deviation from this straight line, the degree of deviation relating to the severity of the erythrocyte haemolysis *(Fig. 17.1)*.

In cases where the mother has previously given birth to a severely affected baby, the level of iso-agglutinins may need to be tested earlier than the 24th week, and if found to be raised, fetal cord blood sampling and the measurement of the fetal haematocrit may be performed, as amniocentesis is inaccurate before the 24th week of pregnancy.

The bilirubin 'peak' is entered on to a graph *(Fig. 17.2)*. If the level is in the high zone (or the high-to-mid zone on a second test), the baby is severely affected, may be hydropic if its haemoglobin is <40g/l and it may die in utero. If the pregnancy has advanced to 32 weeks the pregnancy should be terminated, usually by caesarean section. Earlier than 32 weeks, intrauterine fetal transfusion should be made, either into the peritoneal cavity, or into the umbilical vein under ultrasonic guidance. The latter procedure permits a sample of fetal blood to be checked for the severity of the anaemia and the amount of blood required to correct the anaemia to be assessed. It also produces a higher salvage rate.

If the level is in the mid-zone a second amniocentesis is performed 2–3 weeks later, treatment being based on this result. If the peak lies in the low zone a second tap is made 3–4 weeks later.

THE PREVENTION OF RHESUS ISO-IMMUNIZATION

The following schema would solve the Rhesus problem, provided that no Rhesus negative woman received a transfusion of Rhesus positive blood:

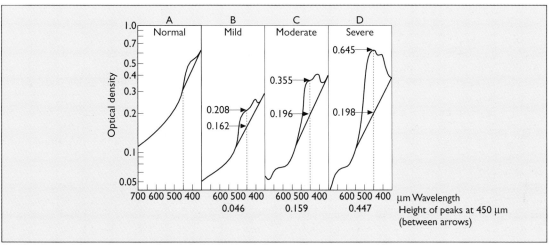

Fig 17.1 Spectral absorption curves of amniotic fluid in (from left) normal late pregnancy, mild, moderate and severe haemolytic disease.

- All Rhesus negative, unsensitized women who abort and require curettage are given an injection of 50–100μg Rhesus anti-D IgG within 72 hours of the abortion.
- All Rhesus negative unsensitized women (whose husband or partner is Rhesus positive or has unknown Rhesus status) who require chorionic villus sampling, amniocentesis, have an ectopic gestation, antepartum haemorrhage, abdominal trauma or who require an external cephalic version are given Rhesus anti-D IgG. The dose before the 20th week is 50μg, and after 20 weeks it is 100μg.
- All Rhesus negative unsensitized women, whose pregnancy progresses to the 28th week, receive an injection of 100μg Rhesus anti-D IgG, repeated at 34 weeks, unless the father of the fetus is Rhesus negative. This recommendation is controversial as only 1–2 per cent of Rhesus negative women are sensitized during pregnancy, but the amount of Rhesus anti-D IgG required is increased at least 4-fold.
- All Rhesus negative unsensitized women who give birth to a Rhesus positive baby are given an injection of 100μg Rhesus anti-D IgG within 72 hours of the birth. An indirect Coombs test is made 24 hours later. If the Coombs test is negative (indicating no circulating anti-D IgG) a test is made on the mother's blood to determine the number of fetal red blood cells present (Kleihauer test). A level of >80 fetal blood cells/50 high-power fields equals a fetal transfusion of >5ml fetal blood. This indicates the need for an additional injection of Rhesus anti-D IgG. The dose is 20μg/ml of fetal red blood cells. In the USA and many European countries, a single injection of 250–300μg is given within 72 hours of the birth and Kleihauser testing is not undertaken.

THE INFANT

At birth the infant is examined to determine the degree of fetal blood haemolysis. A very few infants are hydropic at birth, with ascites, pleural effusion and hepato-splenomegaly. Their outlook is very poor. Most infants appear normal or have mild jaundice.

Blood is taken for haemoglobin concentration, ABO and Rhesus grouping, serum bilirubin assay and Coombs test. The results will enable the neonatologist to decide if exchange transfusion is required. This is usually given within 10 hours of the birth. The objective is to restore the fetal blood haemoglobin level to 148g/l using Rhesus negative, ABO-compatible blood.

Follow-up is essential as the infant may develop jaundice within 48 hours of birth (icterus gravis neonatorum). The infant's liver and spleen are enlarged and its serum bilirubin is >210μmol/l.

Treatment is by exchange transfusion. In the absence of these findings, serum bilirubin measurements are made at frequent intervals during the first 10 days of life, treatment being given depending on the level found. A few babies develop jaundice in the 2nd week of life, when further haemolysis occurs (haemolytic disease of the newborn). The prognosis is good provided that the infant's haemoglobin and serum bilirubin levels are kept within the normal range. The baby is given phototherapy.

OTHER TYPES OF ISO-IMMUNIZATION

Few of the other irregular antibodies detected at antenatal screening cause problems to the neonate, apart from anti-Kell and anti-C iso-immunization, which are managed in pregnancy, during birth and in the neonatal period in the same way as for Rhesus iso-immunization

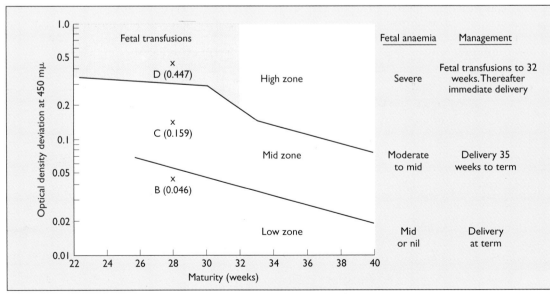

Fig 17.2 The relationship between the size of the amniotic fluid pigment peak at different stages of maturity and fetal anaemia and management. (The peak figures from **Fig 17.1** B,C and D are charted in **Fig 17.2**).

18

ENDOCRINE DISORDERS IN PREGNANCY

DIABETES MELLITUS

Most cases of diabetes diagnosed before or detected in pregnancy are insulin-dependent diabetes mellitus (IDDM) and affect between 0.1 and 0.3 per cent of pregnant women. In addition, between 1.5 and 2.5 per cent of pregnant women develop glucose intolerance during pregnancy (gestational diabetes). The reason for this is that these women are less able to manage the altered carbohydrate metabolism in pregnancy, which leads to a delay in the exchange of glucose between the blood and the tissues. The cause of the delay is not known. It may be due to the raised levels of oestrogen, and rising levels of human placental lactogen (hPL) which mobilizes fatty acids for energy, sparing glucose; or to a placental insulin-degrading system.

The effect of the metabolic changes is that IDDM is made worse and gestational diabetes may appear during the pregnancy.

Until recently certain pregnant women were thought to be more likely to develop gestational diabetes and were classified as potential diabetics. These women had a close family member or members who were diabetic, had given birth to a baby weighing >4500g, had a previously unexplained intrauterine death or were obese. The sensitivity and specificity of these 'markers' for diabetes are poor.

THE DIAGNOSIS OF DIABETES

Expert committees in several countries and the WHO have agreed on criteria to determine if a person has diabetes:

- If diabetes is suspected, random or fasting blood glucose concentrations are measured. A random venous plasma glucose level of 11.0mmol/l or more; or a fasting glucose concentration 8mmol/l or more is diagnostic of diabetes. Random or fasting levels below those mentioned exclude diabetes.
- If the results are equivocal, a glucose load of 75g (mixed in flavoured water) is drunk over a 5-minute period and an oral glucose-tolerance test (OGTT) is performed.
- If diabetic symptoms are present the 2-hour glucose value is sufficient to diagnose diabetes; when there are no symptoms at least one abnormal reading in the OGTT and a raised fasting or a two-hour level are required to establish the diagnosis (Table 18.1).

DETECTION OF GESTATIONAL DIABETES

Many obstetricians screen all pregnant women between the 20th and 28th week of pregnancy for gestational diabetes using a 50g or a 75g OGTT. A venous whole blood glucose level at 1 hour >7.8mmol/l after a 50g glucose load and >8mmol/l after a 75g glucose load indicates that a full OGTT should be made. Other experts, including the authors of *Effective Care in Pregnancy and Childbirth* state that 'the tests are not reproducible at least 50 to 70 per cent of the time, and the mortality and morbidity of gestational diabetes has been exaggerated'. (Gestational diabetes cannot be detected by testing the urine for glucose as glycosuria is common in normal pregnant women because of the lowered renal threshold for glucose).

The Diagnosis of Diabetes: Diagnostic Values for 75g Oral Tolerance Test				
	Glucose concentration mmol/l (mg/dl)			
	Whole blood		Plasma	
	Venous	**Capillary**	**Venous**	**Capillary**
Diabetes mellitus: Fasting value and/or	≥6.7 (≥120)	≥6.7 (≥120)	≥7.8 (≥140)	≥7.8 (≥140)
2 hours after glucose load	≥10.0 (≥180)	≥11.1 (≥200)	≥11.1 (≥200)	≥12.2 (≥220)
Impaired glucose tolerance: Fasting value and	<6.7 (<120)	<6.7 (<120)	<7.8 (<140)	<7.8 (<140)
2 hours after glucose load	6.7–10.0 (120–180)	7.8–11.1 (140–200)	7.8–11.1 (140–200)	8.9–12.2 (160–220)

Table 18.1 The diagnosis of diabetes: diagnostic values for 75g oral tolerance test. From Diabetes Mellitus. Report of WHO Study Group; WHO 1985. Technical Report Series 727.

The Effects of Diabetes Mellitus on Pregnancy	
Condition	**Risk (% of women affected)**
Pregnancy induced hypertension	10–20
Polyhydramnios	20–25
Bacteriuria	7–10
Congenital malformations	6
Perinatal mortality	50–100 per 1000

Table 18.2 The effects of diabetes mellitus on pregnancy.

If gestational diabetes is diagnosed, renal function should be assessed and an ophthalmological examination made.

THE EFFECT OF THE PREGNANCY ON THE DIABETES

Insulin requirements increase, particularly in the fourth quarter of pregnancy and must be monitored regularly by blood glucose measurements. Ketosis is fairly common. It requires to be corrected quickly and its recurrence avoided to reduce the risk of intrauterine death of the fetus. Immediately after the birth, insulin sensitivity increases and the insulin dose should be reduced to avoid hypoglycaemia and coma.

THE EFFECT OF THE DIABETES ON THE PREGNANCY

The effects of IDDM on the pregnancy have been established *(Table 18.2)* , the effect of gestational diabetes is less clear. The frequency of the complications listed depends to a large extent on the quality of the care of a diabetic woman, which should start before pregnancy if possible.

THE MANAGEMENT OF DIABETES
Prepregnancy advice

A known diabetic woman or a woman who has impaired glucose tolerance should avoid becoming pregnant until her glycosylated haemoglobin (HbA$_{1c}$) and her glucose levels have been controlled within the normal range. This will reduce the risk of congenital malformations and makes optimal control of the diabetes easier.

Pregnancy

In pregnancy certain principles obtain:
- Euglycaemia should be maintained for as much of the day as possible, to reduce the risk of intra-uterine fetal death.
- Major congenital defects should be sought by ultrasound examination between the 14th and 18th week of pregnancy, and by alpha fetoprotein measurement at about the 16th week of pregnancy.

- The optimal time for the birth should be determined for each woman.
- The neonate should be born where it can receive optimal intensive care if needed.

These aims can be best achieved if the woman is cared for by a team comprising physician, obstetrician, dietitian and neonatologist. The woman should discuss her diet with the dietitian, and obese women may be given a weight reduction programme.

Insulin-dependent diabetes mellitus

The medical care starts when a general assessment is made early in pregnancy. Admission to hospital may be required for renal function testing, blood lipid estimation, and stabilization of the diabetes. The diabetes is considered stable when the woman's fasting whole blood capillary glucose is <5.5mmol/l and her 2-hourly postprandial level is <4.8mmol/l.

The woman measures her preprandial blood glucose daily and attends weekly for her home glucose monitoring to be reviewed and for her glucose meter to be calibrated. She is given a mixture of a pure short-acting insulin (e.g. Actrapid) and an intermediate-acting insulin (e.g. Monotard) twice daily. The glycosylated Hb level is measured every 4 weeks. If this is greater than 10 per cent or if good control is not obtained, the woman is admitted to hospital to stabilize the diabetic condition. Selective admission to hospital is made from the 35th week of gestation.

The purpose of the additional antenatal care is to seek and detect PIH, urinary tract infection, polyhydramnios and to assess fetal well-being and growth. Assessments are made from the 28th to 30th week of pregnancy and the fetal condition is evaluated weekly by kick counts and perhaps other measures (see Chapter 22). Fetal growth is evaluated by repeated ultrasound examinations at about 2-week intervals.

Gestational diabetes

Most of these women do not require admission to hospital but require the same meticulous care during pregnancy. They are unlikely to have a baby with a congenital malformation, however, the baby may be large. Dietary measures are suggested and if these do not achieve the maintenance of blood glucose in the desired range, the woman is treated with insulin.

The timing of the birth

Most diabetic women whose diabetes in under good control can continue the pregnancy to the 38th week or even later and go into labour spontaneously. Some 'diabetic management teams' prefer to induce labour at about the 37th week of pregnancy provided that the conditions for induction are met (page 185). The reason for this is that as the timing of the birth can be anticipated reasonably well, hospital staff and facilities are prepared for the birth and the care of the neonate. If the labour does not progress quickly as shown on a partogram, it may be accelerated using an oxytocin infusion, or a caesarean section performed. Other teams perform an elective caesarean section at the 38th week of pregnancy, arguing that the control of the diabetes during labour is complex and better results are obtained by caesarean section.

If pregnancy induced hypertension supervenes or the tests on the fetus show that it is at high risk of dying in utero, the pregnancy may need to be terminated by caesarean section or induction of labour.

The management of labour

The patient's blood glucose levels are maintained in the desirable range through the labour by setting up

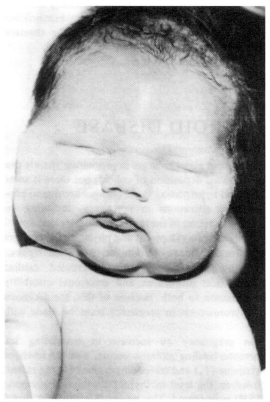

Fig 18.1 Newborn baby of a diabetic mother.

an intravenous infusion of 5 per cent glucose and adding insulin to provide 5.0–7.5u per hour, depending on total daily insulin needs. Blood glucose is monitored every 2 hours. Following the birth of the baby, the infusion rate is reduced by half and continued for 12 hours or longer.

The newborn baby

Most babies of diabetic mothers are large, mainly due to fat deposition from the stimulation of pancreatic beta-cells by transplacental glucose which causes extra insulin production. This in turn leads to fat deposition. The better the control of the diabetes during pregnancy the less is the chance that an excessively large baby will be born. Most of the babies have neuromuscular excitability and a cushingoid appearance *(Fig 18.1)*. Babies of diabetic mothers are likely to develop hypoglycaemia (<1.7mmol/l); hypokalaemia (<1.8mmol/l); polycythaemia (>7.0%); and the respiratory distress syndrome. Early clamping of the umbilical cord reduces the risk of polycythaemia, and intensive neonatal care reduces the risk of the other conditions. Feeding (oral or intragastric) is started early, usually 2–6 hours after the birth, to prevent hypoglycaemia. The babies tend to lose considerable weight and are lethargic in the first week of life, but after this time they progress normally. Because of the risk the women should be advised to take the following measures: avoid becoming obese, take regular exercise, avoid cigarette smoking and be checked annually for hypertension. The woman's general practitioner has a major role in helping the woman meet these measures, and should give advice about life style changes including weight-controlling diets and exercise programmes.

The follow-up of women who have gestational diabetes

Follow-up by annual testing is important as 5 per cent of women with gestational diabetes will continue to have glucose intolerance; 10 per cent will develop diabetes within 10 years, and >20 per cent in 20 years.

THYROID DISEASE

AUTOIMMUNE HYPERTHYROIDISM (GRAVES' DISEASE)

Autoimmune hyperthyroidism (Graves' disease) may precede pregnancy or may arise in pregnancy because of the hypermetabolic state. In pregnancy, treatment with propylthiouracil is to be preferred as it does not readily cross the placenta. The objective is to maintain the free T_4 index in the normal range. If possible the drug should be discontinued in the last 4 weeks of pregnancy to avoid the chance of fetal goitre. Labour is usually uneventful. About 10 per cent of neonates become thyrotoxic in the neonatal period because of the transplacental passage of thyroid stimulating immunoglobulins. The babies can be identified during pregnancy by measuring the level of the long-acting thyroid stimulator protector or LATS-P in the maternal blood.

PARENCHYMATOUS (COLLOID) GOITRE

Although the thyroid gland enlarges in pregnancy, it is uncommon for it to cause symptoms. The cause of the goitre is partly due to decreased absorption of iodine in the first half of pregnancy. A pregnant woman should take iodized table salt to prevent the fetus developing colloid goitre.

PRIMARY HYPOTHYROIDISM

This is an uncommon complication of pregnancy. In early pregnancy an increased need for thyroxine occurs and is associated with a rise in T_3 and T_4 which plateaus at about the 30th week. In women with hypothyroidism this rise cannot occur, and these women need rather more thyroxine than when not pregnant. The extra quantity needed can be estimated from the serum TSH (thyrotropin) level, a fall indicating a need for more thyroxine. In hypothyroid pregnant women TSH should be measured at regular intervals and the dose of thyroxine needed adjusted, above the average daily dose of $100\mu g$, as required. The compliance of the patient should be ensured, as insufficient thyroxine may increase maternal and fetal morbidity.

19

INFECTIONS DURING PREGNANCY

With the exception of poliomyelitis, pregnancy does not alter a woman's resistance to infection. The severity of any infection, however, correlates positively with its effect on the fetus. For example, the more severe the infection and the earlier in pregnancy it occurs, the greater is the risk of miscarriage or of intrauterine death of the fetus.

Infections have an *indirect* and a *direct* effect on the fetus. The indirect effect operates by reducing the oxygenation of the placental blood, and by altering the nutrient exchange through the placenta. The direct effect depends on the ability of the invading organism to penetrate the placenta and infect the fetus. Viruses, being smaller than bacteria, are able to do this more easily. At first the virus multiplies in the trophoblast and subsequently invades the fetus. Most viral infections do not affect the fetus unless the mother's infection is very severe. Four exceptions to this are toxoplasmosis, rubella, cytomegalovirus and herpes simplex virus infections. The infections may cause congenital defects and have been given the acronym TORCH. The clinical effects of TORCH infections are microcephaly, congenital heart disease, eye damage such as cataract, deafness, hepatosplenomegaly (with jaundice) purpura and, later in childhood, mental handicap.

As maternal antibodies cross the placenta, they offer the fetus a degree of immunity, except following a primary infection. The fetus becomes immunologically competent from about the 14th week of pregnancy, but the efficacy of this protection is low until the second half of pregnancy.

URINARY TRACT INFECTIONS

Urinary tract infection is the most disturbing of the bacterial infections. It occurs because the urinary tract dilates owing to the relaxation of the muscles of the ureter and the bladder in pregnancy with consequent urinary stasis.

SYMPTOMLESS BACTERIURIA.

The prevalence of symptomless bacteriuria (defined as >100 000 bacteria per ml of urine) in non-pregnant women is about 2 per cent. In pregnancy it rises to 3–8 per cent because of the physiological changes mentioned, and 30 per cent of pregnant women who have symptomless bacteriuria will develop symptomatic urinary tract infection. Unless the infection is treated these women have a slightly higher chance of developing hypertension in pregnancy and twice the risk of delivering a low birth-weight baby.

Because of this risk, many authorities recommend that all pregnant women are screened for symptomless bacteriuria in early pregnancy. A midstream specimen of urine is sent to a laboratory for culture. In 85 per cent of cases *E. coli* are isolated, and in the remainder a variety of microorganisms are found. As the procedure is costly, other procedures such as dip slides covered with a culture medium and reagent strips have been developed and are reliable screening methods.

Treatment of symptomless bacteriuria is to prescribe amoxycillin 3g or cephalexin 2g as a single dose or in appropriate doses for 5–7 days. Seven days after finishing the antibiotics, a midstream specimen of urine is re-examined. If the symptomless bacteriuria has not been eliminated a longer course of antibiotics is prescribed. Regular follow-up urine cultures must be made, and recurrences treated.

PYELONEPHRITIS

As mentioned, about 30 per cent of women who have untreated bacteriuria will develop pyelonephritis during pregnancy as will 1 per cent of women who do not have the condition.

The infection occurs when bacteria growing in the stagnant urine spread from the bladder to the ureter and then to the renal pelvis. Haematogenous infection is very uncommon.

Pyelonephritis usually begins after the 20th week of pregnancy. In mild cases the woman complains of tiredness and urinary frequency and, occasionally, dysuria. More severe infections start suddenly with chills and rigors, fever, and pain over one or both renal areas. The patient may become rapidly dehydrated. The diagnosis is confirmed by examining a midstream specimen of urine, having excluded other causes of abdominal pain such as acute appendicitis and abruptio placentae.

Treatment is to correct the dehydration and to prescribe appropriate antibiotics having tested for bacterial sensitivity. In most cases a cephalosporin or amoxycillin is appropriate initial treatment. As some women with pyelonephritis are nauseated, the antibiotic may have to given intravenously. Follow-up examinations of a midstream urine culture at 2-week intervals for the remainder of the pregnancy should be instituted. Some authorities recommend prophylactic antibiotics for the duration of the pregnancy.

VAGINAL INFECTIONS

Vaginal infections during pregnancy due to *Candida* spp., *Trichomonas* and *Gardnerella* are discussed on pages 248–249. The diagnosis and treatment are the same as for pregnancy.

GROUP B STREPTOCOCCUS

Colonies of Group B streptococci are harboured in the upper vagina of 0.3 per 1000 pregnant women in Britain and in up to 4 per 1000 women in Australia and the USA, depending on their socioeconomic and sexual status.

If Group B streptococcal infection is present during labour the bacteria may colonize the neonate. Some studies suggest that half the babies born through an infected vagina are colonized, and 1–2 per cent of them develop streptococcal infection.

To prevent this it is recommended that pregnant women should have a vaginal swab taken for culture between the 26th and 28th week of pregnancy. If group B streptococcal infection is detected the woman should be prescribed *intrapartum* intravenous ampicillin (2g initially; 1–2g every 6 hours until delivery) in cases of preterm labour, preterm premature rupture of the membranes, rupture of the membranes for more than 18 hours and multiple gestation. An alternative is to use a rapid latex agglutination test on a vaginal swab taken in early labour. The result is obtained within 20 minutes and if it is positive the woman is given antibiotics.

GONORRHOEA

Depending on the population studied, between 1 and 6 per cent of pregnant women are found to have gonorrhoea on culture studies using the Thayer-Martin medium. Many of these women have no symptoms. In symptomatic gonorrhoea, the woman complains of dysuria and a vaginal discharge which occurs within 5 days of sexual intercourse. If the symptoms suggest gonorrhoea or if the woman's sexual behaviour suggests that she may have gonorrhoea, cervical and urethral swabs should be taken and inoculated directly on to preheated plates of culture medium. In addition, vaginal swabs should be made for other vaginal infective organisms. The management of gonococcal infection is discussed on pages 250.

SYPHILIS

The importance of syphilitic infection in pregnancy is that treponemes are able to penetrate the placenta after the 15th week of pregnancy and infect the fetus. If the fetus survives the initial infection, by the time of the birth it is in the secondary stage of syphilis.

For this reason every pregnant woman should be tested for syphilis using a reagin test (either the VDRL or the Rapid Plasma Reagin (RPR) test),

although the incidence of syphilis in most areas is >0.1 per cent. The test should be made at the first antenatal visit, and in the opinion of some authorities, repeated at the 30th week of pregnancy. False positives may occur, and thus a woman who has had a positive screening test, is investigated using a procedure which detects specific anti-treponemal antibodies in her serum (e.g. the *Treponema pallidum* haemagglutination test [TPHA]; the fluorescent treponemal antibody test [FTA-ABS]; or the *Treponema pallidum* immobilization test [TPI]).

The treatment is that described on page 246 for non-pregnant women. Follow-up serological tests are made monthly for 3 months; every 2 months for the next 6 months and every 3 months for the next year.

The infant. As the signs of syphilis in a neonate are often equivocal and serology inaccurate, the infant of a woman who has been diagnosed as having syphilis whilst pregnant and who has not had a complete course of treatment and follow-up, should be given a full course of antibiotic treatment (aqueous procaine penicillin 50 000u/kg body weight daily for 10 days).

TOXOPLASMOSIS

Toxoplasma gondii infects 3–6 pregnant women per 1000. In 90 per cent there are no clinical signs. Infections acquired in pregnancy may lead to a miscarriage or congenital infection of the fetus, one fetus in 4 being affected. The eyes and the central nervous system may be severely damaged.

Screening tests for toxoplasma are available but are not cost-effective. If chosen they are best made before pregnancy, and seronegative women should be retested in each of the quarters of pregnancy.

Preventive measures taken by a pregnant woman are more cost-effective. A pregnant woman should avoid touching cat faeces. She should avoid touching her eyes or mouth whilst handling raw meat and wash her hands after handling it. She should only eat well-cooked meat. She should wash vegetables and fruit thoroughly before eating them and, if a gardener, should wear gloves.

VIRAL INFECTIONS

Several viral infections need some discussion.

RUBELLA

Rubella infection is widespread. By the age of 19 years, >85 per cent of people have been infected, and 9 out of 10 of those infected have lifelong immunity.

Should rubella occur in a non-immune woman in the first 14 weeks of pregnancy, viraemia and infection of the fetus is almost certain, and >40 per cent of the infected fetuses will be damaged by the virus. The virus invades actively dividing cells and alters the genome. Infection in weeks 4–12 of pregnancy affects the lens of the eyes (causing cataract) or the ears (causing deafness). Infection between the 5th and 12th week damages the chambers of the heart. As well as causing damage to specific organs, rubella infection may cause widespread cellular damage leading to fetal growth retardation, thrombocytopenia, hepatosplenomegaly, and vasculitis, especially renal artery stenosis.

These problems could be avoided if all women were immunized against rubella between the ages of 11 and 13 using a live attenuated strain of the virus (the RA 27/3 strain). Programmes to accomplish this have been developed in many countries.

A woman should be tested for rubella antibodies either when she decides to become pregnant or at the first pregnancy visit. The test used is the Single Radial Haemolysis Test (SRH test). If this test is positive with a titre of >15 000IU/l the woman is immune to rubella. A non-immune woman who is not pregnant may be offered vaccination but should avoid pregnancy for 3 months. If a pregnant woman is inadvertently vaccinated, the risk of the baby being infected is <2 per cent, but the woman should be offered the choice of terminating the pregnancy or continuing it. Either way she should be rechecked after the pregnancy.

A problem arises when a pregnant non-immune woman develops a rubelliform rash, (as in half of women the rash is not due to rubella); or if the woman has been in contact with a case of rubella. A serological test should be made as soon as possible, preferably within 15 days of the appearance of the rash or the contact. An SRH test positive in a titre of >15 000 IU/l is evidence of immunity to rubella and the woman may be reassured that her baby is in no danger of being infected. A second SRH test is repeated in 21 days for confirmation.

If the woman is seronegative, the problems of congenital infection should be discussed with her and a therapeutic abortion may be offered.

GENITAL HERPES

A general discussion on herpes simplex virus (HSV) can be found on pp 245. In pregnancy HSV may cross the placental 'barrier' to infect the fetus, and is more likely to be found in primary than in recurrent infections. Overall the risk is low, only one fetus per 1000 being infected. The risk is greater during childbirth, particularly if the mother has developed a recurrence of the condition or is shedding the virus from her cervix.

These findings suggest:

- A woman with a history of genital herpes need have no anxiety that her baby will be infected and may expect to be delivered vaginally, unless a recurrence of the infection or a new infection occurs during the pregnancy.
- If a first infection or a recurrence of genital herpes occurs during the pregnancy, but has healed by the time labour starts, the woman may give birth vaginally.

- If herpetic lesions are present when the membranes rupture or labour starts, a caesarean section should be performed to avoid the risk that the baby will acquire a herpetic infection during the passage through the birth canal.

The strategy of taking endocervical swabs for viral culture every 2 weeks from the 34th week of pregnancy in women can be abandoned, as positive HSV-infected swabs do not predict the risk of the infant being exposed to herpes infection during birth.

HEPATITIS B

Although fewer than 0.5 per cent of women in the developed nations are hepatitis B carriers, up to 30 per cent of migrants from parts of Africa, East and South East Asia have hepatitis B surface antigen (HB_s Ag) in their blood and are potentially infectious to healthcare workers who may be infected by contact with blood and body secretions. For this reason, screening of pregnant migrant women and drug addicts for Hb_s Ag is now recommended. Precautions are taken when caring for such women in childbirth and most hospitals have developed appropriate protocols.

It is also known that the hepatitis B virus is readily transmitted to the baby, probably during the birth. Babies at special risk are those whose mothers have HB_c Ag as well as HB_s Ag in their blood. If not treated, many of the babies will develop hepatocellular carcinoma when adult. This can be avoided to a large extent if babies at high risk are given hepatitis B globulin together with hepatitis B vaccine $10\mu g$ at birth, and two further injections of the vaccine at the ages of 1 and 6 months.

CYTOMEGALOVIRUS INFECTION (CMV)

Over half of all pregnant women show serological evidence of previous CMV infection. One per cent of women may become infected with CMV during pregnancy, all of whom are asymptomatic. The infection is associated with an increased perinatal mortality and 3–7 per cent of the infants have congenital abnormalities.

Screening has proved to be of no value – there is no vaccine.

HUMAN IMMUNODEFICIENCY VIRUS INFECTION (AIDS)

Although in western countries most cases of HIV infection occur in homosexual or bisexual men, intravenous drug users who share needles are increasingly being infected, as are some heterosexual men and women, who do not abuse drugs. In Subsaharan Africa and South and South East Asia many heterosexual women and men are HIV positive and the numbers are increasing. Infected women who become pregnant have a 20–40 per cent risk of transmitting the virus to the fetus, and all infected fetuses will be antibody positive and develop AIDS. There is a strong argument that screening for

HIV infection should be offered to all pregnant women, particularly as there is evidence that the use of drugs such as zidovudine may delay the progression of the disease. HIV infection has no adverse effect on the pregnancy nor has the pregnancy any adverse effect on the progress of HIV infection. As the HIV infects the amniotic fluid as well as the women's blood, full infectious disease control precautions should be taken by attendant medical staff during labour and child birth. Vaginal delivery may be anticipated and there is no place for caesarean section purely because the woman has HIV infection. Because of all the problems involved, women infected with HIV should be given the opportunity to choose to have an abortion rather than giving birth to a baby who may have HIV infection.

INFECTIONS IN THE TROPICS

HELMINTH INFESTATIONS – HOOKWORM DISEASE

Endemic infections by helminths are almost universal among rural dwellers in the tropics and subtropics, and the most serious of these is hookworm disease. Two types of hookworm are found, *Ancylostoma duodenale* and *Necator americanus*. In the gut the worms attach to the villi by suckers, and feed on blood obtained from the villi which, after passing through their bodies, is excreted into the lumen of the bowel. In studies in Malaysia in the 1950s, we found that the blood loss due to hookworm was found to relate closely to the hookworm load, and varied from 2 to 90ml per day. Hookworm infesta-

tion is a cause of iron deficiency anaemia, and this is particularly serious in pregnancy. Treatment is to eliminate the worms by administering bephenium hydroxynaphthoate (Alcopar) in a dose of 5g, daily for 3 days, and to treat the anaemia with iron.

MALARIA

Exacerbation of malaria or relapse in a partially immune female is particularly common during pregnancy, and each attack may precipitate abortion or the onset of premature labour. The fetus is protected by the placenta in most cases, although large numbers of immobilized parasites may be found in the placenta, particularly if the infection is by *P. falciparum*. Occasionally in non-immune patients, congenital transmission of malaria occurs.

Pregnant women travelling to an area where malaria is endemic should take prophylactic antimalarial drugs. If the strains of *P. falciparum* in the area are chloroquine resistant, problems arise. The alternative drugs, Fansidar and Maloprim, affect folic acid synthesis and may induce a fatal Stevens–Johnson syndrome. They should be avoided. If the risk of chloroquine resistance is low, chloroquine and proguanil should be given. If the risk of chloroquine resistance is high, a pregnant woman should postpone her visit until she has given birth.

Any pregnant woman developing a high fever in a malarial area should be suspected of having the infection, and if this is confirmed by finding parasites in a thick blood film, treatment is given with chloroquine 600mg (base) initially, followed 8 hours later by 300mg, and 300mg daily for the next 3 days.

20

DISEASES OF THE PLACENTA AND MEMBRANES

ABNORMAL PLACENTATION

The shape of the definitive placenta is determined at the time the placenta forms, the variations found *(Fig 20.1)* mostly having no clinical significance.

The umbilical cord may enter the placenta at its mid-point or may join it at an edge (**marginal insertion of the cord**) or the umbilical vessels may run some distance along the membranes (**velamentous insertion of the cord**). Should the vessels run across the cervix, they may be compressed by the fetal head during labour, or bleed causing fetal anaemia. In some cases the placenta is smaller than the chorionic plate and the trophoblast invades the decidua laterally more deeply, giving a ridged appearance on the placental surface (**placenta circumvallata**). In most cases this has no clinical significance but occasionally may be found in women who have antepartum or intrapartum haemorrhage. In other cases the placenta has an accessory lobe separated by membranes from the main placenta (**placenta succenturiata**)

In a few cases the trophoblastic invasion is not regulated by maternal immune defenses and the myometrium is invaded causing **placenta accreta, increta or percreta**. **Haemangiomata** occur in 1 per cent of placentae. In most cases they are small and of no clinical significance, but larger haemangiomata may be associated with hydramnios, antepartum haemorrhage or preterm labour.

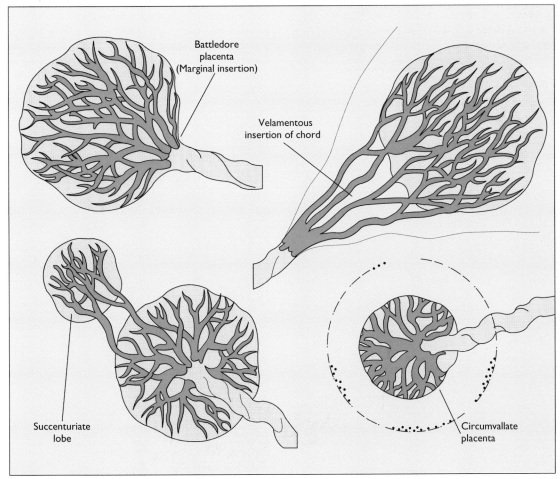

Battledore placenta
(Marginal insertion)

Velamentous insertion of chord

Succenturiate lobe

Circumvallate placenta

Fig 20.1 Abnormal placentation.

Classification of Trophoblastic Neoplasms
1. Benign trophoblastic disease (hydatidiform mole) Complete hydatidiform mole Partial hydatidiform mole Hydropic degeneration of the trophoblast
2. Persistent trophoblastic disease (often malignant) Apparently confined to the uterus (invasive mole) Usually with extra-uterine spread (choriocarcinoma)

Table 20.1 Classification of trophoblastic neoplasms.

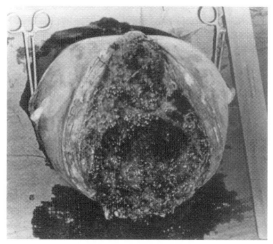

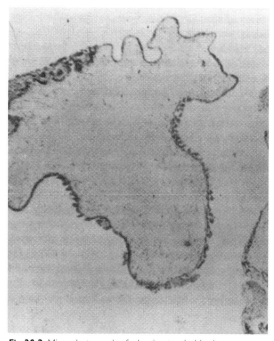

Fig 20.2 Benign trophoblastic tumour (hydatidiform mole) – gross specimen. Note the grape-like masses.

Fig 20.3 Microphotograph of a benign trophoblastic tumour (hydatidiform mole), showing the distended villi and irregular trophoblastic proliferation.

GESTATIONAL TROPHOBLASTIC DISEASE

Gestational trophoblastic disease is uncommon. It is discussed here as it is potentially lethal, but with treatment a 90 per cent cure rate is attainable. The disease occurs in two forms *(Table 20.1).*

HYDATIDIFORM MOLE

The tumour may have completely or partially replaced the placenta. In the complete form, hydropic swelling and vesicle formation is associated with trophoblastic proliferation and a paucity or absence of blood vessels within the villi *(Fig 20.2 and 20.3).* No fetus can be found. Five per cent of complete moles undergo malignant change.

In the partial form a fetus is present but areas of the placenta show the changes described for the complete mole. Partial moles become malignant less frequently (0.05 per cent).

MALIGNANT TROPHOBLASTIC DISEASE

The tumour may be confined to the uterus (**invasive mole**) or spread via the bloodstream to distant organs (**choriocarcinoma**).

In the invasive mole the trophoblastic covered villi penetrate the myometrial fibres and may extend to other organs, the appearance of the villi remaining that of the benign tumour.

In choriocarcinoma, the tumour is characterized by sheets of trophoblastic cells, both syncytio- and cytotrophoblast with few or no villi formed *(Fig 20.4).*

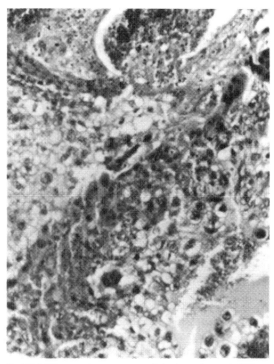

Fig 20.4 Microscopic appearance of choriocarcinoma (×160).

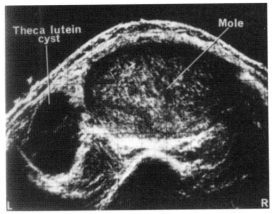

Fig 20.5 The echogram shows the characteristic vesicular pattern of a hydatidiform mole (by kind permission of Dr W. J. Garrett).

Aetiology

Gestational trophoblastic disease is caused by a genetic disorder in which a spermatozoon enters an ovum which has lost its nucleus, or in which two sperms enter the ovum. In over 90 per cent of complete moles, only paternal genes are found and in 10 per cent the mole is heterozygous. In contrast, partial moles usually have a triploid chromosomal constitution suggesting dispermy as the cause.

The development of gestational trophoblastic tumours is thought to be due to a defective maternal immune response to the invasion by the trophoblast. In consequence the villi become distended with nutrients. The primitive vasculature within each villus does not form properly with the result that the embryo 'starves', dies and is absorbed, whilst the trophoblast continues to thrive and in certain circumstances invades maternal tissues.

The increased syncytiotrophoblast activity leads to an increased production of hCG, chorionic thyrotrophin and progesterone. A fall in oestradiol secretion occurs, as oestradiol synthesis requires enzymes from the fetus, which does not exist. The raised hCG levels may induce the development of theca-lutein cysts of the ovary.

THE DIAGNOSIS OF BENIGN GESTATIONAL TROPHOBLASTIC DISEASE

The first sign is bleeding per vaginam, which tends to persist. The bleeding may be followed fairly soon by uterine contractions and the expulsion of grape-like material. In other cases the tumour grows without symptoms. During this time examination will show the following features:

- The uterus is usually larger than expected from the gestational dates and is 'doughy' to the touch.
- Fetal heart sounds cannot be heard.
- Ultrasonic scanning shows a distinct speckled appearance *(Fig 20.5).*
- If serum hCG is measured it is found to be unexpectedly high *(Fig 20.6).*

Treatment

If the patient is admitted expelling the tumour, no immediate treatment is needed unless the expulsion slows down, at which time a digital evacuation of the uterus is carried out. Blood is obtained for possible transfusion, as the expulsion is often accompanied by marked blood loss.

If the diagnosis is reached before the expulsion of any vesicles, the uterus may be evacuated using a suction curette or by the administration of prostaglandins to induce uterine contractions (this method has the disadvantage that it may lead to the intravascular dissemination of trophoblast). Gentle curettage is performed about 7 days later to remove any residual trophoblast.

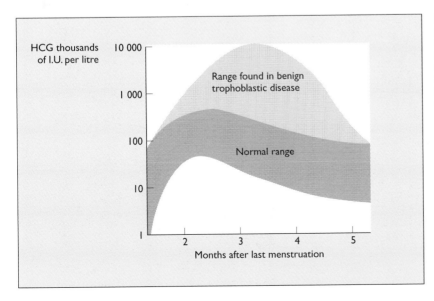

Fig 20.6 Chorionic gonadotrophin excretion in trophoblastic disease. The normal range is shown darkly shaded; levels found in trophoblastic disease are shown in the lightly shaded area.

The Follow-up of Benign Trophoblastic Disease Using a Specific Radio-immuno-assay

1. Radio-immuno-assay of serum βhCG at 7–10-day intervals. If the level falls serially no drug treatment is needed. Complete disappearance of βhCG takes 12 to 14 weeks on average.

2. When βhCG level has been normal for 3 consecutive weeks, test monthly for 6 months.

3. If the assay shows normal βhCG levels for 6 consecutive months, follow-up can be discontinued.

4. During the follow-up period pregnancy should be avoided. Oral contraceptives may be prescribed.

5. If the serum βhCG level plateaus for more than 3 consecutive weeks, or rises, or if metastases are detected, treat with methotrexate or actinomycin D.

Table 20.2 The follow-up of benign trophoblastic disease using a specific radio-immuno-assay.

If bleeding persists for more than 21 days a further curettage may be indicated.

Women over the age of 40, or women who have completed their family may prefer to have a hysterectomy, to avoid potential malignancy.

Follow-up

Follow-up is important as the disease persists in between 5 and 10 per cent of cases, often developing a malignant form. Follow-up includes vaginal examinations at 2-weekly intervals to evaluate uterine involution and the presence or absence of theca-lutein cysts. Alternatively ultrasound examinations

may be made at 2-weekly intervals. HCG assays should be made according to a schedule *(Table 20.2 and Fig 20.7).*

MALIGNANT GESTATIONAL TROPHOBLASTIC DISEASE

Malignancy follows a benign trophoblastic tumour in 1 in 10 cases, usually within 6 months of the expulsion of the benign tumour. It follows a spontaneous abortion in 1 in 5 000 cases and a viable pregnancy in 1 in 50 000 cases.

Women who have had a benign gestational trophoblastic tumour are at greater risk of developing a malignancy if the woman:
- Is over the age of 40.
- Secretes large amounts of βhCG (> 1000IU per ml).
- Has theca-lutein cyst(s) more than 6cm in diameter.

Malignant gestational trophoblastic disease is best managed at special centres, where meticulous follow-up is conducted. Treatment is by chemotherapy *(Table 20.3).* Follow-up is shown in *Table 20.4.*

ABNORMALITIES OF THE AMNIOTIC FLUID

Amniotic fluid is secreted into the amniotic sac by the amniotic cells which lie over the placenta. This fluid is 99 per cent water and increases in quantity during pregnancy. In the amniotic sac it is swallowed by the fetus. Most of the swallowed fluid is absorbed by the fetal intestinal villi and enters the fetal circulation. From the circulation most is exchanged in the placenta, but some is returned to the amniotic sac by

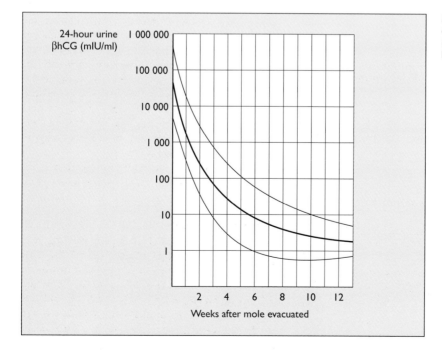

Fig 20.7 Hormone follow-up of benign trophoblastic disease (mean and 95% confidence limits).

Chemotherapy in Malignant Trophoblastic Disease		
Initial course	**Non-metastatic**	**Metastatic**
Methotrexate at 48-hour intervals for 4 doses	1mg/kg IM	1.5mg/kg IM
Folinic acid (citrovorum factor) on alternate days 24 hours after the injection of methotrexate	0.1mg/kg IM	0.15mg/kg IM
Subsequent courses		
A. If response, that is a fall in the βhCG level <20%, repeat the regimen B. Without response, increase methotrexate by 0.5mg/kg and folinic acid by 0.05mg/kg C. If no response after two consecutive courses change to actinomycin D D. If no response to actinomycin D after two courses change to three chemotherapeutic drugs used in combination		
Laboratory tests		
Full blood count, platelet count, SGOT on day 1 (before starting therapy) days 3, 5, 7, 11, 15, 18, 21		

Table 20.3 Chemotherapy in malignant trophoblastic disease.

transudation through the fetal skin. In the last quarter of pregnancy fetal urination adds to the amniotic fluid.

POLYHYDRAMNIOS

Polyhydramnios is caused by increased secretion of amniotic fluid because of a large placenta or by a fetal malformation which prevents the fetus swallowing the fluid, or prevents its absorption through the fetal intestinal villi. Examples of the former are multiple pregnancy and diabetes and of the latter, anencephaly, spina bifida and atresia of the upper gastrointestinal tract.

The fluid may accumulate rapidly (**acute polyhydramnios**) which causes considerable distress to the mother. She may develop dyspnoea, tachycardia, vomiting and severe abdominal pain.

Principles of the Management of Malignant Trophoblastic Disease
1. During treatment the serum levels of the βhCG are assayed each week
2. Provided that the βhCG level continues to fall after a course of chemotherapy, withhold further courses
3. When the βhCG level is normal for 3 consecutive weeks, assay each month for 6 months
4. If the βhCG level remains normal for 12 months, discontinue follow-up. Patients should avoid pregnancy throughout this period
5. Repeat the course of chemotherapy if the βhCG level plateaus for more than 3 consecutive weeks or rises, or if new metastases are detected
6. If the βhCG level plateaus after 3 consecutive courses of a chemotherapeutic agent, or if it rises during a course, change to another chemotherapeutic regimen

Table 20.4 Principles of the management of malignant trophoblastic disease, using a specific βHCG assay.

Treatment is to remove amniotic fluid by amniocentesis, repeated if necessary. The outlook for the fetus, even if normal, is poor.

The slow accumulation of amniotic fluid is more commonly found (**chronic polyhydramnios**). Symptoms similar to those of acute polyhydramnios may be experienced by the expectant mother and examination shows a distended uterus from which a fluid thrill can be obtained. Ultrasound scanning will confirm the diagnosis and identify the presence of either a multiple pregnancy or a fetal abnormality (in most cases).

Treatment

A patient who has a minor degree of polyhydramnios may be relieved by sedation at night. If the symptoms become worse between 30 and 35 weeks of pregnancy, an amniocentesis using a spinal needle to remove no more than 500ml at any one time (to reduce the onset of preterm labour) may be performed, although half the women go into labour. After the 35th week labour may be induced by vaginal amniocentesis if the symptoms become worse, or if a gross fetal malformation is present. The liquor should be released slowly to prevent cord prolapse. Postpartum haemorrhage is likely and prophylactic oxytocin should be given.

The baby or babies should be examined carefully to detect fetal malformations including oesophageal and duodenal atresia.

OLIGOHYDRAMNIOS

Oligohydramnios occurs if the liquor-secreting cells are defective or, in late pregnancy, is caused by renal tract malformations which prevent fetal urination; it also occurs in postdatism. If oligohydramnios occurs early in pregnancy abortion is usual. Should the pregnancy continue, amniotic bands may occur which may damage the fetus. In late pregnancy, oligohydramnios may cause pressure deformities such as wry neck, altered shape of the skull or club foot, and the fetal skin is dry and leathery.

ABNORMALITIES OF THE UMBILICAL CORD

A normal umbilical cord is 45–60cm long, but extremes of 200cm and 2cm have been recorded. The umbilical cord usually contains one vein and two arteries set in Wharton's jelly. In 1 per cent of cords, only one artery is formed and half the fetuses with such cords are malformed. Long cords have no clinical significance unless they form a coil or coils around the fetal neck. A cord of normal length may be shortened by coiling around the fetus. During childbirth the cord may be pulled tight as the fetus descends, reducing the oxygen supply and occasionally causing fetal death. Knots may occur in the umbilical cord. They may be true knots or false knots. True knots may lead to a reduced fetal circulation. False knots are accumulations of Wharton's jelly and have no clinical significance.

21

VARIATIONS IN THE DURATION OF PREGNANCY

The duration of human pregnancy averages 260 days from conception and 280 ±14 days from the first day of the last menstrual period. In 5 per cent of pregnancies the duration of pregnancy is curtailed and a preterm birth (<36 completed weeks) occurs. In 10 per cent of cases the pregnancy is prolonged and the woman does not give birth until more than 41 weeks have been completed.

CURTAILED PREGNANCY: PRETERM BIRTH

There are some problems inherent in defining preterm birth as one which occurs before the 36th completed week of pregnancy. This is because the survival of the neonate depends not only on the duration of the pregnancy, but also on the birth-weight of the baby.

By definition a preterm baby born to a mother living in an industrialized country weighs less than 2500g. This includes two populations of babies: those who are really preterm and those whose growth has been retarded during the pregnancy (dysmature babies) but who are delivered after the 36th week of pregnancy.

Dysmature babies account for 6 per cent of all babies born with a low birth-weight (<2500g) and are at greater risk of dying.

Studies of preterm births show that curtailed pregnancy (preterm labour) may be due to medical complications which developed during the pregnancy (pregnancy-induced hypertension, antepartum haemorrhage) or which existed before the pregnancy (anaemia); to multiple pregnancy; to fetal malformations; or to spontaneous rupture of the membranes from unknown causes *(Table 21.1)*.

PREVENTION OF PRETERM BIRTH

There are no effective ways of preventing preterm birth. Increased contact with health professionals to provide better social support (France), the prophylactic use of tocolytic agents such as terbutaline (Germany) and bed rest in early pregnancy have been tried and have not been shown to be effective. At present a multicentre trial of low-dose daily aspirin is being conducted in Britain, Australia and the USA.

Regular antenatal examinations will detect medical conditions complicating pregnancy and pregnancy-induced hypertension (PIH) at an early stage of their development but it is uncertain if this will reduce the incidence of preterm birth. Cervical circlage increases the duration of pregnancy in women who have a diagnosis of incompetent cervix but not in other cases.

PRETERM LABOUR

The diagnosis of preterm labour must be made carefully or women who are having mild contractions which do not cause cervical dilation will be included. The criteria for diagnosis are:
- The gestational period is less than 36 completed weeks.
- Uterine contractions, preferably recorded on a tocograph, occur every 5–10 minutes, last for at least 30 seconds and persist for at least 60 minutes.
- The cervix is more than 2.5cm dilated and more than 75 per cent effaced.

Using these criteria, two-thirds of women presenting with presumed preterm labour will not be in labour. They need reassurance, not drug treatment.

If the criteria are met, the woman is in preterm labour. If the pregnancy is less than 35 completed weeks' gestation and the woman is not in a facility with a neonatal intensive-care unit, she should have uterine contractions suppressed and be transferred as soon as possible to such a facility. If she has access to neonatal intensive care, the choice is to attempt to suppress uterine activity or to permit labour to proceed. In some third-level hospitals women who start preterm labour at or after the 32nd week of gestation are permitted to proceed, as the low birth-weight infant can be competently cared for with no increase in perinatal mortality.

The greatest challenge is the management of a woman whose labour starts when the gestation period is less than 32 completed weeks.

Causes of Curtailment of Pregnancy and Prematurity	
	(%)
No cause found (including premature rupture of the membranes)	35 – 45
Hypertensive disorders	18 – 30
Multiple pregnancy	12 – 18
Maternal disease	5 – 15
Abruptio placentae	5 – 7
Placenta praevia	3 – 4
Fetal malformations	1 – 2

Table 21.1 Causes of curtailment of pregnancy and prematurity.

Tocolytic drugs in the Management of Preterm Labour		
Drug	**Dose**	**Side effects**
Beta agonists		
Salbutamol	Infused at 4µg/min, increasing by 4µg/min every 20min until uterine contractions suppressed; dose maintained for 6 hours and then reduced. Oral salbutamol started 8mg 6hrly for 5 days	Tachycardia Palpitations Increase in cardiac output Pressure in the chest. Pulmonary oedema and myocardial ischaemia in 5% Fluid retention in all women
Ritodrine	Infused at 50ug/min increased by 50ug every 10 min. until the contractions cease. Maximum dose:350ug/min. Run for 24hr then oral ritodrine 10-20 mg 2-6hrly.	
Calcium channel blocker		
Nifedipine	10mg sublingually, repeated 20min later if contractions persist (max 40mg in first hr). If contractions cease, 20mg by mouth 4-6 hourly.	Limited experience but side effects said to be less than with beta agonists.
Note: beta agonists and calcium channel blockers are relatively ineffective if the cervical dilation is >5cm		
Maintenance of labour inhibition		
NSAIDs	This class of drugs is not effective in suppressing labour but may have a place in maintaining inhibition of labour. The most experience has been with indomethacin. More data needed for evaluation	May cause ductus arteriosus constriction. Inhibits platelet aggregation, esp. in the fetus

Table 21.2 Tocolytic drugs in the management of preterm labour.

MANAGEMENT OF PRETERM LABOUR OF LESS THAN 32 COMPLETED WEEKS

The main treatment is bed rest, which may reduce the risk of premature rupture of the membranes and prolong the pregnancy. Because of the uncertainty that bed rest is effective, various tocolytic drugs have been tried in order to suppress the uterine contractions (Table 21.2).

The side effects of the tocolytics (especially the beta-agonists) means that only some women are suitable to be treated with the drugs. These women include those in whom:

- The pregnancy is advanced to less than 35 weeks.
- There has been confirmation of preterm labour.
- The cervix is less than 5cm dilated.
- The patient is not hypertensive, has no cardiac disease, is not diabetic, does not have abruptio placentae and is not infected.
- The fetus is alive and no evident malformations have been detected by ultrasound scanning.

These exclusions mean that fewer than 25 per cent of women in preterm labour can receive tocolytic drugs. The few randomized trials of tocolytic drugs show that the only significant effect is to delay childbirth by a mean of 24 hours, although in a few instances, labour may be delayed for 2 weeks or more. The studies show that statistically the drugs do not reduce the frequency of delivery before the 37th week nor the proportion of preterm babies born, nor the incidence of hyaline

membrane disease. It would appear that their main value is to enable a woman in preterm labour to be transferred to a hospital with a level-3 nursery.

Because of the risk that labour will start and that the infant may develop hyaline membrane disease of the lungs due to lack of surfactant, the woman should be given betamethasone (celestone chronodose) 24mg in two doses, 12 hours apart. To be effective, corticosteroids have to be given >24 hours and <7 days before the birth. They have no value if the pregnancy has advanced to >34 weeks' gestation.

The membranes should be kept intact for as long as possible and when they rupture a vaginal examination is made to exclude a prolapsed cord. If labour starts it may either be allowed to proceed or a caesarean section may be made. If vaginal delivery is chosen, and proceeds normally, an episiotomy should be made in the late second stage, because of the effect of pressure on the head of the premature infant. If there is delay when the infant's head is in the pelvic outlet, a forceps delivery may be appropriate.

The place of caesarean section in the management of preterm labour is controversial. Most obstetricians believe that if labour starts when the pregnancy is 26–31 weeks' gestation, caesarean section should be performed if:

- The fetus does not present cephalically.
- There is associated antepartum haemorrhage.
- The labour fails to progress normally.
- Fetal distress develops.

While there can be little disagreement about these indications, the *routine* use of caesarean section to deliver babies weighing less than 1500g is controversial. In 1990, the US Institute of Child Health and Human Development examined the available data and concluded that routine caesarean section did not improve survival rates.

PRELABOUR RUPTURE OF THE MEMBRANES

Prelabour (premature) rupture of the membranes may lead to the onset of preterm labour, with or without other causal factors. In most cases the baby is born within 7 days of the prelabour rupture. Rupture of the membranes after the 35th week is of no clinical significance, and if labour does not start quickly it may be induced by the use of prostaglandins or syntocinon (see page 185) depending on the state of the cervix. A woman whose cervix is 'not favourable' (see page 185), may prefer to delay induction for 48 to 72 hours in the anticipation that during this time the cervix will ripen and induction will be easier and more successful.

The real problem occurs when the membranes rupture between the 26th and the 35th week, as the longer the birth is delayed the more mature does the baby become. Against this is the risk of ascending intra-uterine infection occurring.

The woman should be admitted to or transferred to a hospital with a level-3 nursery. If the diagnosis is not obvious, it should be confirmed by taking a sample of fluid from the posterior vaginal vault. This is tested using a monoclonal alphafetoprotein antibody test which has a sensitivity of 98 per cent. A high vaginal swab is also taken for bacteriological examination.

Regular assessments of maternal temperature and pulse are made to detect intra-uterine infection and observations are made to see if the amniotic fluid continues to leak. An ultrasound examination may be made to determine if oligohydramnios has occurred.

The use of prophylactic tocolytics has been suggested, but studies show them to be of little value. Prophylactic corticosteroids should be given as the risk that they will increase the chance of intra-uterine infection is less than their beneficial effect on fetal lung maturation.

The main dilemma is whether prophylactic antibiotics should be given to the mother. Although controlled trials of their use show no reduction in maternal infection before delivery or in neonatal infection (particularly pneumonia), many obstetricians give antibiotics prophylactically, either before labour or when labour starts. This applies particularly if Group B streptococci are grown in vaginal culture (see page 134).

If antibiotics are not given and the mother develops signs of intra-uterine infection (chorioamnionitis), i.e. tachycardia, fever (>38°C), leukocytosis. and an offensive vaginal discharge, antibiotics should be prescribed. In most cases the infection is polybacterial, with anaerobes and Group B streptococci predominating. Antibiotics are chosen which take these findings into account.

If labour does not start within 48 hours, the patient may ambulate, and provided her home conditions are suitable and she lives near the hospital, may go home. At home she should rest as much as possible, avoid sexual intercourse, and return to hospital if she develops a fever or an offensive vaginal discharge.

FETAL MATURITY

As more women attend for antenatal care early in pregnancy and with the increasing use of ultrasound, the degree of maturity of the fetus is generally known to within 2 weeks. In a few cases the woman does not seek medical attention until the fourth quarter of pregnancy, at which time the estimation of fetal maturity is less exact. If the fetal maturity is uncertain and labour starts prematurely, if an elective caesarean section is contemplated, or if the pregnancy appears to have become postdate, it is helpful to know the stage of maturity of the fetus. Ultrasound helps but the main concern is about the maturity of the fetal lungs and the likelihood that hyaline membrane disease will be developed. Fetal lung maturity can be tested by measuring the ratio between lecithin and sphingomyelin in a sample of amniotic fluid. As pregnancy advances the L/S ratio increases *(Figs 21.1 and 21.2)*.

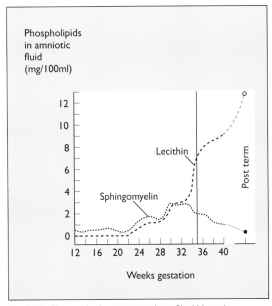

Fig 21.1 Changes in the concentration of lecithin and sphingomyelin in amniotic fluid.

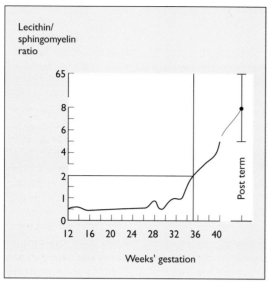

Fig 21.2 Mean L/S ratios during normal gestation.

POST-TERM PREGNANCY OR POSTDATISM

In 10 per cent of cases the pregnancy lasts for more than 42 weeks. In some cases there may be a genetic cause for postdatism, but for most the aetiology is not known. The diagnosis is established by scrutinizing the woman's antenatal record and confirmed, if needed, by an ultrasound examination in which the fetal abdominal circumference, the length of the femur and the length of the longest column of amniotic fluid are compared with a nomogram.

The risk of a post-term pregnancy is that the perinatal mortality rate increases, especially if the duration of the pregnancy exceeds 43 weeks. At least one-third of the increased mortality is due to the death of a malformed fetus.

MANAGEMENT

If the woman is an older primigravida, has a history of infertility or has PIH, diabetes mellitus or other pregnancy complications, the pregnancy should be terminated before it becomes post-term. In other cases three options are available and they should be discussed with the patient and her partner.

The first option is to monitor the welfare of the fetus and permit the pregnancy to continue in the expectation that labour will start spontaneously. The second is to induce labour at the 42nd week. Studies show that there is no difference in fetal morbidity or mortality whichever option is chosen, but caesarean section is less likely if labour is induced. The third option is to perform an elective caesarean section.

If monitoring is chosen the mother records fetal movements daily, non-stress cardiotocography is made twice weekly and ultrasound examinations are made to measure the volume of the amniotic fluid. Abnormalities in these tests (see Chapter 22) may indicate the need for induction of labour or caesarean section.

The possible development of cephalopelvic disproportion (determined by the descent of the fetal head into the pelvis) and the state of the cervix are checked each week.

In most cases labour will start spontaneously. But if the mother becomes anxious or distressed that the baby has not been born, induction of labour or caesarean section should be discussed.

22

THE AT-RISK FETUS

The birth-weight of an infant depends on its genetic growth potential which may be retarded or enhanced by the growth support provided by the mother, the functional integrity of the placenta and the ability of the fetus to use the nutrients provided.

Most fetuses grow normally throughout pregnancy *(Fig. 22.1)*. Some fetuses are genetically programmed to have a low growth potential. They are healthy, but small at birth. Some fetuses have a genetic defect which reduces their growth potential and causes slow intra-uterine growth which may not become apparent until some time in the second half of pregnancy. Some fetuses grow normally initially, but in the last quarter of pregnancy their growth is retarded by alterations in the uteroplacental function. This has lead to the descriptive term *placental dysfunction* or *placental insufficiency*.

Within genetically set limits, the actual fetal growth depends on:
- An adequate supply of nutrients (especially glucose) and oxygen from the mother.
- An adequate placental transfer of the nutrients, which depends on a good blood supply reaching the placenta.
- A good fetal circulation.
- Functioning fetal pancreatic beta cells, as insulin is the main regulator of fetal growth, provided that nutrients are available.

Of all these factors, an adequate blood supply reaching the placenta so that exchange of nutrients across the placenta can take place seems the most important.

With this background the identified causes of fetal growth retardation can be listed *(Table 22.1)*. The degree to which these causes affect fetal growth depends on the amount of placental functioning reserve, so that not all women having these complications will give birth to a growth-retarded fetus.

A growth-retarded fetus is more likely to develop metabolic disturbances, such as acidosis, hypoglycaemia, hypercapnia and erythroblastosis. If the disturbances are severe the fetus may die in the uterus.

Aetiological Factors in Fetal Growth Retardation (Placental Dysfunction)	
Maternal Causes	**Per cent**
Hypertensive disorders	60
Prolonged pregnancy	5
Maternal diseases (esp. renal disease and severe anaemia)	5
Fetal Causes	10
Malformations, transplacental infections	
Multiple pregnancy	
Unknown	20

Table 22.1 Aetiological factors in fetal growth retardation (placental dysfunction).

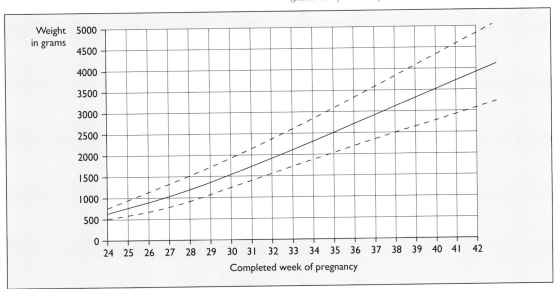

Fig 22.1 Fetal weight at various weeks of gestation (from 24 weeks).

'At-risk fetus' Scoring System	
Variable	Weighted value
1. Previous birth of baby weighing ≤2500g, stillbirth or first week neonatal death	1
2. Blood pressure ≥140/90	1
3. History of renal disease repeated urinary tract infection (UTI) or UTI in present pregnancy	1
4. Bleeding in current pregnancy	1
5. Weight gain >0.5kg in any week after 20 weeks	1
6. Decrease or no increase in girth	1
7. Smoking	2
8. Decrease or no increase in fundal height	3

Table 22.2 'At-risk fetus' scoring system.

Less severe disturbances tend to become worse during labour, causing clinical or monitor-detected 'fetal distress', or the baby may be born with signs of severe hypoxia.

Thus the fetus in an affected pregnancy is at greater risk of dying in utero or if born alive of needing resuscitation and possibly of being brain damaged (cerebral palsy). The pregnancy is 'high risk'. Not all high-risk pregnancies have a growth-retarded fetus, but many do.

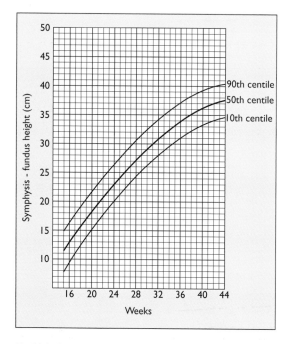

Fig 22.2 Gestational age estimated from symphysis-fundal height.

HIGH-RISK PREGNANCY

Women who have a high-risk pregnancy should be identified early, if this is possible, and given more intensive antenatal care, particularly after the 30th week of pregnancy. No reliable tests have been developed to identify high-risk pregnancies early, but an indication can be obtained by scoring as shown in *Table 22.2*. A score of 4 or more will identify all growth-retarded (small-for-dates) babies, but the positive predictive value is only 34 per cent. As mentioned, in some high-risk pregnancies the fetal growth rate is normal or, in the case of pregnancy in a diabetic woman, the baby may be large (macrosomic). In other words a large number of normal size for dates babies occur in high-risk pregnancies, and their morbidity and mortality is less than if the fetus is growth retarded.

A second method of detecting fetal growth retardation is to measure the symphysio-fundal height with a tape measure and refer to a chart *(Fig. 22.2)*.

A third test is to use ultrasound to determine the size of the fetus and to estimate its maturity, although doubt has been expressed about the value of this test.

TESTS FOR FETAL WELL-BEING IN HIGH-RISK PREGNANCIES

Having identified that the pregnancy is high risk for the fetus, tests to determine fetal well-being should be started after the 30th week. In the past 10 years, biophysical tests to determine fetal well-being have superseded biochemical tests. The tests are:

• Fetal movement (fetal kick) counts.
• Cardiotocography.
• Serial ultrasound examinations.
• Doppler flow velocity wave forms.

None of these tests has a high positive predictive value, but each has a high negative predictive value.

A note of caution should be made. The authors of *Effective Care in Pregnancy and Childbirth* point out that although the tests may provide 'a minimum level of care and attention in settings where these are adequate', in other settings their use may result in 'a variety of unwarranted interventions'.

FETAL MOVEMENTS

The patient counts the number of times the fetus kicks until she has recorded 10 kicks. Usually this number of kicks occur in a 3-hour period, but as fetuses have different patterns of activity, the woman may have to check the number of kicks during another 3-hour period that day. The test is performed 3 or more times a week. If the fetus fails to kick 10 times in a day, the patient should contact her doctor or hospital.

CARDIOTOCOGRAPHY – THE NON-STRESS TEST

Cardiotocography depends on the assumption that a healthy fetus will normally be more active than an 'at risk' fetus and that its heart will respond to a uterine contraction by accelerating. An external cardiotocograph is applied to the woman's abdomen, as she sits in a reclining position (not on her back as this may result in erroneous findings). If spontaneous contractions do not occur over a 30-minute period, they may be provoked by nipple stimulation. The heart beat variations in relation to the contraction are recorded. If the fetus is lethargic, it may be stimulated to move by tapping the uterus gently. Cardiotocography is usually done in hospital but can be done at home using domiciliary fetal heart monitoring and a telephone link.

Four cardiotocographic patterns may occur. These are:

- Normal.
- Suboptimal.
- Decelerative.
- Preterminal.

A normal pattern indicates that the fetus is not at risk of dying in the next 7–10 days *(Fig. 22.3)*. Such a fetus is termed *reactive (Fig. 22.4)*. If the suboptimal pattern is found the fetus is at slightly increased risk and the test should be repeated in 3–4 days. The decelerative pattern indicates that the test should be repeated the next day, unless conditions for delivery are suitable, in which case labour should be induced. The preterminal pattern indicates that the fetus is at considerable risk of dying in utero and should be delivered quickly *(see Table 22.3)*.

A problem with cardiotocography is that normal patterns predict that the fetus is in no danger, and an abnormal pattern does not give an accurate prediction of fetal danger.

SERIAL ULTRASOUND EXAMINATIONS

The growth of the fetus, as a measure of its health, may be monitored by examining it using real-time ultrasound at 2-weekly intervals. The fetal abdominal circumference and the longest column of amniotic fluid are measured. The relatively long

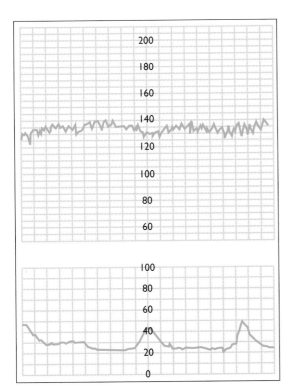

Fig 22.3 Normal fetal heart rate pattern.

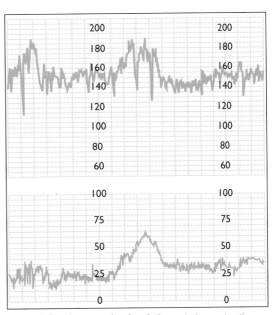

Fig 22.4 Fetal heart acceleration during a uterine contraction (reactive).

Patterns Found on Antepartum Cardiotocography				
	Pattern			
	Normal	**Suboptimal**	**Decelerative**	**Preterminal**
Variation in baseline FHR beats per min	>10	>10	<10 >5	<5
Acceleration on fetal movement (over a 30-45 min period)	At least 2 of 15 bpm	At least 2 of 10 bpm	At least 1 episode of acceleration (10 bpm) every 20 min	None
Deceleration (in relation to Braxton Hicks contractions)	None	None	Variable	Late

Table 22.3 Patterns found on antepartum cardiotocography.

interval between tests limits the value of ultrasonography in monitoring fetal well-being.

FETAL BLOOD FLOW VELOCITY

Uteroplacental and fetoplacental circulations are low-resistance systems in which the flow of blood towards the placenta continues throughout the cardiac cycle, causing wave forms. If fetoplacental vascular resistance increases because of acute uteroplacental atherosclerosis, fetal disease or unknown causes, the wave forms are altered. In the umbilical artery the difference between the peak systolic flow (A) and end diastolic flow (B) can be measured *(Fig. 22.5)*. The greater the A/B ratio the more likely is the fetus to be compromised. This potentially valuable *screening* method of determining fetal well-being in high-risk pregnancies should be restricted to controlled clinical trials, according to a Consensus Conference held in Australia in 1991.

It is not a diagnostic test and abnormal A/B ratios should be followed by a non-stress test.

BIOPHYSICAL PROFILE

Some obstetric units, especially in the USA, believe that the at-risk status of a fetus can be detected with greater accuracy if a biophysical profile is obtained. This consists of monitoring fetal movements, fetal breathing, tone, reactivity and amniotic fluid volume by real-time ultrasound. The procedure is costly and time consuming and at present there is no evidence that it is superior to non-stress testing.

THE MANAGEMENT OF A HIGH-RISK PREGNANCY

Although fetal growth may be retarded at all stages of pregnancy (commonly in malformed fetuses), it is unusual for problems to arise before the 30th week of pregnancy. The effects of placental dysfunction are observable between the 30th and 35th week and become more marked after that time. In three-quarters of cases the expectant mother has a clinical disorder.

There are no known preventive measures, although a multicentre trial is taking place to determine if daily low doses of aspirin (75mg) will reduce the risk of the development of severe pregnancy-induced hypertension (PIH) and of fetal growth retardation among women who have previously had a compromised pregnancy.

All that can be done is to monitor the maternal disease if it is present, to detect deterioration and to check fetal well-being *(Fig. 22.6)*. If the maternal condition worsens, for example, PIH deteriorates or if the fetus appears likely to die in utero, the pregnancy should be terminated either by inducing labour or by caesarean section.

MONITORING THE AT-RISK FETUS IN LABOUR

When caesarean section is not chosen to perform an immediate delivery, the health of the mother and fetus should be monitored during the labour. The care of the woman in labour has been described in Chapter 10. In this section the care of the fetus will be described.

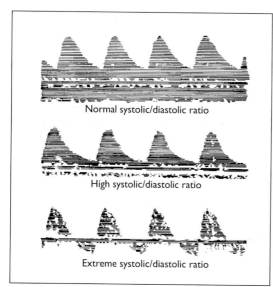

Normal systolic/diastolic ratio

High systolic/diastolic ratio

Extreme systolic/diastolic ratio

Fig 22.5 Blood flow in pregnancy.

An at-risk fetus, particularly growth retarded, has fewer reserves on which it can draw for energy should placental gas and glucose transfer be reduced further during labour. Normally the fetus converts glucose (released from glycogen stores) by anaerobic pathways into ketopyruvic acid and then, in the presence of oxygen, into carbon dioxide and water via the Krebs cycle. The process releases '30 high-energy bonds' per molecule of glucose. When the supply of oxygen is limited, the conversion cycle stops before the Krebs cycle is initiated and only the anaerobic cycle operates. Anaerobic glycolysis releases far less energy and leads to the accumulation of lactic acid in the fetal blood, causing acidaemia. In addition if the fetus is growth retarded and has limited glycogen and fat stored, it is at greater risk of developing acidaemia and may die.

Fetuses which are at particular risk of developing hypoxia and acidaemia are those whose mother has had a pregnancy complication or who have been

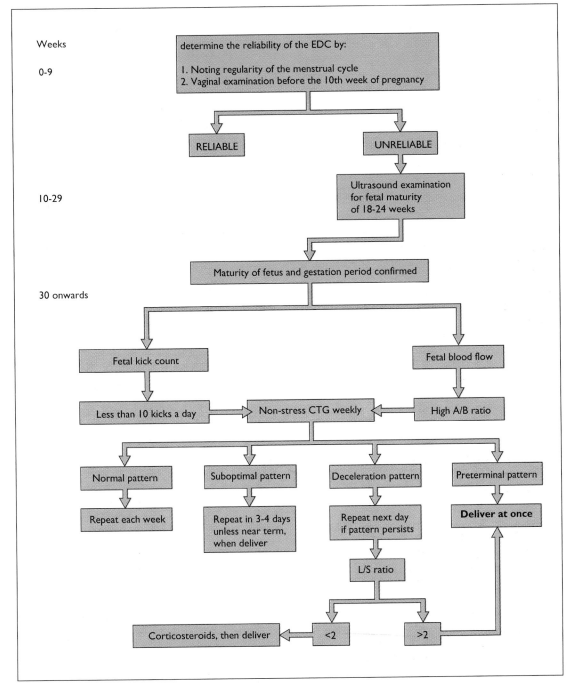

Fig 22.6 A scheme for monitoring the 'at-risk' fetus.

compromised either before labour or during the birth process *(Table 22.4)*.

During labour the well-being of the fetus may be monitored by listening to the fetal heart at regular intervals. A problem arising is that counting the fetal heart rate between contractions misses three-quarters of early signs of fetal hypoxia (fetal distress).

This problem has been overcome by the development of fetal heart monitors (cardiotocograph (CTG) machines), which monitor the fetal heart continuously throughout the labour. There is little clinical or statistical justification for *routinely* monitoring normal labour with a CTG. Its value is to monitor labour in which the fetus is at high risk of developing hypoxia.

The physiological basis of fetal heart monitoring is that when fetal hypoxia occurs, the altered composition of the blood causes a rise in sympathetic and vagal tone, which differ in character and effect. In mild hypoxia, the sympathetic response predominates with resulting tachycardia; the onset of the tachycardia is delayed and it persists for 10–30 minutes after the cause of the hypoxia has ceased. In moderate or severe hypoxia the vagus response predominates. Bradycardia is rapid in onset and lasts as long as the hypoxic episode and then disappears rapidly.

The fetal heart monitor records these changes in the fetal heart rate in relation to uterine contraction. The abnormal patterns are shown in *Fig. 22.7*:

- *Persistent tachycardia* (>160bpm). This indicates that the fetus has mild hypoxia and more careful monitoring is demanded.
- *Early decelerations* (Type 1 dips). The dip occurs in the early part of a uterine contraction and has a V shape. Early decelerations are probably due to pressure on the fetal head during a contraction and have no prognostic significance.
- *Variable decelerations* (Type 2a dips). The decelerations are variable in time of onset and severity. The deceleration pattern is U-shaped. Variable decelerations are probably caused by compression of the umbilical cord and are only prognostically significant if the dip is severe and prolonged.
- *Late decelerations* (Type 2b dips). The deceleration of the fetal heart rate starts late during the contraction and persists after the contraction has ceased. The deceleration is V-shaped. Late decelerations, particularly if severe (<100 bpm) indicate impairment of the uteroplacental blood flow and consequent fetal hypoxia.

A further piece of information can be obtained from the heart monitor tracing, and this is *beat-to-beat variation (baseline variability)*. Normally the beat-to-beat heart rate shows variations of >5 bpm, leading to a wavy line on the trace. The diminution or absence of beat-to-beat variation indicates some degree of fetal hazard.

If in addition to abnormal fetal heart tracings, the fetus passes thick, green meconium, the probability of severe fetal hypoxia is increased.

Fetuses at High Risk of Developing Intrapartum Hypoxia and Acidaemia
Maternal factors
Hypertensive diseases in pregnancy Diabetes Multiple pregnancy Severe anaemia Severe malnutrition
Placental factors
Abruptio placentae
Fetal factors
Growth retardation (small for dates) Malpresentations Cord complications Clinical 'fetal distress'*
* Clinical fetal distress is diagnosed if the fetal heart rate is >160 or <110 beats per minutes sustained for 5 minutes; and/or meconium-stained liquor is seen

Table 22.4 Fetuses at high risk of developing intrapartum hypoxia and acidaemia.

THE BENEFITS AND PROBLEMS OF FETAL HEART MONITORING

Fetal heart monitors are available in most obstetric units and it is believed that their use 'saves' 1–2 infants per 1000 births. There are problems with their use. These include the fact that the interpretation of the trace may be difficult and although the sensitivity of the test is high, its specificity is low. There is also a medico-legal problem. An obstetrician who observes an abnormal trace and does not take action to deliver the baby before it dies from possible hypoxia, may be sued by the parents should be baby be born dead or have physical or mental damage; whilst an obstetrician who operates and delivers a healthy baby may be accused of carrying out unnecessary surgery.

These problems add weight to the belief that if the baby cannot be delivered vaginally expeditiously, a trace showing late decelerations (Type 2 dips) should be followed by fetal scalp blood sampling.

FETAL SCALP BLOOD SAMPLING

You will recall that if fetal hypoxia persists, after a time acidaemia develops. The more severe the acidaemia, the higher the risk of fetal death. The degree of fetal acidaemia can be detected by sampling the fetal scalp blood. A tubular speculum is introduced through the cervix and pressed on the fetal scalp, which is made hyperaemic. (If the membranes have not already ruptured, they are deliberately broken). A

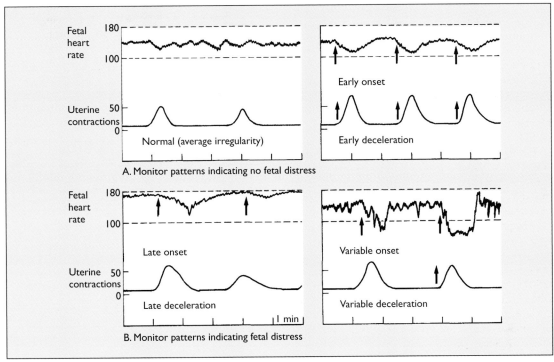

Fig 22.7 Abnormal fetal heart patterns in labour.

small incision is made into the scalp. The blood obtained is drawn by capillary action into a specially prepared tube and its pH is measured. A pH of <7.20 indicates severe fetal hypoxia and the need to deliver the baby expeditiously. A reading of >7.20 suggests that if no other indication to deliver the fetus quickly is present, the labour may continue and vaginal birth may be expected.

THE MANAGEMENT OF MONITOR-DETECTED 'FETAL DISTRESS'

If the patient is in the second stage of labour, the baby should be delivered by forceps or caesarean section. In the first stage of labour the problems are greater. The patient should be placed in a different position, preferably on her side or well propped up to reduce any pressure by the uterus on the major blood vessels; she may be given oxygen via a face mask, although the benefit of this has not been proven. If an oxytocin infusion causes very strong uterine contractions, the drip should be slowed or stopped. (In the past, maternal acidoketosis was corrected; maternal acidoketosis is now uncommon and should not be corrected, as to do so may lead to a fall in the pH of the fetal blood and a rise in lactate, which may precipitate oedema of the fetal brain).

After these actions have been taken, the monitor tracing is observed to see if the fetal heart pattern reverts to normal. If it does not the baby must be delivered.

23

ABNORMAL FETAL PRESENTATIONS

Abnormal presentations include occipito-posterior presentations, breech presentations, face presentations, transverse presentations and brow presentations in order of frequency.

OCCIPITO-POSTERIOR PRESENTATIONS

In about 10 per cent of pregnancies, the fetal head enters the maternal pelvis with its occiput in one of the posterior segments of the pelvis (see *Fig. 10.5* p 71). In most cases the pelvic architecture is normal, but in a few it is classified as long oval (page 175).

The diagnosis may be made on abdominal palpation when the fetal back is felt in one of the mother's flanks, the fetal heart being loudest here *(Fig. 23.1)*. In labour, vaginal examination provides more information, the occiput and the anterior fontanelle being identified *(Fig. 23.2)*.

During labour, the fetal head is forced deeper

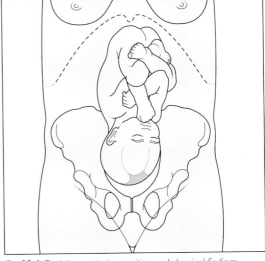

Fig 23.1 Occipito-posterior position – abdominal findings.

Fig 23.2 Possible modes of rotation of the head.

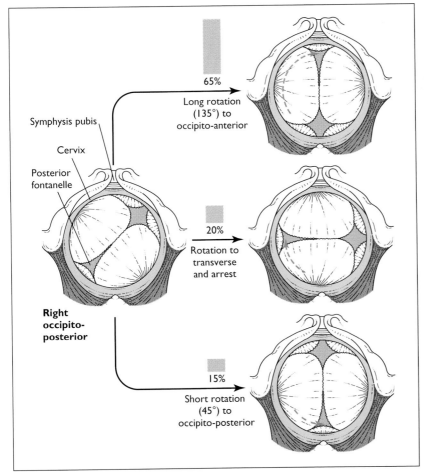

65%

Long rotation (135°) to occipito-anterior

Symphysis pubis

Cervix

Posterior fontanelle

20%

Rotation to transverse and arrest

Right occipito-posterior

15%

Short rotation (45°) to occipito-posterior

into the pelvis, and usually flexes on the fetal neck. Once full dilation of the cervix has occurred its progress may be in one of three ways *(Fig. 23.2)*:

- In 65 per cent of cases the head rotates through

135° so that the occiput lies behind the symphysis pubis.

- In 20 per cent of cases rotation of the fetal head

Long-Rotation

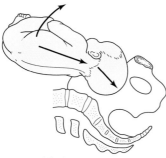

(A) The uterus and fetal axis move forward, and the head flexes as it is forced down into the pelvis

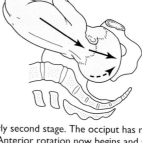

(B) Early second stage. The occiput has reached the pelvic floor. Anterior rotation now begins and the head flexes still more.

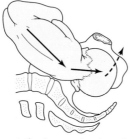

(C) Anterior rotation is occurring through 135°

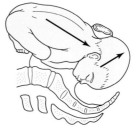

(D) Anterior rotation is complete and the remainder of the delivery is as for an occipito-anterior position

Short-Rotation

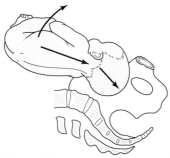

(E) The uterus and fetal axis move forward, and the head enters the pelvis

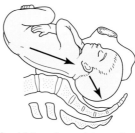

(F) The head fails to flex and descends into the pelvis in the posterior position

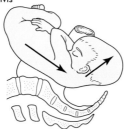

(G) The occiput rotating backwards through 45° when it reaches the pelvic floor to lie in the hollow of the sacrum

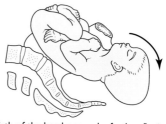

(H) Birth of the head occurs by further flexion to permit the occiput to crown and escape over the perineum. Then by extension, the brow, nose, face and chin appear from behind the symphysis

Fig 23.3 Occipito-posterior. Long rotation (A–D); short rotation (E–H).

ceases and it becomes arrested in a transverse diameter of the pelvis.

- In 15 per cent of cases the fetal head rotates posteriorly.

Thus in most cases the fetal head undergoes a long or a short rotation *(Fig. 23.3)*.

MANAGEMENT OF OCCIPITO-POSTERIOR PRESENTATIONS

There is no management before labour starts. Once begun, the duration of labour tends to be longer in occipito-posterior positions, and the mother requires more support, analgesia and hydration. Progress is monitored using a partogram. The descent of the head and its position are checked regularly. Any marked delay in the first stage of labour leads to prolonged labour (see page 172) and a decision has to be made whether to continue or to perform a caesarean section. Delay in the second stage stage of labour of longer than 1.5–2 hours' duration indicates the need for help to deliver the baby. If the fetal head undergoes the long rotation a spontaneous vaginal delivery may be expected. This occurs in 65 per cent of cases. If the fetal head undergoes the short rotation and descends to the pelvic floor in the posterior position the infant may be born spontaneously (8 per cent of all cases) or may need to be helped by forceps (7 per cent). On the other hand the fetus may not descend much beyond the ischial spines and a manual rotation and forceps delivery or Kjelland's forceps delivery may be necessary (see page 189). These procedures are also required if the fetal head arrests in a transverse diameter of the pelvis. Between 5 and 10 per cent of babies who are occipito-posterior are delivered by caesarean section.

BREECH PRESENTATION

The frequency of breech presentation falls as pregnancy advances. At the 30th week of pregnancy 15 per cent of fetuses present as a breech; by the 35th week the proportion has fallen to 6 per cent and by term only 3 per cent present as a breech. Most of these babies spontaneously turn to become cephalic. If the presentation is still a breech at the 34th week, many obstetricians attempt a cephalic version, which is described on page 194. Version is easier if the breech has flexed legs, one of the three types of breech presentation *(Fig. 23.4)*.

The presentation of the fetus is of no clinical importance before the 32nd–35th week. At this stage of pregnancy the diagnosis of a breech presentation is made by finding on palpation that the lower pole of the uterus is occupied by a soft irregular mass and that in the fundal area a firm, smooth, rounded mass is present which bounces between the fingers if gently pushed. On auscultation the fetal heart beat is loudest above the umbilicus. If any doubt exists after palpation and a vaginal examination, an ultrasound image will clarify the diagnosis.

PROBLEMS WITH BREECH PRESENTATION

Few problems occur during pregnancy, although some expectant mothers complain of pressure beneath the diaphragm. Since breech births frequently require operative delivery, there is an increased risk to the fetus, which is minimized by skilled attention and decision making. In the absence of any other complication of pregnancy, preterm breech births (weight <2 500g) carry a mortality of 12 per cent, as do large postmature babies

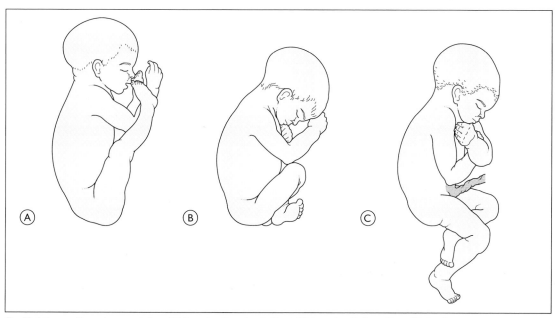

Fig 23.4 Types of breech presentation. (A) Breech with extended legs; (B) breech with flexed legs; (C) footling.

(weight >3500g). Mature fetuses whose weight is in the 'normal' range have a mortality of 3 per cent.

The main causes of morbidity are intracranial haemorrhage, asphyxia and fracture of the humerus, femur or clavicle.

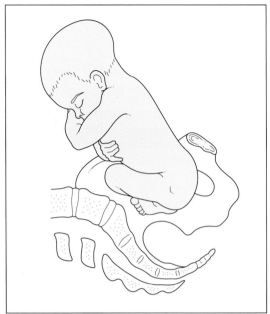

Fig 23.5 In this illustration, the breech is presenting as a right sacro-anterior. The bitrochanteric diameter of the buttocks has entered the pelvis in the transverse diameter of the pelvic brim. With full dilatation of the cervix, the buttocks descend deeply into the pelvis.

THE MANAGEMENT OF BREECH BIRTH

Elective caesarean section at term. Because of risks mentioned, an increasing number of breech presentations at term are being delivered electively by caesarean section. In some institutions the caesarean section rate is >60 per cent; the average rate is about 30 per cent.

The arguments in favor of caesarean section are:
- Possible damage to the fetus and the perinatal mortality is less than that following a vaginal birth.
- Couples are having fewer children, demand a 'perfect child' and may sue if a damaged child is born.
- 30–40 per cent of trials of vaginal breech birth end as a caesarean birth.
- Caesarean section is a safe operation.

Counter arguments are:
- The maternal morbidity is greater after caesarean section.
- 5–15 per cent of breech fetuses have a congenital malformation, and might be better delivered vaginally.
- Some expectant mothers prefer to attempt to give birth vaginally.

Vaginal breech birth. The success of the vaginal birth of a breech depends on the skill of the doctor, which in turn depends on experience.

To understand the management of breech birth, a description of the mechanism of the birth of a breech is needed. This is shown in the sequence of illustrations (*Figs 23.5–23.14*) and described in the captions.

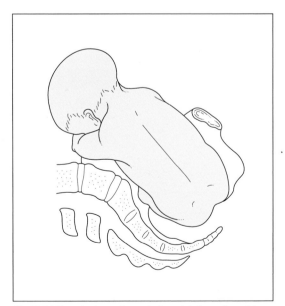

Fig 23.6 When the buttocks reach the pelvic floor, the pelvic 'gutter' causes the buttocks to rotate internally so that the bitrochanteric diameter lies in the anterior posterior diameter of the pelvic outlet.

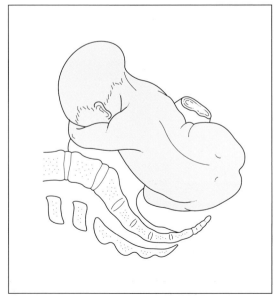

Fig 23.7 The anterior buttock appears at the vulva. With further uterine contractions the buttocks distend the vaginal outlet. Lateral flexion of the fetal trunk takes place and the shoulders rotate so that they may enter the pelvis. At this stage the attending doctor or nurse–midwife has donned gown and gloves and is prepared to aid the delivery.

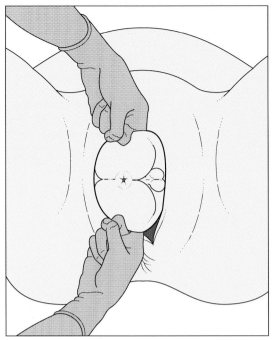

Fig 23.8 If the buttocks make no advance during the next several contractions, an episiotomy is made and the buttocks are born by groin traction.

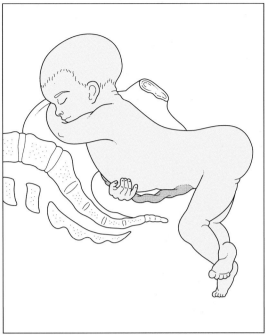

Fig 23.9 The buttocks have been born and the shoulders have entered the pelvis in its transverse diameter. This causes the external rotation of the buttocks so that the fetal back becomes uppermost.

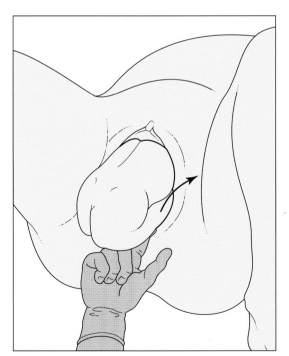

Fig 23.10 If the fetus has extended legs, the attendant may have to slip a hand along the anterior leg of the fetus and deliver it by flexion and abduction, so that the rest of the birth may proceed.

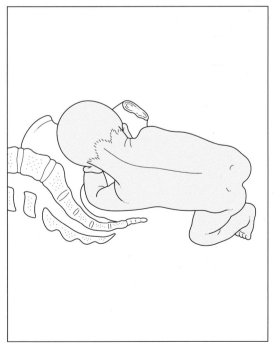

Fig 23.11 The fetal shoulders have reached the pelvic `gutter' and have rotated internally so that the bis-achromial diameter lies in the antero-posterior diameter of the outlet. Simultaneously the buttocks have rotated anteriorly through 90°. The fetal head is now entering the pelvic brim, its sagittal suture lying in the the brim's transverse diameter. Descent into the pelvis occurs with flexion of the fetal head.

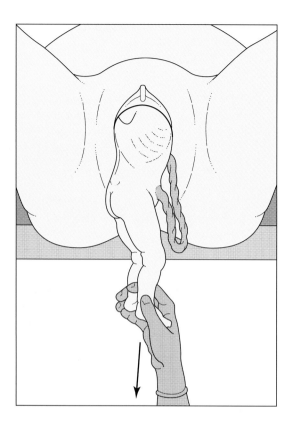

Fig 23.12 The baby has been born to beyond its umbilicus. A loop of umbilical cord is pulled down to make sure that it is not holding back the birth. Gentle traction downwards and backwards is made by the attendant, so that the anterior shoulder and arm are born. The baby is now lifted upwards in a circle so that the posterior shoulder and arm may be born. Sometimes one arm is extended and has to be dislodged downwards. The procedure requires skill or a fractured clavicle or humerus may result. Once the anterior arm has been born the baby's body and the posterior arm are freed in a similar manner.

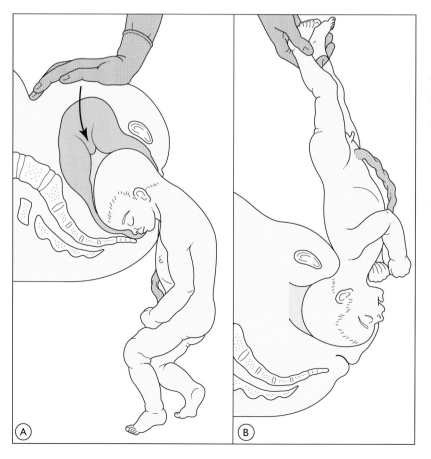

Fig 23.13 A: The baby hangs unsupported from the mother's vulva. The doctor applies slight suprapubic pressure to encourage further flexion of the head. When the nape of the baby's neck has appeared, the attendant holds it by the feet and swings it upwards through an arc. B: This manoeuvre, by using the lower border of the sacrum as a fulcrum, pulls the head down and rotates it through the pelvic outlet so that the chin, nose and forehead appear.

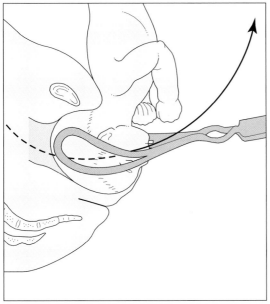

Fig 23.14 An alternative is to deliver the fetal head by forceps.

AN ALGORITHM FOR THE MANAGEMENT OF BREECH PRESENTATION

In *Fig. 23.15* an algorithm for the management of breech presentation is given. Not included is breech extraction. In breech extraction the baby is delivered by the doctor. The main use of breech extraction is for the birth of a second twin, or if the breech is impacted in the mid pelvic cavity. Unless the obstetrician is very skilled, caesarean section is probably safer.

TRANSVERSE LIE, OBLIQUE LIE, AND SHOULDER PRESENTATION

Shoulder presentation, unstable lie, transverse lie and oblique lie may be detected in late pregnancy. These conditions occurs in 1 in 200 births, usually among multiparous women. The aetiology is varied. They may occur in a lax multiparous uterus with no other complication of pregnancy, but may be associated with polyhydramnios, placenta praevia or a uterine malformation (see page 266). An ultrasound examination is helpful in excluding placenta praevia.

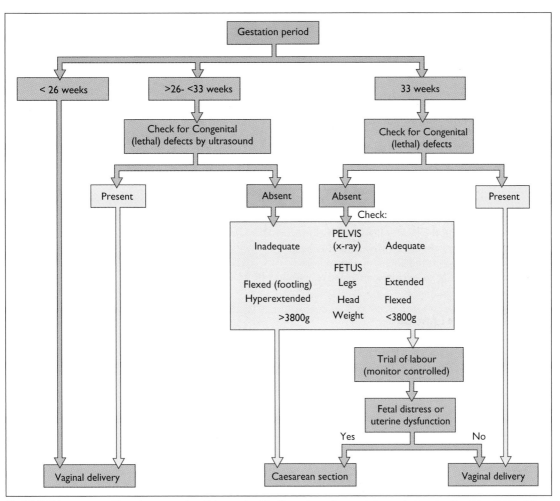

Fig 23.15 Management of breech presentation. If detected at 33–35 weeks confirm gestation period by checking date of LMP, visits during pregnancy, ultrasound examination. Attempt external cephalic version (ECV) without anaesthesia, ? using tocolytics and real-time ultrasound. If failure of ECV wait for labour.

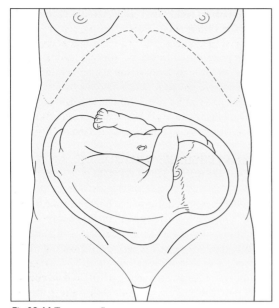

Fig 23.16 Transverse lie.

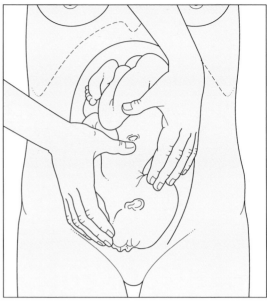

Fig 23.17 Abdominal palpation in face presentation.

The diagnosis is made by finding a broad asymmetrical uterus with a firm ballotable round head in one iliac fossa, and a softer mass in the other *(Fig. 23.16)*.

MANAGEMENT IN PREGNANCY

When placenta praevia has been excluded, a gentle cephalic version may be attempted, but in many cases the fetus returns after some time to its previous presentation. If the lie remains unstable the expectant mother should be advised to report to hospital immediately labour starts, or if the social conditions are unfavourable may be admitted to hospital to await labour. In some cases the presentation is corrected to cephalic and the head is held over the brim. The membranes are then ruptured and the head pressed into the pelvis as the liquor amnii is released.

Another choice is to perform an elective caesarean section.

MANAGEMENT IN LABOUR

If the shoulder presentation is not detected until labour has been established, caesarean section is the preferred option, although the manoeuvre of guiding the fetal head to lie above the pelvic brim and rupturing the membranes has some advocates.

FACE PRESENTATION

Face presentation occurs in 1 in 500 births, usually by chance but in 15 per cent of cases the baby is anencephalic, has a tumour of the neck or shortening of the neck muscles.

Face presentation is rarely diagnosed before labour, and even then may be missed until a face

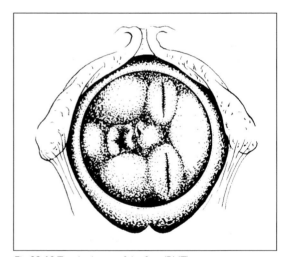

Fig 23.18 Touch picture of the face (RMT).

with swollen distorted lips appears at the vulva. Abdominal palpation may reveal a peculiar S-shaped fetus with feet on the opposite side to the prominent occiput. The fetal head has not usually entered the pelvis *(Fig. 23.17)*.

Vaginal examination during labour may clarify the presentation *(Fig. 23.18)*, but in late labour when much facial oedema has occurred a breech may be misdiagnosed.

MECHANISM AND MANAGEMENT OF LABOUR

In most cases the face enters the transverse diameter of the pelvis with the fetal chin in a mento-transverse position. Descent into the pelvis is delayed until late in the first stage or the second stage of

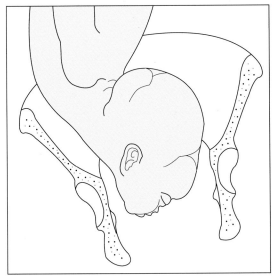

Fig 23.19 Diagram of engagement. In the face presentation engagement occurs late as the parietal prominences do not enter the brim until the face has reached the pelvic floor.

labour *(Fig. 23.19)*. Rotation usually occurs anteriorly so that the chin lies behind the pubis, and delivery occurs spontaneously by flexion of the head or may be aided by forceps. In a few cases the fetal chin rotates posteriorly, impacting the fetal head and preventing vaginal delivery. The impacted fetal head may be rotated using Kjelland's forceps or, preferably, the fetus may be delivered by caesarean section.

BROW PRESENTATION

Brow is the most unfavourable and the least common (1 in 1500 births) of all malpositions and malpresentations. It may occur during late pregnancy (when it usually converts into a cephalic presentation). An ultrasound examination should be made to exclude fetal malformations, especially hydrocephaly.

The patient should be seen each week to check the presentation and told to come into hospital as soon as contractions start or the membranes rupture.

In labour, brow presentation is diagnosed when the fetal head is high and a sulcus can be identified between the head and the back

Treatment is to perform a caesarean section, unless the baby is grossly abnormal or dead, when a destructive operation may be chosen (see p. 194).

MULTIPLE PREGNANCY

Multiple pregnancy occurs when two or more ova are released and fertilized (dizygotic) or when a single fertilized ovum divides early to form two identical embryos at the inner cell mass stage or earlier (monozygotic). The incidence of twins is 1 in 90 pregnancies and that of triplets of 1 in 90×90 pregnancies. Since the introduction of assisted reproductive technology, the incidence of multiple pregnancies has increased. Ultrasound examination in early pregnancy has also identified more twins but in half of those identified one fetus dies and disappears before the second half of pregnancy, the so-called 'vanishing twin'.

In dizygotic multiple pregnancy, each fetus is a separate individual with its own placenta, amnion and chorion. In monozygotic multiple pregnancy, the two fetuses have a single placenta and chorion, but each twin has its own amniotic sac. As there is vascular communication between the two parts of the placenta it is not unusual for one twin to obtain a reduced supply of nutrients and grow more slowly than the other. Occasionally one fetus dies early in pregnancy, becoming mummified (fetus papyraceous).

Because of the greater demands for nutrients, a fetus in a multiple pregnancy tends to be smaller than a singleton fetus, as its growth in utero is slower *(Fig. 23.20)*.

Fig 23.20 The intra-uterine growth of multiple and single pregnancies as assessed by ultrasound fetometry

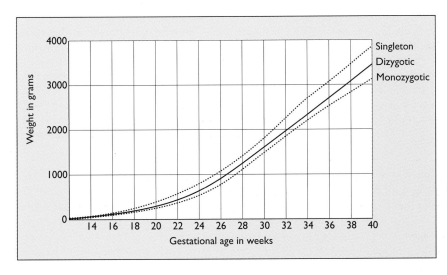

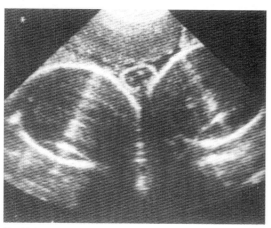 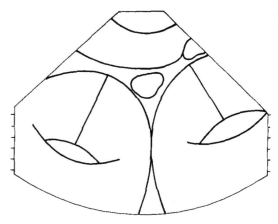

Fig 23.21 Multiple pregnancy. Transverse scan at 32 weeks – two heads visible.

THE DIAGNOSIS OF MULTIPLE PREGNANCY

Few multiple pregnancies are diagnosed in the first half of pregnancy except by ultrasound scanning. In the second half of pregnancy, a multiple pregnancy can be suspected if:

- The abdominal girth and uterine size are greater than expected from the period of amenorrhoea.
- Palpation shows an excess of fetal parts, and two fetal heads can be detected.

Multiple pregnancy is confirmed by an ultrasound examination *(Fig. 23.21)*.

THE MANAGEMENT OF MULTIPLE PREGNANCY

Compared with a singleton pregnancy, a multiple pregnancy is likely to be associated with more pregnancy complications *(Table 23.1)*. For this reason the expectant mother requires additional antenatal care. She should be seen at 2-weekly intervals from the time of diagnosis. Maternal anaemia should be sought and treated, and there is a strong argument for insisting that the patient takes folic acid 5mg and an iron salt each day. When a woman carrying twins goes into preterm labour, the decision whether to deliver the twins by caesarean section or to attempt a vaginal birth has to be made. There is no consensus about the safest method.

A woman carrying a multiple pregnancy has an increased blood volume and an extra burden on her cardiovascular system. Traditionally the doctor recommends that an expectant mother carrying a multiple pregnancy takes extra rest, for example 2 hours in the afternoon, supposedly to reduce the risk of PIH and preterm labour. There are no accurate data to support this belief, and the woman should be given the opportunity to make up her own mind.

A few obstetricians monitor fetal growth every 2 weeks from the 30th week using ultrasound. If growth ceases, they consider intervening. The value of this approach has not been established.

MANAGEMENT IN LABOUR

The position of the leading fetus should be checked on admission. In a twin pregnancy, both fetuses present as cephalic in 45 per cent of cases; as cephalic and breech in 25 per cent; and as breech and cephalic or breech and breech in 10 per cent each. If the first twin presents transversely, caesarean section is the preferable approach. In other cases a vaginal birth may be expected. The management of the labour is conducted in the way already described (Chapter 10). When the membranes rupture a vaginal examination is made to check if the umbilical cord has prolapsed.

Complications of Pregnancy in Singleton and Multiple Pregnancies		
Complication (per cent)	**Singleton**	**Multiple**
Pregnancy induced hypertension	5	15
Anaemia	3–5	15
Polyhydramnios	<2	>5
Preterm labour (birth before 37th week)	<5	>25

Table 23.1 Complications of pregnancy in singleton and multiple pregnancies.

The first baby is usually born without difficulty, if necessary following an episiotomy. Immediately following the birth, the doctor makes an abdominal examination to determine the presentation of the second twin. If it is transverse the doctor may attempt external version to bring the fetus into a longitudinal position. A vaginal examination is then made to confirm the presentation and if it is longitudinal the second amniotic sac is artificially ruptured. The fetal presenting part is led into the pelvis. A second twin which remains in the transverse presentation should be delivered either by caesarean section or by internal podalic version, depending on the skill of the obstetrician.

Following the birth of the first twin, uterine contractions may diminish for a few minutes. If they do not return soon, an intravenous oxytocin infusion may be set up.

The birth of the second twin is usually uncomplicated, but postpartum haemorrhage may be expected and should be anticipated by managing the third stage actively.

THE RISK TO MOTHER AND FETUSES

There is no increased risk to a mother who has received appropriate antenatal care. The risk to a fetus of a multiple pregnancy is higher than to a singleton, mainly because of the increased incidence of preterm birth. The perinatal mortality of twin births is 50 per 1000, five times that of a singleton birth. The risk to a second twin is greater than that to the first born, because it often has a lower birth-weight and has been subjected to intra-uterine hypoxia during the birth. The death of one of the twins during the birth or the neonatal period presents the parents with unique problems, as they have to adjust to having one living baby who no longer has a same-age sibling.

THE PSYCHOLOGICAL EFFECTS OF TWINS ON THE PARENTS

The knowledge that she is carrying twins may have a considerable psychological effect on the mother and, her partner and the attending health professional needs to help and counsel the couple. If the multiple pregnancy has been diagnosed in the early weeks of pregnancy by ultrasound scanning, the first matter to be discussed is the problem of the 'vanishing twin'. After the 20th week of pregnancy the woman and her partner should be made aware that there is a higher chance of developing complications during the pregnancy which may require admission to hospital, and may lead to a premature birth. If the woman already has a child or children her absence from the home may require help from partner or relatives, and studies have shown that she has an increased chance of developing depression in late pregnancy. She also has a greater chance that the birth will be by caesarean section, which may cause anxiety and the issue should be discussed. In the postnatal period, the demands of caring for two small babies adds to the problem of adjusting to parenthood (see page 92), and usually means that the couple have little time to be with each other to enhance their general and their sexual relationship. In the period after childbirth more women who have given birth to twins report anxiety and depression and often need support and help. Women report that discussion of these matters during pregnancy and the availability of support both during and after pregnancy reduce the 'stress' of having twins. Fortunately, in the community there are 'self help' groups whose support and counselling are invaluable. However, the doctor or nurse attending the woman during and after pregnancy should be aware of the problems and of the need to talk with the woman and her partner.

PROLAPSE OF THE UMBILICAL CORD

Although prolapse of the umbilical cord is not a malpresentation, it is more likely to occur when there is a fetal malpresentation or position. For this reason it is included in this chapter. Prolapse of the umbilical cord occurs in 1 in 300 deliveries. The cord may be contained within the forewaters, when it is said to be presenting, or may have prolapsed to lie in front of the fetal presenting part after the membranes have ruptured (Fig. 23.22).

AETIOLOGY

The umbilical cord is more likely to prolapse if anything prevents the snug application of the presenting part in the lower uterine segment or its

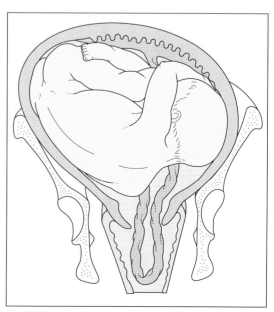

Fig 23.22 Prolapse of the umbilical cord.

descent into the maternal pelvis. For this reason, fetal malpresentations and positions, cephalopelvic disproportion and preterm births are more likely to be associated with cord prolapse. The cord may also prolapse at amniotomy, during version of the fetus and in other obstetric manipulations.

DIAGNOSIS

Presentation of the umbilical cord is rarely diagnosed. When prolapse of the cord occurs after the membranes have ruptured it can be detected by a vaginal examination. This should be made in all cases of preterm labour or if a fetal malpresentation or position is present. If the cord is felt on the vaginal examination its pulsations should be sought and the fetal heart sounds checked to determine if they are within the normal range or show tachycardia or bradycardia.

MANAGEMENT

The management of prolapsed cord depends on the condition of the fetus and the degree of cervical dilatation. If the fetus is dead its birth may be awaited. If the fetus is alive and the cervix is not fully dilated a caesarean section is safest for the baby. Whilst arranging for the section, it may help to relieve pressure on the cord by placing the woman in the knee–chest position.

If the cervix is fully dilated and the fetal head or breech is deep in the pelvis a forceps delivery or breech extraction may be performed if an experienced obstetrician is present.

24

ABNORMAL LABOUR (DYSTOCIA) AND PROLONGED LABOUR

If the duration of labour exceeds the accepted norm or if intervention has to be made either before or during labour, the condition is defined as dystocia. Dystocia may result from:
- 'Faults' in fetus.
- An abnormal size or shape of the pelvis.
- Inefficient uterine contractions.

These matters are discussed in this chapter.

'FAULTS' IN THE FETUS (THE PASSENGER)

The presentation of the fetus may cause prolongation of labour (for example, an occipito-posterior position), as may the size of the fetus. A large fetus (>4000g) may not be able to be born vaginally easily even if the pelvis is of normal size. Some genetically programmed mothers habitually produce large babies as do some diabetic mothers. Some babies have congenital defects which may make vaginal birth difficult or impossible, for example a fetus who has hydrocephaly or a tumour of the neck or abdomen. A 'fault' in the fetus may be anticipated if an abdominal examination in late pregnancy reveals a large fetus, whose head has not entered the maternal pelvis. The diagnosis can be established by an ultrasound examination.

ABNORMAL SHAPE OR SIZE OF THE PELVIS (THE PASSAGES)

The ideal obstetric pelvis is described on page 52. If any of the two main diameters, particularly those of the pelvic brim, is reduced by 2cm or more the pelvis is considered to be contracted. The shape of the pelvis may also be affected, for example the sacral curve may be replaced by a straight sacrum, or the pelvis may have been damaged by a serious accident .

In many cases an abnormal size or shape of the pelvis is detected in primigravidae by determining the woman's height (women less than 150cm in height may have a small pelvis) and by making a pelvic examination at the 36–38th week of pregnancy, particularly if the biparietal diameter of the fetal head has not entered the maternal pelvis. If the woman has previously given birth and there is concern about her ability to deliver vaginally, the doctor should scrutinize her obstetric history and assess if the fetal head is able to enter the pelvis, by pressing on it in a downwards and backwards direction, or by performing the examination shown in *Fig. 7.24* (p 46).

If the doctor has any doubt after these investigations about the capacity of the pelvis to permit the fetus to be delivered vaginally, an x-ray pelvimetry should be carried out *(Fig. 24.1)*. The use of x-ray pelvimetry has decreased in recent years, as better maternal nutrition during childhood has led to a substantial reduction in the incidence of contracted pelvis and as it has become realized that, provided that the pelvis is not too small or the fetus too large, the quality of the uterine contractions is the final arbiter of a successful vaginal delivery.

The results of x-ray pelvimetry enable a prognosis regarding the likelihood of vaginal delivery to be made, but this prognosis is not particularly accurate, as different observers attach different prognostic values to the measurements and the shape of the pelvis. For example, if the anteroposterior diameter of the pelvic brim is <9cm, nearly all obstetricians would perform a caesarean section; whilst if the anteroposterior diameter is between 9cm and 10.5cm, an obstetrician might attempt a 'trial' of labour, provided the woman was agreeable, unless the sacrum was straight, when a caesarean section would be performed. If the anteroposterior diameter is >10.5cm a vaginal delivery would be anticipated, unless the fetal head was very large.

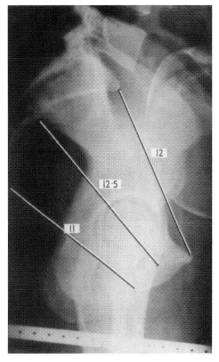

Fig 24.1 Lateral view of pelvis.

CEPHALOPELVIC DISPROPORTION

Apart from the quality of the uterine contractions, the main issue with regard to vaginal birth is the size of the fetus *relative* to the size of the maternal pelvis, thus the concept of cephalopelvic disproportion (CPD) has arisen. The term cephalopelvic is used rather than fetopelvic as any presentation other than cephalic would be treated by caesarean section.

In cases of CPD if the fetal head has not entered the pelvic brim by term, a caesarean section is likely to be performed because of risks to the fetus should labour proceed. On the other hand if the fetal head has entered the pelvic brim the choices are between an elective caesarean section and a 'trial of labour'. The decision will depend on the woman's preference and the doctor's experience. For example, a woman over the age of 35, or one who had had a long history of infertility would generally be delivered by caesarean section, as would women with medical complications.

If a trial of labour is attempted, the patient should be told that she has about a 30 per cent chance that she will require a forceps delivery and a 30 per cent chance that the trial will be abandoned and that a caesarean section will be performed.

In a trial of labour the aim is to determine what the woman can accomplish, not how much she can endure. As operative delivery is likely, an intravenous infusion should be established and no food permitted by mouth. The progress of the labour is monitored using the partogram, particular attention being paid to the speed of the descent of the fetal head and the dilatation of the cervix. A vaginal examination is made when the membranes rupture, to exclude cord prolapse. Special attention is paid to the woman's response to the trial. The trial should be abandoned if:
- There is no increase in cervical dilatation over a period of 4 hours (or 2 hours after rupture of the membranes) in spite of strong uterine contractions.
- Fetal distress develops.
- Full dilatation of the cervix is not achieved within 12 hours of labour.

ABNORMALITIES OF UTERINE ACTION

Labour will only progress normally if the contractile wave is propagated over the entire uterus in a triple descending gradient of activity (see page 61).

If the normal pattern of uterine activity fails to occur, the progress of labour will be abnormal, usually prolonged. Until the 1940s, prolonged labour was considered to be caused by 'uterine inertia'. Research since that time has shown that several patterns of uterine activity may lead to delay in the birth of the child. The patterns are designated 'inefficient uterine activity' and are divided into subgroups of abnormal uterine activity *(Table 24.1)*. In some cases of labour the reverse occurs and the uterus is overactive, leading to a precipitate birth.

Classification of Abnormal Uterine Activity
Inefficient uterine activity

1. Hypoactive states
2. Hyperactive, incoordinate states
    (a) hyperactive lower uterine segment
    (b) colicky uterus
    (c) constriction ring dystocia
3. Cervical dystocia

Over-efficient uterine activity
1. Precipitate labour 2. Tetanic uterine activity

Table 24.1 Classification of abnormal uterine activity.

Changes in the management of labour in recent years, with the increasing use of epidural anaesthesia and of caesarean section have rendered the description of the patterns of uterine activity less useful. They are worth recording, however, as they form the physiological basis of the modern classification.

INEFFICIENT UTERINE ACTIVITY
The two main types of inefficient uterine activity are:
- Hypoactive uterine activity.
- Hyperactive incoordinate activity, which includes incoordinate uterine activity, 'colicky' uterus and its end result, and constriction ring dystocia.

It is difficult to determine exactly how often labour is complicated by inefficient uterine activity, but the most reliable estimates suggest that this condition is predominantly found among primigravidae, affecting 4–6 per cent of such labours; and about 1 per cent of all labours.

Aetiology. The aetiology of inefficient uterine action is not clear. In some cases cephalopelvic disproportion is present, in others, psychological factors have been postulated, as the uterine dysfunction is predominantly a disorder of primigravid labours which is not repeated in a subsequent labour.

TYPES OF ABNORMAL UTERINE ACTION
Hypoactive states (uterine inertia). The uterine resting tone is low and the intensity of the contractions is reduced so that only a feeble contractile wave is propagated *(Fig. 24.2)*. The contractions occur at longer intervals than usual and do not cause the patient much distress.

Hyperactive incoordinate states (incoordinate uterine action). In normal labour the perception of pain is usually only reached when the uterine tone exceeds 25 torr. In hyperactive, incoordinate uterine activity the resting uterine tone is increased; in consequence the pain threshold is reached earlier during the contraction and the pain persists for longer *(Fig. 24.3)*. In spite of the strong contractions, cervical

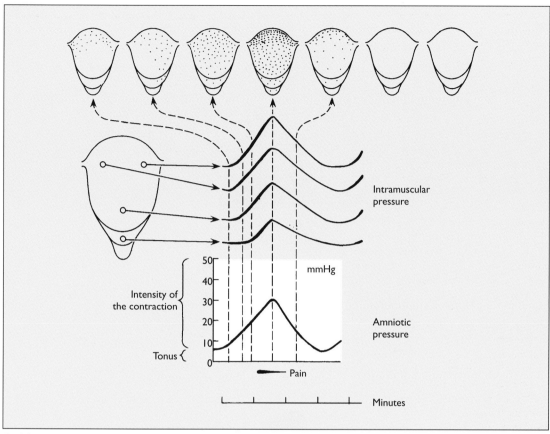

Fig 24.2 Hypoactive uterus. Note that the intensity of the contraction is diminished and the tone lowered slightly (drawn from information from the writings of R. Caldeyro-Barcia).

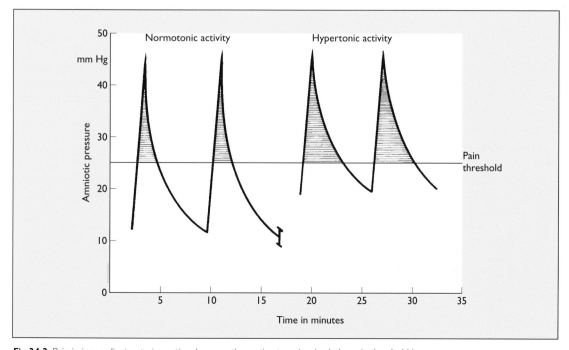

Fig 24.3 Pain in incoordinate uterine action. because the resting tone is raised, the pain threshold is reached earlier in the contraction, and remains above the threshold for longer (redrawn from Caldeyro-Barcia).

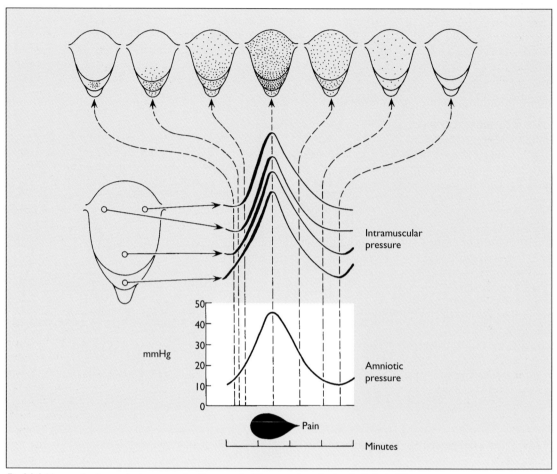

Fig 24.4 Hyperactive lower uterine segment, with reversal of the normal gradients of activity. In this case the uterine tone is still normal but the cervix fails to dilate (redrawn from Caldeyro-Barcia).

dilatation is slow, because the triple gradient is reversed *(Fig. 24.4)*.

If the patient has not been given an epidural anaesthetic, she will complain of severe backache which increases during each contraction when the pain radiates into her lower abdomen.

Two variations of hyperactive uterine activity may occur. Both are uncommon today and are the result of action not being taken to relieve the problem. They are colicky uterus and constriction ring dystocia. In colicky uterus, various parts of the uterus contract independently and the pain of the contrac-

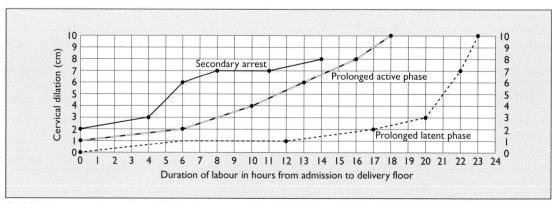

Fig 24.5 Abnormal patterns of cervical dilatation.

tion is generalised and severe. Constriction ring dystocia occurs when an annular spasm arises at the junction between the upper uterine segment and the lower uterine segment, usually late in the first stage of labour or early in the second stage. It may follow the injudicious use of oxytocin or intrauterine manipulations.

THE MODERN CLASSIFICATION OF INEFFICIENT UTERINE ACTIVITY

As the clinical diagnosis of the two main types of inefficient uterine activity depends on the patient's perception of the severity of the pain, its distribution and the findings on uterine palpation, the increasing use of epidural anaesthesia has limited the value of the classification.

With the introduction of the partogram, a different classification has been developed *(Fig. 24.5)*.

Prolonged latent (quiet) phase. The duration of the latent phase of labour is increased. In most cases the pattern of uterine activity shows hypoactivity.

Prolonged active phase. This can be equated to the hyperactive incoordinate state of uterine activity, usually involving a hyperactive uterine lower segment (i.e. a reverse gradient of uterine activity).

Secondary arrest of cervical dilatation. This pattern can be equated to incoordinate uterine activity or to the end result of obstruction to the birth in a primigravida.

MANAGEMENT OF INEFFICIENT UTERINE ACTIVITY

Before any specific treatment is considered the course of the labour thus far must be reviewed by scrutinising the partogram, to identify, if possible, the abnormality of uterine action. The physical and psychological condition of the patient must be assessed. Dehydration and acidoketosis should be sought and if present corrected by infusing 500ml of Hartmann's solution rapidly. After this, Hartmann's solution is alternated with 5 per cent glucose infused at a rate of 50–100ml per hour. Fluids by mouth are avoided.

Specific treatment
Prolonged latent phase. Having established that there is no major degree of cephalopelvic disproportion and that the woman is prepared to continue with the labour, two approaches are possible. In the

first, no treatment beyond reassurance is given and the onset of the active phase is awaited. The alternative is to rupture the membranes and to set up a dilute oxytocin infusion which is increased incrementally (see page 186). Abdominal palpation and a vaginal examination are made at 2-hourly intervals. There are no reliable data to show that the invasive approach shortens the duration of labour significantly.

Prolonged active phase. If cephalopelvic disproportion is excluded, and the woman's condition is good, the membranes are ruptured if they are still intact and a dilute oxytocin infusion is set up, the rate of which is increased incrementally. Progress of labour is monitored as in the management of the prolonged latent phase. Failure of the cervix to dilate by more than 2cm over a 4 hour period may be an indication for caesarean section.

Secondary arrest of the active stage. In this pattern of uterine activity it is essential to exclude cephalopelvic disproportion. If the woman does not have an epidural anaesthetic, this should be established and a dilute oxytocin infusion set up. (If it is not possible to provide epidural anaesthesia, an alternative is to sedate the woman with an intravenous infusion containing pethidine 300mg and diazepam 10mg in normal saline. The rate of the infusion is adjusted so that the woman sleeps between uterine contractions). Monitoring the progress of labour is essential, and preparations for caesarean section are made if the cervix has not dilated by more 2cm over a 4-hour period.

THE OUTCOME OF LABOUR
The outcome of labour treated in the above way has been reported in several studies of which a representative is shown in *Table 24.2*. Since the date of that study the proportion of women delivered by caesarean section has increased but this has not led to a reduction in the perinatal mortality or morbidity, which is low.

UTERINE OVER-EFFICIENCY

PRECIPITATE LABOUR
The birth occurs within 2 hours of the contractions starting. The contractions are intense and frequent.

Table 24.2 Type of uterine activity and method of delivery in 684 British primigravidae (Cardozo, L.D. et al. Brit. J. Obstet. Gynecol., 1982: 89, 33–8).

		Outcome		
Pattern	Per cent of all cases	Spontaneous per cent	Forceps per cent	Caesarean per cent
Normal pattern	65–70	80	18	2
Prolonged latent phase	2–5	75	10	15
Prolonged active phase	20–30	55	30	15
Secondary arrest	5–10	40	35	25

Classification of Abnormal Uterine Activity

The problems are that the baby may be born in an inappropriate place without adequate care; the baby may be anoxic in utero because of the frequent intense contractions; may suffer intracranial haemorrhage during its rapid descent through the birth canal; or may be injured by falling on the floor.

Management. If the baby has been born before the arrival of a medical attendant, it and the mother should be examined for any injury.

Since precipitate birth tends to recur, the expectant mother should be admitted to hospital before the estimated date of birth in her next pregnancy.

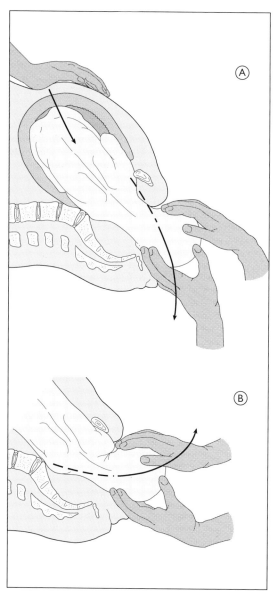

Fig 24.6 Shoulder girdle dystocia. (A) The anterior shoulder is brought into the pelvis by backward traction; (B) the posterior shoulder is brought lower in the pelvis by anterior traction.

TETANIC UTERINE ACTIVITY

This follows the uncontrolled use of oxytocin. The treatment is to stop the oxytocin infusion. It should not occur in today's obstetric practice.

SHOULDER DYSTOCIA

Occasionally, following a trial of labour or when a large baby was not diagnosed before labour, the fetal head may be born, but the shoulders cannot be delivered. The delay occurs because the bis-achromial diameter of the fetus fails to rotate to enter the transverse diameter of the pelvic brim. The baby must be delivered quickly or it will die *(Fig. 24.6)*. Shoulder dystocia occurs rarely and the delivery requires considerable experience: damage to the lower genital tract is usual and damage to the baby not uncommon. Most often the damage is to the brachial plexus, or a fractured clavicle or humerus occurs.

PROLONGED LABOUR

By convention a labour which has lasted for more than 12 hours after the woman has been admitted to hospital in labour, is considered to be prolonged. Between 5 and 8 per cent of labours are classified as prolonged; and the incidence is twice as common among primigravidae than among multigravidae.

Cephalopelvic disproportion and inefficient uterine action are the usual causes of prolonged labour, but in a few cases no cause can be identified.

Forty years ago, labour was defined as being prolonged if it had lasted for >48 hours. Labours of this length were associated with increased maternal morbidity. During labour dehydration often occurred, infection was not uncommon and the risk of postpartum haemorrhage was increased. These problems should not arise in the developed countries today, but they still occur in some developing countries. Perinatal morbidity and mortality also increase in prolonged labour. The main causes are pneumonia following intra-uterine infection, increased fetal acidaemia and trauma from an operative delivery.

Earlier intervention has reduced or eliminated these problems, but care must be taken to monitor women in labour to ensure that they do not become dehydrated, acidoketotic or infected. If the woman is anxious and distressed this should be attended to by reassurance and explanation of the progress of the labour.

THE PSYCHOLOGICAL EFFECTS OF DYSTOCIA AND PROLONGED LABOUR

The memory of a difficult labour, attended by unsympathetic, uncommunicative medical personnel and terminated by an operative delivery, may leave a deeper scar on the woman's mind than the scar on her abdomen or perineum.

The woman and her partner need explanation and reassurance. Most couples are anxious to know if the next childbirth will be as difficult or painful as the last one. As inefficient uterine action is the only identified cause in many cases of prolonged labour, and as this is less likely to occur in a subsequent labour, the woman can be given some reassurance. When she becomes pregnant again the doctor or nurse responsible for her antenatal care needs to listen to her concerns, to reduce her anxieties and to communicate with her, so that she reaches labour in a positive frame of mind. The use of adequate anaesthesia should be discussed and the patient given the choice of having an epidural anaesthetic if she wishes it.

OBSTRUCTED LABOUR

Obstructed labour is the end result of a badly managed or neglected labour, in which cephalopelvic disproportion or a shoulder presentation has not been detected early and intervention made.

During an obstructed labour uterine contractions attempt to overcome the obstruction. In a first labour, the uterus contracts strongly for a while and then, failing to overcome the obstruction, becomes hypoactive, developing secondary arrest. In contrast, if the obstruction occurs in a subsequent labour, the uterus continues to contract strongly in an attempt to push the fetus through the maternal pelvis. With each contraction there is some myometrial shortening (retraction) so that the upper uterine segment becomes progressively thicker and shorter, and the lower segment of the uterus becomes progressively stretched and thinner. The junction between the two segments becomes obvious, forming a pathological retraction ring – Bandl's ring *(Fig. 24.7)*. The pathological retraction ring may be confused with a distended urinary bladder, but the oblique line is diagnostic. The patient is dehydrated, with a coated tongue and dry lips. She has tachycardia and concentrated urine. She faces the risk of ruptured uterus at any time.

Treatment is urgent. The dehydration should be corrected rapidly and a caesarean section performed under antibiotic cover as soon as possible, even if the fetus is dead.

RUPTURE OF THE UTERUS

The end result of obstructed labour, unless intervention is made, is rupture of the uterus. Rupture may also occur in late pregnancy when it may follow trauma to the uterus, or be of a caesarean scar. In labour, as well as following an obstructed labour

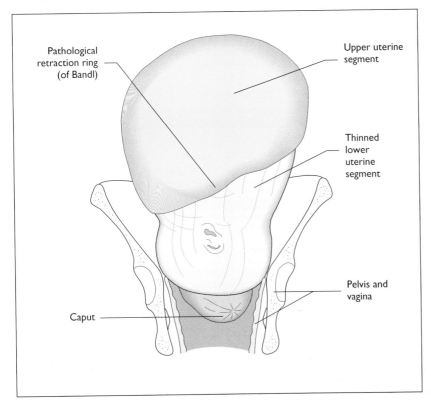

Pathological retraction ring (of Bandl)

Upper uterine segment

Thinned lower uterine segment

Pelvis and vagina

Caput

Fig 24.7 Threatened rupture of the uterus in a case of cephalopelvic disproportion and obstructed labour.

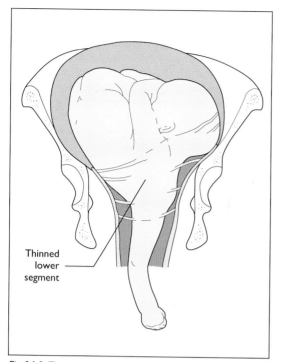

Fig 24.8 Threatened rupture of the uterus in a neglected shoulder presentation.

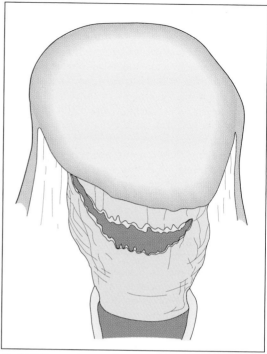

Fig 24.9 Ruptured uterus, from a case of obstructed labour (redrawn from Martin, *Atlas of Obstetrics and Gynaecology*, Lewis, London, 1881).

(Fig. 24.8), rupture of the uterus may be caused by the inappropriate use of oxytocics and the dehiscence of a caesarean section scar.

In modern obstetric practice, the most common cause of uterine rupture is caesarean scar. Three per cent of classical scars rupture, most of them during labour, which is the reason for performing an elective caesarean section on a woman who has a classical caesarean scar. Rupture of a lower segment caesarean scar is less common, 0.25 per cent rupturing, most doing so during labour.

In cases of uterine rupture following trauma or obstructed labour, the rupture usually involves one or other lateral wall and extends into the upper uterine segment *(Fig. 24.9)*.

Rupture of a lower segment caesarean scar is usually quiet. Slight vaginal bleeding may occur and the patient complains of pain which becomes constant. The patient's pulse begins to rise and shock supervenes in some cases. In some patients no symptoms or signs occur and the ruptured uterus is only detected by routine intra-uterine palpation following the birth.

TREATMENT

Rupture following obstructed labour or trauma generally requires hysterectomy, although in a few cases the uterine tear can be sutured. Rupture of a caesarean scar generally can be sutured, but the woman should be consulted to find out if she prefers this or to have a hysterectomy.

APPENDIX
A CLASSIFICATION OF PELVIC ABNORMALITIES

In the developed nations of the world, contracted pelvis has diminished as a cause of dystocia. However, among the less privileged groups in the rich nations and among the urban poor in the developing nations, contracted pelvis still occurs and may lead to a difficult labour. Of the many classifications of pelvic abnormalities available, that suggested by

Baird is one of the most helpful. Studies by his group in Aberdeen found that nutritional influences in infancy and childhood were the major factors in causing minor alterations from the normal, whilst gross alterations were due to disease or injury. The classification is based on brim size and shape, as it has been found that mid-pelvic or outlet contraction

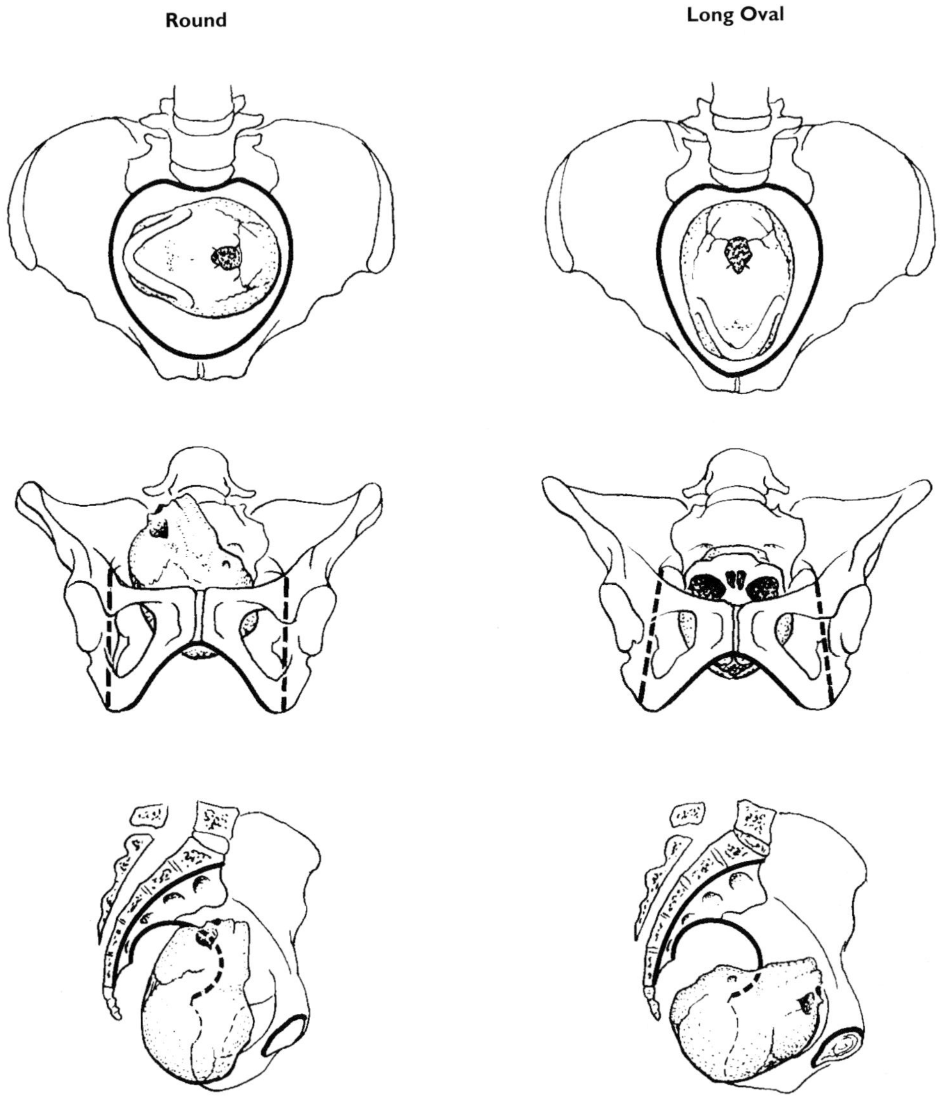

	Round	Long oval
Shape of inlet	Round	Long oval
Forepelvis	Wide	Narrow
Antero-posterior (cm)	12	13
Transverse (cm)	13	12
Brim index	85–100	85–100
Side walls	Straight	Divergent
Ischial spines	Not prominent	Not prominent
Sciatic notch	Wide	Wide
Subpubic angle	Wide	Wide
INCIDENCE (per cent)		
European women	50–70	15–30
Asian women	80	15

(Modified from Danforth and Ivy. *Amer. J. Obst. Gynecol.* 1963, **86**, 29, by kind permission)

Fig 24.10 Pelves with normal shape and bone development.

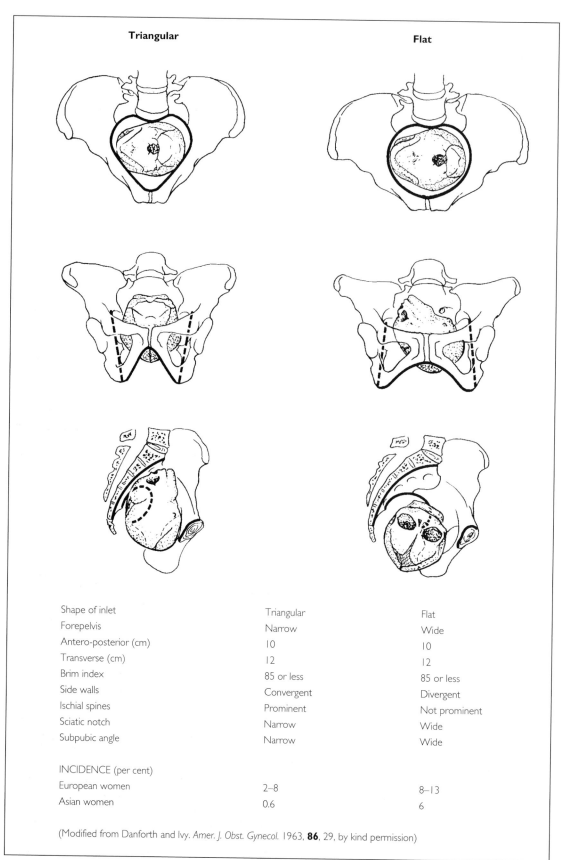

	Triangular	Flat
Shape of inlet	Triangular	Flat
Forepelvis	Narrow	Wide
Antero-posterior (cm)	10	10
Transverse (cm)	12	12
Brim index	85 or less	85 or less
Side walls	Convergent	Divergent
Ischial spines	Prominent	Not prominent
Sciatic notch	Narrow	Wide
Subpubic angle	Narrow	Wide
INCIDENCE (per cent)		
European women	2–8	8–13
Asian women	0.6	6

(Modified from Danforth and Ivy. *Amer. J. Obst. Gynecol.* 1963, **86**, 29, by kind permission)

Fig 24.11 Pelves with abnormal shape and bone development.

Pelvic Classification
1. Pelves with normal shape and bone development
(Measurements usually normal, may be small) Round ('gynaecoid') Long oval ('anthropoid')
2. Pelves with abnormality of shape and bone development

(Measurements usually decreased)
a. Defects of nutrition and environment
  1. Minor defects—Triangular brim (android)
                    Flat brim (platypelloid)
  2. Major defects—Rachitic
                   Osteomalacic
b. Disease or injury
  1. Spinal (kyphosis, scoliosis, spondylolisthesis)
  2. Pelvic (tumours, fractures, caries)
  3. Limbs (poliomyelitis in childhood, congenital
    dislocation of the hip)
c. Congenital malformations
  1. Naegele's pelvis and Robert's pelvis
  2. High assimilation pelvis

3. Mid-pelvic contraction

Table 24.3 Pelvic classification (after Baird).

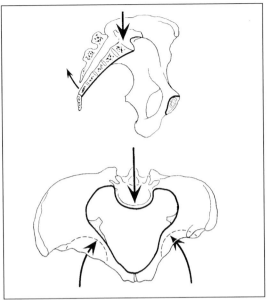

Fig. 24.12 The rachitic pelvis. Tracing from a radiograph showing the antero-posterior diameter of 8cm, the widest transverse diameter of 11.7 and a brim index of 69. The arrows show how pressure on the softened bones alters the shape of the pelvis.

is rare if the brim shape and size are normal *(Table 24.3)*. There is one exception to this: tall thin girls, whose growth has spurted during puberty, may have mid-pelvic narrowing with no brim contraction.

PELVES WITH NORMAL SHAPE AND BONE DEVELOPMENT

The *round* brim is obstetrically ideal *(Fig. 24.10)* and in the developed countries is found in 70 per cent of women whose height exceeds 163cm, the percentage dropping to 55 in women less than 153cm tall. The factor of height does not apply in Asian countries, where the overall incidence of the round pelvis is more than 80 per cent.

The *long oval* brim *(Fig. 24.10)* is relatively uncommon and is found in about 15 per cent of women; in Asia the incidence is smaller.

PELVES WITH ABNORMALITY OF SHAPE AND BONE DEVELOPMENT

MINOR DEFECTS OF NUTRITION OR ENVIRONMENT

The *triangular* brim, with some degree of funnelling of the pelvis, is relatively uncommon, and in a British study was found in only 2 per cent of women. It appears to have a higher incidence among women from Southern Europe, but is not particularly common is Asia. The mid-pelvis is also likely to be narrowed *(Fig. 24.11)*.

The *flat* brim is the commonest minor abnormality of pelvic shape and the incidence increases from less than 5 per cent in tall European women to more than 30 per cent in Europeans whose height is less than 150cm. It is even more common among Africans *(Fig. 24.11)*.

MAJOR DEFECTS OF NUTRITION OR ENVIRONMENT

Rickets and osteomalacia

In the past 40 years most developed countries have paid increasing attention to social and preventive medicine, and rickets – a disease of poor nutrition, particularly a lack of vitamin D and calcium – has largely disappeared. Since the developing countries have an abundance of of sunshine (which converts ergosterol in the skin into vitamin D), and in most the drinking water is rich in calcium, rickets is not common among children, although protein deficiency is usual.

In a young child suffering from rickets the weight of the upper body presses down through the spine on to the softened pelvic bones. The sacral promontory is pushed forwards and downwards, whilst the sacrum itself pivots backwards. At the same time the ligaments of the back draw the spinous process medially do that the ilia flare outwards, as do the ischial tuberosities. In extreme cases the softened acetabulae may be forced inwards. The main alteration in pelvic shape is a marked reduction of the antero-posterior measurement of the brim, with some irregular widening of the cavity *(Fig. 24.12)*.

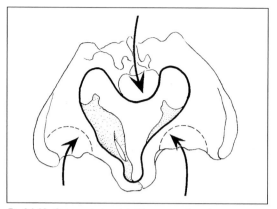

Fig 24.13 Osteomalacic pelvis. The arrows show how pressure deforms the softened bones.

Osteomalacia, due to an acquired deficiency of calcium and encountered in adult life, causes the same deformities as rickets but is rare, except in certain inland parts of Northern India and China *(Fig. 24.13)*.

DISEASE OR INJURY
Spinal
Kyphosis of the lower dorsal or lumbar region which started in childhood may alter the shape of the brim of the pelvis, as the weight of the body pushes the

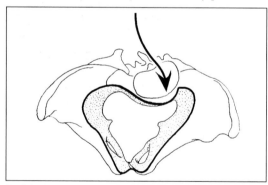

Fig 24.14 Scoliosis and kyphosis.

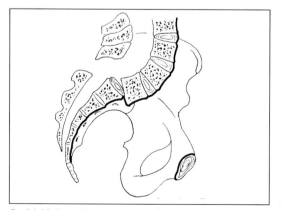

Fig 24.15 Spondylolisthesis; tracing from the radiograph showing the subluxation of the fifth lumbar vertebra upon the sacrum. The diagnosis can only be made by radiography.

upper part of the sacrum backward and the lower part forward. The side walls of the pelvis converge forming a funnel. In scoliosis the altered pressure distribution on the soft bones may cause bays on each side of the sacral promontory, so that the shape of the brim is asymmetrical *(Fig. 24.14)*. Spondylolisthesis, which means slipping forward of the fifth lumbar vertebra so that it projects beyond the sacral promontory, is rare *(Fig. 24.15)*.

Pelvic
Osteomata may develop, or an injury may lead to excessive bone formation over the site of the fracture. If all patients are examined vaginally at the first visit these abnormalities will be detected.

Limbs
Poliomyelitis in childhood, or congenital dislocation of the hip, may cause pelvic deformity. The child puts most of its weight on the stronger leg, and on this side the pelvis is pressed in, with flattening of the brim on the same side.

CONGENITAL MALFORMATIONS
Naegele's pelvis and Robert's pelvis
These are due to the defective development of one or both sacral lateral masses so that the sacrum fuses with the ilium on one or both sides *(Fig. 24.16)*. The *high assimilation pelvis* occurs when the fifth lumbar vertebra is fused to the sacrum, thus increasing the inclination of the pelvic brim. This hinders engagement of the fetal head.

MID-PELVIC CONTRACTION
The incidence of this condition in the absence of brim abnormality is difficult to estimate. As has been mentioned the condition is found in certain women over 163cm in height, who have had a sudden 'spurt' of growth at about the time of puberty. Another type of woman in whom the abnormality is found, often in association with some degree of triangular brim, is the short, squat, hirsute woman who is frequently obese and occasionally has reduced fertility. These women have heavy bones and the pelvic cavity and outlet resembles that of the male.

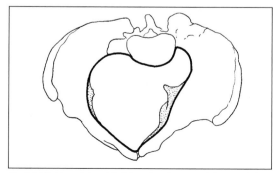

Fig 24.16 Naegele's pelvis. Note the absence of the sacral ala.

25

DISORDERS OF THE PUERPERIUM

During the puerperium four main problems may arise. These are:

- Postpartum haemorrhage.
- Puerperal infection.
- Thromboembolism.
- Postpartum depressioin.

POSTPARTUM HAEMORRHAGE

Postpartum haemorrhage, that is, a blood loss per vaginam of >500ml, may occur in the first 24 hours after the birth when it is defined as primary postpartum haemorrhage or later in the puerperium when it is defined as secondary postpartum haemorrhage.

PRIMARY POSTPARTUM HAEMORRHAGE (PPH.)

Better obstetric care and the appropriate use of oxytocic drugs after birth has reduced the incidence and the severity of primary postpartum haemorrhage to <4 per cent.

Aetiology

In normal labour following the birth of the baby, a blood loss of 200–400ml of blood occurs before myometrial retraction supplemented by strong uterine contractions causes shortening and kinking of the uterine blood vessels and a retraction of the placental bed. These changes prevent further blood loss *(Fig. 25.1)*.

If the uterus does not contract effectively (atonic uterus) or if placental remnants prevent good placental site retraction, haemorrhage may occur ('an empty contracted uterus does not bleed!'). These two causes account for 80 per cent of cases of PPH.

In 20 per cent of cases the cause is a laceration of the genital tract, usually of the vagina or cervix, but rarely following uterine rupture (page 173).

In a few instances PPH follows a blood coagulation defect, such as may occur following abruptio placentae.

Primary postpartum haemorrhage is more likely to occur following a prolonged labour; overdistension of the uterus (multiple pregnancy or polyhydramnios); antepartum haemorrhage; and deep general anaesthesia. In these cases action is taken to prevent PPH, either prophylactic oxytocics are given following the birth, or if the third stage is managed traditionally, 'fundal fiddling' is avoided.

Diagnosis

The diagnosis is usually obvious, excessive blood loss

occurring before the placenta has been delivered (third stage bleeding), or following its expulsion. After the delivery of the placenta, blood may clot inside the uterus and not be expelled so that the fundus rises in the abdomen and, if a contraction is 'rubbed up', it contracts and blood clots are expelled. The bleeding tends to be intermittent, as the uterus contracts periodically.

Management
PPH must be dealt with expeditiously, as it is a cause of maternal death. The management differs depending whether the placenta is still in the uterus or if it has been expelled.

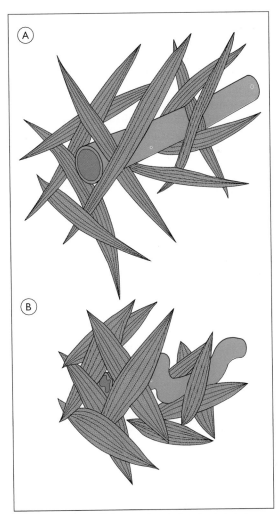

Fig 25.1 Diagram of 'living tourniquet' of contracted uterine muscle.

THIRD STAGE BLEEDING (PLACENTA IN THE UTERUS)

Two stages are involved:

- A contraction is rubbed up and fundal pressure combined with controlled cord traction is generated with the aim of delivering the placenta. If bleeding continues in spite of a contracted uterus, the lower vaginal tract should be inspected to see if there is any damage.
- If the placenta cannot be delivered or if, when it is delivered, inspection shows that it is incomplete, the uterine cavity must be explored. Unless the patient already has an epidural anaesthetic, a general anaesthetic is given and manual removal of the placenta is effected by inserting a gloved hand into the uterine cavity and controlling its actions with the other hand placed on the fundus *(Fig. 25.2)*. The umbilical cord is followed to its insertion and the lower placental edge is identified. With the palm of the intra-uterine hand facing the uterine cavity, the doctor separates the placenta from its attachments with a sawing motion. When the placenta has been completely separated, the remainder of the uterine cavity is explored for further placental remnants and damage. This completed, the placenta is grasped by the hand in the uterus and the membranes are pulled out of the birth canal, whilst the external hand massages the fundus. The placenta is inspected carefully to ensure that it is complete. Ergometrine 0.5mg is then injected intravenously and 0.5mg is given intramuscularly.

TRUE POSTPARTUM HAEMORRHAGE (PLACENTA EXPELLED)

Several stages are involved:

- Check the placenta to determine if it is complete.
- Massage the uterus with a slow rotary movement.
- Set up an infusion of Hartmann's solution and give 0.25mg of ergometrine IV or Syntocin by continuous infusion (10IU in 500ml Hartmann's solution. (an alternative is to use a prepared solution of $PGF_{2\alpha}$ called Haemabate).
- If the blood loss is >1000ml, give blood.
- Check a blood sample for coagulation defects and if present treat.
- If bleeding continues in spite of firm uterine contractions induced by the oxytocics mentioned, inspect the genital tract for lacerations.
- If bleeding persists, try manual compression of the uterus *(Fig 25.3)*. This is painful to the patient and tiring to the obstetrician.
- If bleeding persists, internal iliac artery ligation or hysterectomy may have to be performed.

SECONDARY POSTPARTUM HAEMORRHAGE

The most common causes of secondary postpartum haemorrhage are:

- Poor epithelialization of the placental site (80 per cent of cases).
- A retained placental fragment and/or blood clots.

An ultrasound scan of the uterus will identify placental tissue or clots. The uterus may be bulky and tender and the cervix open. The initial treatment is to give ergometrine 0.5mg intramuscularly, repeated if

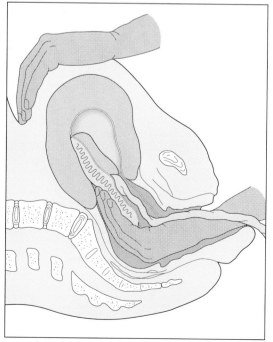

Fig 25.2 Manual removal of the placenta.

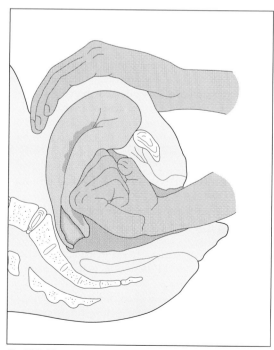

Fig 25.3 Bimanual compression of the uterus.

needed; and antibiotics are given to control any infection present. Curettage is only needed if placental tissue or clots are found in the uterus by ultrasound scanning or if bleeding persists in spite of the oxytocics.

PUERPERAL INFECTION

Puerperal infection (puerperal pyrexia) is defined as a rise in temperature to 38°C or over, maintained for 24 hours or recurring during the period from the end of the 1st to the end of the 10th day after childbirth or abortion. In recent years because of better obstetric care, better hygiene and better control of infection within the hospital, the incidence of puerperal pyrexia has fallen to 1–3 per cent of all births or abortions.

The infection may be genital or nongenital. The main causes and the probable infecting agent are shown in *Table 25.1*.

SITE AND SPREAD OF THE INFECTION

Most cases of puerperal infection arising in the genital tract are ascending infections from the vagina or cervix which infect the placental bed. Spread from here is either into the parametrium or via the uterine cavity to the Fallopian tubes and in some cases onwards to cause pelvic peritonitis.

The severity of the infection depends on the virulence of the infective agent and the patient's immune response.

Diagnosis

Any woman who develops puerperal pyrexia should be investigated and may require to be isolated. The breasts are examined for signs of mastitis and a midstream urine specimen is examined to exclude urinary tract infection. An abdominal examination may reveal a tender bulky uterus. The lower genital tract is inspected for infected lacerations, tears or episiotomy wound. A high vaginal swab is made for bacteriological examination, and the lochia smelt for an offensive odour.

Treatment

Treatment is to give broad spectrum antibiotics appropriate for the infecting agent and metronidazole for 5 days. As the preferred antibiotic depends on the institution and on local knowledge, the hospital infection disease control officer should be consulted, whether the woman is in hospital or is being treated by her general practitioner at home.

THROMBOEMBOLISM

Thrombosis of a vein may occur in pregnancy (see page 124) or more commonly in the puerperium, usually between day 5 and 15 of the puerperium. With better obstetric care and early ambulation, fewer women nowadays develop thromboembolic disorders in the puerperium. The incidence is <0.5 per cent and the condition is more likely to occur among women who are overweight, over the age of 35 and women who have had a caesarean section.

The thrombotic process usually starts in the deep veins of the lower leg but may extend into the femoral or pelvic veins before being detected, or may arise de novo in the pelvic veins. If these veins are involved, pulmonary embolism may occur. Pulmonary embolism affects one puerperal woman in 6000 births in most developed Western nations, and one affected woman in five dies.

DIAGNOSIS OF DEEP VEIN THROMBOSIS (DVT)

The clinical signs are the presence of a low grade pyrexia, a raised pulse rate and a feeling of uneasiness. The clinical signs are a poor guide to the diagnosis of

Table 25.1 The main bacterial causes of infection in the puerperium.

The Main Bacterial Causes of Infection in the Puerperium	
Genital infection	**Proportional Per cent**
1. Potential pathogens which normally inhabit the vagina	
Anaerobic streptococci	65 to 85
Anaerobic Gram-negative bacilli	5
Haemolytic streptococci (other than Group A)	1
2. Bacteria introduced from adjacent viscera	
E. coli	5 to 15
Cl. welchii	Rare
3. Bacteria introduced from distant organs or from outside	
Staphylococci	5 to 15
Streptococcus haemolyticus (Group A)	3
4. Mycoplasma hominis	Rare
Non-genital infection	
1. Urinary tract infection	
E. coli	
2. Breast infection	
Staphylococci (mainly from the baby)	

DVT and do not give any indication whether the thrombus is stationary, lysing or progressing. If the calf muscles are examined and are found to be tender and painful on firm palpation, DVT may be suspected. The diagnosis should be confirmed by ultrasound scanning, preferably using colour-enhanced Doppler imaging, in which the tibial and femoral veins are imaged in longitudinal and lateral planes and the lumen of each vein is inspected.

DIAGNOSIS OF PULMONARY EMBOLISM

The woman complains of dyspnoea and, later, pleural pain. Cyanosis may develop. Examination of the chest shows a friction rub. A lung scan will confirm the clinical diagnosis. It should be made urgently as two-thirds of the number of woman dying from pulmonary embolus do so within 2 to 4 hours.

TREATMENT OF DVT AND THROMBOEMBOLISM
Deep venous thrombosis

Heparin is given by an intravenous infusion pump (20 000U in 500ml normal saline at 25ml per hour). This provides 25 000U/ day. The rate is adjusted to provide a blood heparin concentration of 0.6–1.0U per ml, as assessed by the active partial thromboplastin time (APTT). Heparin is continued for 5 days. Warfarin is started at the same time as the heparin, which is continued until warfarin has prolonged the international normalized ratio into the therapeutic range (> 2.5 – 2.6). Warfarin is continued for 6–12 weeks in cases of proved DVT and for 12–24 weeks in cases of pulmonary embolism.

The patient remains in bed with her leg elevated until fully heparinized and until the limb ceases to be tender. She may then walk about but should wear a properly fitted elastic stocking.

Pulmonary embolism

A bolus of heparin 25 000U is given intravenously and followed by an infusion as in the treatment of DVT. The idea of the heparin bolus is to reverse the bronchoconstriction and vasoconstriction which follows the release of serotonin from platelets. An alternative is to give streptokinase. Pulmonary embolism is so serious that expert help should be obtained.

THE LONG-TERM CONSEQUENCES OF DVT

The long-term follow-up of women who had DVT in pregnancy or the puerperium, which was adequately treated, showed that after a median time of 10 years, only 25 per cent of the women were without symptoms of deep vein insufficiency. Half of the women had a swollen leg, 40 per cent had leg cramps, 25 per cent leg discolouration and 4 per cent leg ulceration.

POSTPARTUM PSYCHIATRIC PROBLEMS

Three psychiatric conditions affect women after childbirth. The first is 'third-day blues', the second is postpartum depression and the third is postpartum psychosis.

THIRD DAY BLUES

Between 50 and 70 per cent of mothers become emotionally labile, becoming irritable, with episodes of crying, and feel miserable. The cause is not known. The symptoms start between the third and fifth day after the birth of the baby. The emotional lability usually lasts for less than a week but may persist for a month. This is discussed under the heading Adjustment to Childbirth on page 91–92.

POSTNATAL DEPRESSION

Between 8 and 12 per cent of women develop clinically diagnosed depression in the first 3 months after childbirth, and twice that number have psychometric evidence of depression. Women at increased risk are:

- Those who have a family history or a personal history of depressive episodes.
- Those who lacked experience in 'parenting' when a child or an adolescent (for example, having no siblings to care for).
- Those who had an unstable or abusive family during childhood and adolescence.
- Those who lacked positive support from husband or partner during and after pregnancy.
- Those who are cut off from a near relative or friend who could care for the baby from time to time.
- Possibly those who had negative experiences in their contact with health professionals during the pregnancy (for example, lacking communication and information).
- Those who have experienced a complicated pregnancy (for example PIH, placenta praevia, preterm birth, multiple birth).

In other words, women are more likely to develop postnatal depression if they are socially and emotionally isolated or have had recent stressful life events.

There is no persuasive information, however, that postnatal depression is related to any hormonal or biochemical change or to any nutritional deficiency. But it is likely that women who develop postnatal depression may develop problems in maternal-infant relationships and adverse effects on infant cognitive development may occur.

Because of potential problems to the mother and infant, signs of postnatal depression should be sought early and help provided.

Women developing postnatal depression show the symptoms of ordinary depressive illness, although fatigue, irritability and anxiety are more common than in most clinically depressed women.

Management

The woman needs support and encouragement initially, not drugs. The doctor should listen to what she is saying, help her resolve her anxieties and con-flicts about her ability to be a parent and arrange for assistance in caring for the baby so that she may have 'time out'. In some cases admission to hospital for a few days for support and group therapy may help; in others, psychotrophic medications may be needed (but rarely as a first treatment). In more severe cases, psychiatric consultation should be obtained.

POSTNATAL PSYCHOSIS

Between 1 and 3 per 1000 women develop postnatal psychosis, usually manic or depressive illness, but occasionally a schizophrenic episode. The illness starts abruptly between the 5th and 15th day of the puerperium. In the beginning, the woman is confused, anxious, perplexed, restless and sad. Delusions (that the baby has died or is deformed) or hallucinations develop rapidly and the melancholia deepens.

Management

Admission to hospital is essential, preferably with the baby so the woman's delusions may decrease. This throws a considerable strain on the staff who have to make sure that the baby will not be harmed. Psychotrophic drugs are given, haloperidol being currently preferred. Most women respond well and relatively quickly. About 15 per cent develop the illness in a subsequent pregnancy, and one women in three develops a non-puerperal psychosis.

26

OBSTETRIC OPERATIONS

INDUCTION OF LABOUR

Induction of labour may be required to 'rescue' the fetus from a potentially hazardous intra-uterine environment in late pregancy for a variety of reasons or because continuation of the pregnancy is danger-ous to the expectant mother.

The method adopted depends on:

- The duration of the pregnancy.
- The condition of the cervix (i.e. favourable or unfavorable) *(Fig. 26.1)*.
- The position of the fetal head in relation to the pelvis.

The highest rate of success, (i.e. that the induc-tion is followed by a vaginal birth within 24 hours) occurs in a woman whose cervix is favourable and whose Bishop score is 5 or more *(Table 26.1)*.

If the chances of success are evaluated as low, the doctor may recommend caesarean section.

THE TECHNIQUES OF INDUCING LABOUR

Labour may be induced by drugs or by the surgical technique of amniotomy, which is also known as 'artificial rupture of the membranes' (ARM).

INDUCTION OF LABOUR USING DRUGS

Two methods are available: the use of prostaglandins and the use of oxytocin.

Prostaglandins. Three prostaglandins with different properties are available.

PGE_1 (gemeprost, cervigem) is available in pessary form or as an intracervical injection system. It is the preferred prostaglandin for the termination of pregnancy in the second quarter of pregnancy and for the induction of labour in the third quarter. It should be avoided in the fourth quarter of preg-nancy as cases of uterine hypertonicity have been reported.

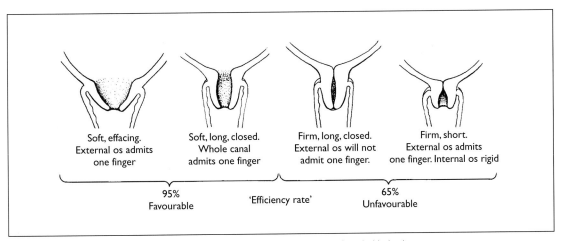

Soft, effacing. External os admits one finger

Soft, long, closed. Whole canal admits one finger

Firm, long, closed. External os will not admit one finger.

Firm, short. External os admits one finger. Internal os rigid

95% Favourable

'Efficiency rate'

65% Unfavourable

Fig 26.1 The relationship between the condition of the cervix and success rate of surgical induction.

A Method of Cervical 'Scoring'				
	Scoring rating			
Factor	**0**	**1**	**2**	**3**
Cervix				
Length (cm)	>4	>2	1–2	<1
Dilatation (cm)	<1	<2	2–3	>4
Consistency	Firm	'Average'	Soft	–
Position	Posterior	Other (mid, anterior)	–	–
Fetal head				
Position relative to ischial spines (cm)	–3	–2	–1 or 0	+1 or more

Table 26.1 A method of cer-vical 'Scoring'. Score: unfavourable 0–4; favourable 5+.

The Relationship Between Concentration of the Oxytocin Solution, mU of Oxytocin Infused per minute and Rate of the Infusion			
Strength	**2u/l**	**7.5 u/l** Oxytocin infusion (mU/minute)	**10u/l**	**Rate drops /min***
0.7	2.5	5	5
2	5.0	10	10
	10	20	20
4	15	30	30
	20	40	40
6		45	45
	25	50	50
8	30	60	60
* if an infusion pump not available			

Table 26.2 The relationship between concentration of oxytocin solution, mU of oxytocin infused per minute and rate of th e infusion.

PGE_2 is available as a gel or in pessary form which may be introduced intravaginally or intracervically. The gel appears to be more effective and is associated with a lower risk of producing uterine hypertonicity. As well as producing uterine contractions, PGE_2 softens the cervical connective tissue and relaxes cervical muscle fibres, 'ripening' the cervix. It is the preferred prostaglandin to produce cervical ripening when the cervical (Bishop) score is <5 and amniotomy is indicated. PGE_2 is available in a prefilled syringe, in a dose of 1–2mg, which is introduced into the posterior vaginal fornix. The patient's pulse rate and uterine activity are monitored for 30 minutes after which time she may walk about if she wishes, provide that the pregnancy is not at high risk. If labour is not established within 6 hours a further dose is administered. Some obstetricians perform an ARM at this time if the cervix is favourable.

(Mifepristone is being investigated an an alternative cervical ripening drug).

$PGF_{2\alpha}$ is available as a vaginal gel or as an intravenous infusion. Its main place is in the augmentation of uterine contractions.

Some patients receiving prostaglandins may have side effects, mainly nausea, vomiting or diarrhoea, but these are unusual in the doses recommended.

Oxytocin (syntocinon). Oxytocin should always be administered by intravenous infusion, preferably using an infusion pump. Used alone 50 per cent of women will be in labour within 12 hours. Induction is more effective if preceded by prostaglandin PGE_2 vaginal pessaries or following amniotomy.

The infusion is made by dissolving a number of units of syntocinon in normal saline *(Table 26.2)*. The rate is increased by 5mU/minute every 20 minutes until contractions lasting >60 seconds recur at 3–5 minute intervals. The maximum concentration used is 60mU/minute. Because of the risk of water intoxication and possible neonatal jaundice, the quantity of fluid infused should not exceed 1500 ml in 10 hours and the infusion should be stopped after this time.

Surgical induction of labour (amniotomy)
Surgical induction of labour (amniotomy) is more effective if the cervix is favourable (Bishop score 5+). The patient is put in the lithotomy position and the vagina swabbed with antiseptic. Two of the doctor's fingers are inserted to reach the cervix and if practicable one is inserted through the cervix to 'sweep' the membranes. An amnihook or a Kocher forceps is introduced along the intravaginal fingers and the membranes below the fetal head (the forewaters) are broken with the instrument.

The problems following amniotomy are:
- Prolapse of the umbilical cord (0.5 per cent).
- Infection, if the induction – delivery interval is more than 24hours.
- Haemorrhage, which is usually slight.
- Postpartum haemorrhage (relative risk 2 compared with no induction of labour).
- Neonatal hyperbilirubinaemia (bilirubin >250 μmol/l) which appears to be related to the maximum dose and duration of an oxytocin infusion following amniotomy.

A suggested schema (flow chart) for the induction of labour is shown in *Fig. 26.2*.

AUGMENTATION OF LABOUR

In cases where the quality of the uterine contractions is poor (see p. 171), their strength may be augmented either by performing an ARM or by setting up an incremental oxytocic infusion, or by both methods. A few obstetricians use $PGF_{2\alpha}$ vaginal pessary form in preference to oxytocin infusion.

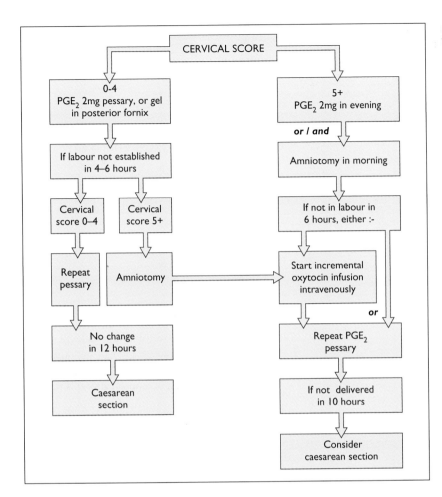

Fig 26.2 Induction of labour flow chart.

OBSTETRIC FORCEPS

In the 400 years since the obstetric forceps was invented as a 'secret instrument', it has developed into a precision instrument, which must be used with great skill.

INDICATIONS
The indications for the use of the obstetric forceps are:
- *Delay in the birth of the baby* when the second stage of labour has exceeded 1.5 hours or the fetal head has been delayed on the perineum for >30 minutes. The delay is usually because:
  (i) The fetal head has not rotated and is arrested in the transverse diameter of the mid pelvic cavity (deep transverse arrest of the head);
  (ii) The head has rotated into the posterior position in the mid cavity or in the lower pelvic strait (posterior arrest of the head);
  (iii) A minor degree of cephalopelvic disproportion is present;
  (iv) The uterine contractions have become weaker.
- *The fetus shows signs of distress* (i.e. bradycardia and/or the passage of meconium).

- *The mother has become distressed*, either physically or mentally, in the second stage of labour.
- *The mother has an existing obstetric or medical condition* (e.g. PIH, chronic hypertension, cardiac disease) which may deteriorate during the expulsive stage of labour.
- *To aid in the delivery of the aftercoming head in a breech presentation.*

TYPES OF FORCEPS DELIVERY
(Fig. 26.3).

Mid-forceps
The forceps are applied to the sides of the fetal head, whose biparietal diameter has entered the pelvis but has not advanced much beyond the ischial spines. Usually the occiput lies in one or other transverse diameter of the maternal pelvis.

Low forceps
The forceps are applied to the sides of the fetal head, whose biparietal diameter has advanced to or beyond the ischial tuberosities and has rotated so that the sagittal suture lies in the anteroposterior diameter of the maternal pelvis.

Outlet forceps

The fetal head distends the vaginal introitus, but the perineum is holding it back.

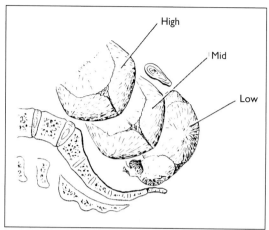

Fig 26.3 Types of forceps deliveries – showing the station of the head when the forceps are applied.

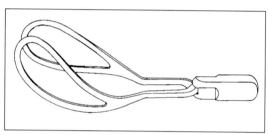

Fig 26.4 Wrigley's forceps (scale × 2 that of Figs 26.5 and 26.6).

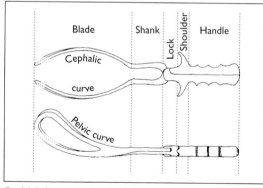

Fig 26.5 Simpson's obstetric forceps.

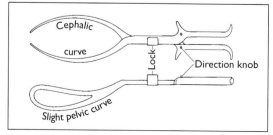

Fig 26.6 Kjelland's forceps.

THE INCIDENCE OF FORCEPS DELIVERY

The incidence of forceps delivery varies widely depending on the belief and practice of the woman's doctor. In Britain and Australia about 10 per cent of all births are effected by forceps, of which 2 per cent are mid-forceps and 8 per cent are low or outlet forceps.

CONDITIONS FOR FORCEPS DELIVERY

These are:
- The greatest diameter of the fetal head must have passed the pelvic brim.
- The cervix must be fully dilated; the blades of the forceps must be applied along the sides of the fetal head.
- The membranes must have ruptured and the bladder must be empty.
- The mother must receive adequate anaesthesia or analgesia.

Women requiring a midforceps should have an epidural block, a general anaesthetic or a pudendal block (although this does not always make the birth pain-free). Women requiring a low or outlet forceps require a pudendal nerve block at the least.

TYPES OF FORCEPS

Three types of forceps are available today. The *short shanked forceps* is used for low or outlet forceps *(Fig. 26.4)*. The *long-shanked forceps* is used for mid-forceps delivery after manually rotating the fetal head if it is arrested in the transverse diameter of the pelvis *(Fig. 26.5) Kjelland's forceps* has a sliding lock and can be used to rotate the fetal head and deliver it *(Fig. 26.6)*.

All forceps compress the fetal head to some extent and apply traction to effect the birth.

TECHNIQUE OF FORCEPS DELIVERY

The technique of forceps delivery is shown in the following series of illustrations and described in the captions.

Low or outlet forceps
Figs. 26.7–26.10

Mid-forceps
The technique for applying the long-shanked curved forceps is the same as that used to apply the short-shanked forceps. As the forceps have to be introduced further into the vagina, great care must be exercised to avoid damaging the vaginal wall and to ensure that the forceps are correctly applied along the sides of the fetal head.

Because the head has to be pulled through the pelvic curve, the mother should be positioned correctly, with her legs in stirrups and her buttocks projecting over the end of the bed *(Fig. 26.11)*. This is because the pull required to deliver the baby has to be downward initially and then curving

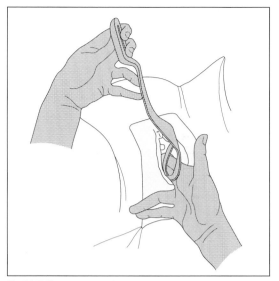

Fig 26.7 The assembled forceps are held in front of the woman's vulva, the pelvic curve uppermost. The left blade is introduced without force into the vagina between the fetal head and the vaginal wall, which is protected by the doctor's fingers; the blade is steered to lie along the left side of the baby's head.

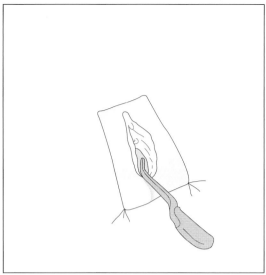

Fig 26.8 When correctly applied the shank will press on the mother's perineum.

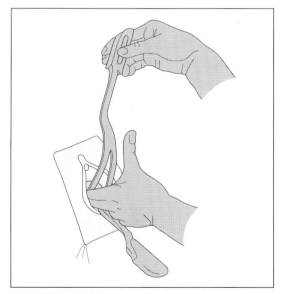

Fig 26.9 The right blade is introduced in a similar manner and the two are assembled in the lock. If they do not fit easily into the lock, there is a malapplication and if they cannot be made to adjust easily, the forceps are removed and the procedure is repeated.

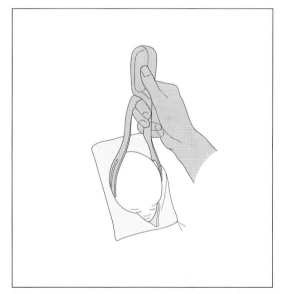

Fig 26.10 The forceps are held as shown and the baby's head is delivered in a smooth curve using controlled traction, preferably during a uterine contraction. An episiotomy is often needed to prevent a perineal tear.

upwards (*Fig. 26.12*). Some obstetricians use the axis traction device but skill is required to use it properly (*Fig. 26.13*).

If the baby's head is arrested in the transverse diameter of the mid-pelvis, manual rotation may be attempted (*Fig. 26.14*) followed by mid-forceps delivery. Alternatively Kjelland's forceps may be chosen or a caesarean section performed.

Kjelland's forceps

This instrument is used to rotate a head arrested in the transverse diameter of the mid pelvis. It requires considerable skill and the woman should be delivered in an operating theatre so that if any difficulty is experienced, a caesarean section can be done immediately.

The forceps are held in front of the woman's vulva and positioned so that the dot on the shoulders

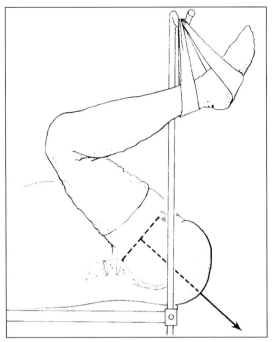

Fig 26.11 Position of the patient for mid-forceps delivery.

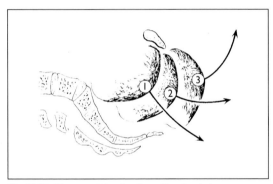

Fig 26.12 Diagram of the direction of traction in forceps delivery. In mid-forceps delivery (1) the initial direction of pull is downwards, in low forceps (2) horizontal and in outlet forceps (3) slightly upwards.

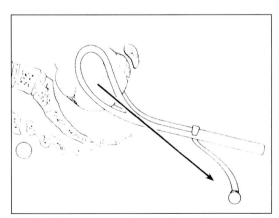

Fig 26.13 The mechanics of forceps delivery. Mid-forceps; with axis traction the force is resolved and the pull is in the axis of the birth canal.

of the instrument points to the side of the pelvis where the baby's occiput lies. The remainder of the application of Kjelland's forceps is shown in *Fig. 26.15*. Usually a wide episiotomy is made as perineal damage is almost inevitable.

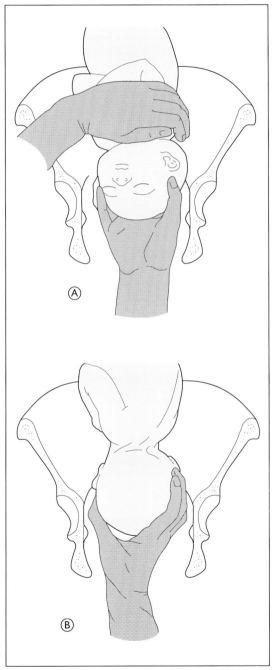

Fig 26.14 Manual rotation of the head from a left occipito-posterior position. (A) The left hand is placed on the abdomen and pulls the right shoulder of the baby towards the mother's right side. Simultaneously the right hand, in supination, holds the head by its biparietal diameter and rotates it through 180 degrees to a position of pronation; (B) The occiput becomes anterior at the end of the manoeuvre.

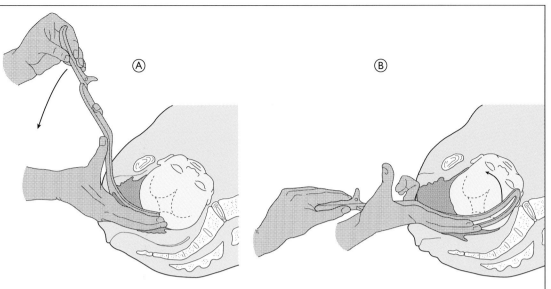

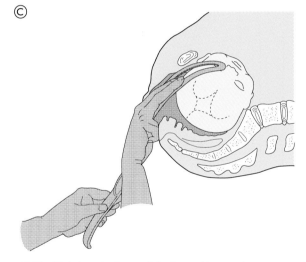

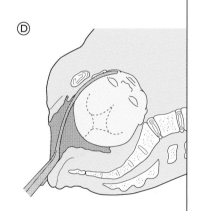

A. The forceps blade is inserted posterolaterally on the same side as the fetal face between the head and the fingers protecting the vaginal wall.

B. The internal fingers, resting behind the blade guide it anteriorly around the fetus's face. The external hand steadies the handle of the forceps.

C. The blade 'wanders' around the face and is now almost anterior. The external hand tilts it slightly so that it presses more on the head than on the pelvic wall.

D. The forceps blade is now completely anterior. The handle is elevated to bring the blade to its correct position over the ear and malar bone of the fetus

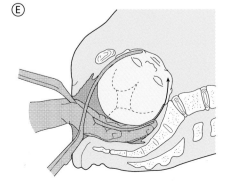

E. The posterior blade is introduced directly along the curve of the sacrum, the tip being applied closely to the fetal head. To make locking easier the blade is inserted on the same side as the lock.

Fig 26.15 Application of Kjelland's forceps in cases of deep transverse arrest.

THE DANGERS OF A DIFFICULT FORCEPS DELIVERY

The vagina and cervix may be damaged, causing haemorrhage. Following a mid-forceps the entire vagina should be inspected with good illumination, and lacerations looked for and sutured.

The dangers to the fetus are trauma, compression of the brain and tentorial tearing caused by too strong compression and traction. Fracture of the fetal skull and facial paresis may occur if the forceps have been incorrectly applied and compress the nerve as it emerges in front of the mastoid process.

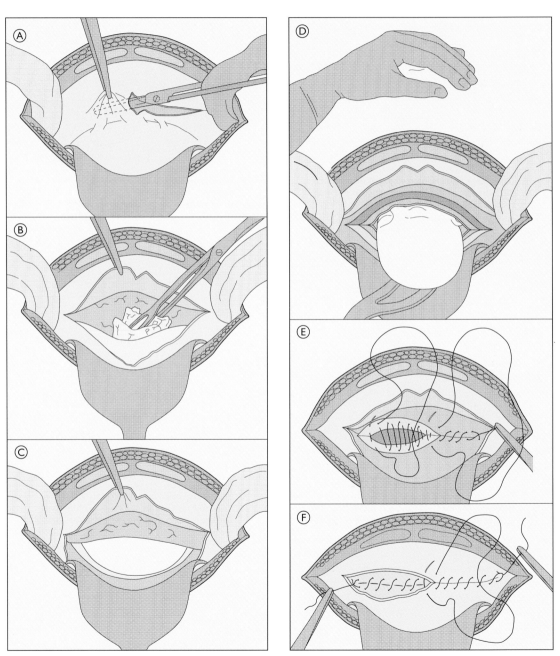

Fig 26.16 The technique of caesarean section.
(A) and (B) The loose peritoneum covering the lower uterine segment is divided and pushed down.
(C) The exposed muscle of the lower segment is incised so that the membranes bulge into the wound. The incision may be extended with a knife, or the muscle fibres separated with the fingers.
(D) The membranes are ruptured and the head delivered using a forceps blade as an inclined plane, counter pressure being exerted on the fundus.
(E) The placenta has been expelled and the wound sutured in layers. Great care must be taken at the angles.
(F) The peritoneum is sutured.

THE VACUUM EXTRACTOR OR VENTOUSE

An alternative to forceps delivery is to extract the baby from the birth canal by applying a cup to the occipital region of the head, and slowly producing a vacuum within the cup. The cup is attached to a chain and a handle. Having obtained the vacuum slowly, traction is applied. Skilled, experienced operators use the vacuum extractor both for low and mid-forceps deliveries.

The advantages are:
* That less is inserted into the vagina which is less distended and less likely to be damaged.
* The mother needs less anaesthesia.

The disadvantages are that delivery is slower; the ventouse may slip off; the baby develops a large artificial caput (chignon) which subsides within 48 hours; and may have scalp lacerations.

CAESAREAN SECTION

Caesarean section means that the baby is removed from an intact uterus by abdominal operation. In many developed countries the caesarean section rate has risen from 5 per cent 25 years ago to over 15 per cent. The increase is in part due to fashion, in part due to fear of litigation if a 'perfect' baby is not born; in part due to the changing pattern of conception: women are delaying the conception of their first child and are limiting the number of children they have.

THE INDICATIONS FOR CAESAREAN SECTION

These have broadened in recent years and are listed in *Table 26.3*.

THE TECHNIQUE OF CAESAREAN SECTION

There are two types of caesarean section. In the first a transverse incision is made through the stretched lower uterine segment. In the second – the classical section – a vertical incision is made through the myometrium. The classical section is now rarely used, except when the lower uterine segment is excessively vascular, or cannot be reached because of extensive adhesions, or if the fetus presents as a transverse lie, with an impacted shoulder. Caesarean hysterectomy may be required if intractable bleeding occurs, for placenta accreta or if the uterus has ruptured.

The operative technique is shown in *Fig. 26.16*. As blood loss is unpredictable, cross-matched blood should be available.

Post operative care is no different from any other abdominal operation. Early ambulation is encouraged, especially since in many hospitals the neonate is kept in the nursery for 24 to 48 hours. Maternal morbidity varies between 3 and 12 per cent depending on the reason for the caesarean section. Endometritis accounts for two-thirds of morbidity. For this reason prophylactic antibiotics are routinely given following the operation. Women at higher risk of developing thromboembolism are prescribed prophylactic anticoagulants.

Caesarean section is a very safe operation, the overall mortality rate being about 0.4 per 1000 sections and 0.1 per 1000 sections performed electively.

VAGINAL BIRTH AFTER PREVIOUS CAESAREAN SECTION

When a caesarean section is performed for a non-recurrent condition, the next baby may be born vaginally or by caesarean section depending on the wishes of the woman and the advice of the obstetrician. Studies from countries outside North America show that nearly half of the women who had had a previous caesarean section deliver their next baby vaginally. In North America less than one-third deliver vaginally.

If a woman chooses a vaginal birth after a caesarean section (VBAC), the birth should take place in a well-equipped hospital staffed by experienced obstetricians. The reason for this is that the trial of vaginal delivery is terminated by caesarean section in one-fifth of all cases 0.25 per cent of women suffering a ruptured uterus.

Indications for Caesarean Section

1. Failure of labour to progress (dystocia)
   abnormal uterine action
   cephalopelvic disporportion

2. Malpresentations or malpositions
   breech — IN PRIMI
   face and brow
   transverse lie
   occipito-posterior
   prolapse of umbilical cord
   multiple pregnancy

3. Antepartum haemorrhage
   abruptio placentae
   placenta praevia

4. Hypertensive disease in pregnancy

5. Diabetes mellitus

6. Fetal conditions
   fetal distress
   iso-immunization
   very low birth-weight

7. Older primigravidae

8. Failed induction of labour

9. Repeat caesarean section

Table 26.3 Indications for caesarean section.

If an elective caesarean section is chosen, the maturity of the fetus must be established so that the operation is performed when the gestation period is >37 weeks.

VERSION

External cephalic version may be chosen when a fetus presenting as a breech has not turned cephalically by the 35th week of pregnancy. Before attempting the version the doctor must be sure that the pelvis has normal dimensions and that the placenta is not praevia. The mother should not have hypertension or a multiple pregnancy.

Some doctors give a tocolytic drug intravenously before the attempt, and a few perform external version with the woman anesthetized. The version is performed gently. The breech is mobilized and the version attempted by lifting it with one hand and pushing the fetal head down with the other *(Fig. 26.17)*. The fetal heart rate is either monitored continuously or every 2 minutes during and for 30 minutes after the version. If the fetal heart falls <90 beats per minute during the version, the attempt is abandoned.

Problems associated with version are uncommon. They include rupture of the membranes, cord entanglement around a limb of the fetus and the onset of premature labour.

Internal podalic version in which the doctor's hand is introduced into the uterus to grasp a limb and pull it through a fully dilated cervix is rarely performed today. It may find use in cases of the delayed birth of a second twin, which is lying transversely in the uterus, but caesarean section is safer in most cases.

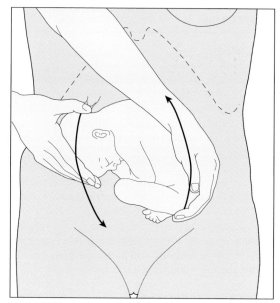

Fig 26.17 External version–the obstetrician has lifted the buttocks out of the pelvis, his right thumb controls the baby's head and the direction in which the child is moved encourages flexion.

DESTRUCTIVE OPERATIONS ON THE FETUS

There is very little place for these procedures in modern obstetric practice. An exception may be when a hydrocephalic fetus has died during labour. In this case the head is perforated with a perforator and fluid allowed to drain, making the fetus easier to deliver.

THE EPIDEMIOLOGY OF OBSTETRICS

The quality of obstetric care in a country can be measured by the maternal and the perinatal mortality rates. The death of a woman in pregnancy or childbirth is one of the greatest tragedies which can befall a family.

MATERNAL MORTALITY

A maternal death is defined by the International Federation of Obstetricians and Gynaecologists as 'the death of any woman dying whilst pregnant or within one year of the termination of the pregnancy, from any cause related to or aggravated by the pregnancy or its management but not from accidental or incidental causes'. The maternal mortality rate is the number of such deaths per 100 000 maternities.

In most developed countries the maternal death rate remained about the same from 1850 to 1934 when it began falling. In the period before the mid 1930s it was about 500 per 100 000; by the mid 1980s it had fallen in many industrialized countries to less than 10 per 100 000 maternities *(Fig 27.1)*. The initial fall was due to the control of infections by better obstetric care and the introduction of antibiotics. The second factor was that most women availed themselves of good-quality antenatal care which enabled complications to be detected early and treatment to be offered, usually in well equipped hospitals, staffed by trained medical attendants. Blood became increasingly and quickly available from blood banks, which reduced considerably the deaths due to haemorrhage. Sociological changes have also occurred in the past 60 years: fewer women now have more than 3 children, and most have their pregnancies before the age of 35. Higher parity and advancing age increase the risk of maternal death.

In the developing countries the maternal mortality rate is much higher. In sub-Saharan Africa it averages 600 per 100 000 live births; in South Asia, 500 per 100 000 births; in Southeast Asia and Latin America 300 per 100 000 live births. The reasons for these high maternal mortality rates are: frequent pregnancies, with short intervals between them; the resort to unsafe abortion performed in unhygienic surroundings; a relative lack of prenatal care and a lack of the perception of its value by poorly educated and poorly informed women; a lack of access to skilled medical help; and a lack of Government support to make changes to the status, education and empowerment of women.

THE CAUSES OF MATERNAL DEATH

Several developed countries publish the results of confidential inquiries into maternal deaths at intervals of about 3 years. In these reports the causes of the deaths are analyzed and suggestions are made which might prevent these deaths occurring.

These reports have been published in the UK since 1952 and in Australia since 1965. In 1990 a report was published analyzing all maternal deaths which had occurred in the USA between 1979 and 1986. Study of the three reports shows that the main causes of maternal death are similar in the three countries. In

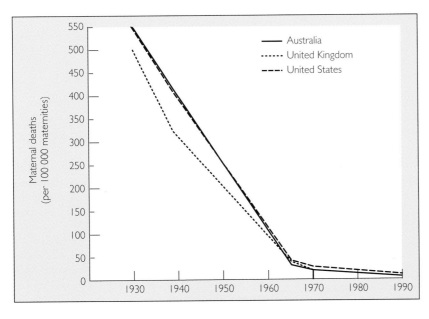

Fig 27.1 The secular trend of maternal mortality in Australia and the United Kingdom.

Most Common Causes of Maternal Deaths (Australia, England and Wales, The USA)		
Cause	Percentage of deaths	Proportion avoidable
Hypertensive disease of pregnancy	10–25	50
Pulmonary embolism	5–20	30
Abortion	5–10	25
Ectopic gestation	5–15	20
Haemorrhage	5–15	50
Sepsis	5–10	30
Cardio-respiratory (including anaesthetic)	5–15	30

Table 27.1 Most common causes of maternal deaths (Australia, England and Wales, and USA).

Table 27.1 the most common causes of death are shown. In *Fig 27.2* the decline in the major causes of maternal death in England and Wales is shown. Maternal deaths can be reduced further, particularly those associated with anaesthesia, ectopic gestation and pulmonary embolism.

PERINATAL MORTALITY

The death of a fetus in utero or its death in the neonatal period causes much distress to the parents and is a measure of the quality of obstetric care.

Before perinatal mortality can be discussed, some terms need to be clarified. In 1979 the World Health Organization published some international definitions.

Live birth is the complete expulsion or extraction from its mother of a product of conception, irrespective of the duration of the pregnancy, which after such separation, breathes or shows any evidence of life, such as beating of the heart, pulsation of the umbilical cord, or definite movement of the voluntary muscles: whether or not the umbilical cord has been cut or the placenta is attached, each product of such a birth is considered live born.

Fetal death is death prior to the complete expulsion or extraction from its mother of a product of conception, irrespective of the duration of pregnancy; the death is indicated by the fact that after such separation the fetus does not breathe or show other evidence of life, such as beating of the heart, pulsation of the umbilical cord, or definite movement of voluntary muscles.

Early fetal deaths equate to abortions, and *intermediate fetal deaths* are those occurring between the 22nd and 27th completed gestational weeks, the fetus weighing 500 – 999g (also called stillbirth).

Late fetal death is fetal death at 28 completed weeks of gestation and over. The fetus usually weighs 1000g or more (also called stillbirth).

In 1975, the following definitions recommended by the World Health Organization, were accepted by the International Federation of Gynaecologists and Obstetricians (FIGO):

Neonatal deaths are deaths of live born infants occurring before 28 completed days of life. Neonatal deaths can be divided into two groups: *early neonatal deaths* and *late neonatal deaths*.

Early neonatal, or *postnatal death* is the death of a live born baby in the first seven completed days (168 hours) of life.

Late neonatal death is the death of a live born infant after seven completed days but before 28 completed days of life.

Two definitions of perinatal mortality are therefore possible: the extended perinatal mortality rate; and the basic, or standard, perinatal mortality rate.

The *extended perinatal mortality* is the sum of all fetal deaths (excluding pregnancies terminating before the 22nd week of pregnancy in which the conceptus weighed less than 500g) and all neonatal deaths per 1000 births.

The *standard perinatal mortality* is the sum of late fetal deaths and early neonatal deaths, or, put in another way, it is the number of stillbirths and first-week deaths of babies weighing 1000g or more at birth per 1000 births.

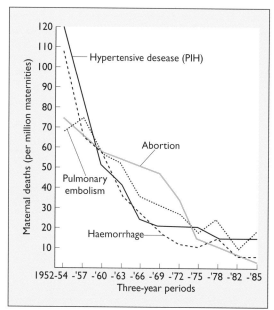

Fig 27.2 Main causes of maternal death directly due to pregnancy or childbirth (England and Wales, 1952-85) per 1 000 000 maternities.

From these data mortality rates can be inferred and should be used for purposes of international comparison.

Standard perinatal mortality rate. The ratio of stillborn infants plus early neonatal deaths of infants weighing 1000g and over × 1000, *divided* by the total births of infants stillborn and live born weighing 1000g and over.

Stillbirth rate. Stillborn infants weighing 1000g and over × 1000 *divided* by the total births of infants (stillborn and live born) weighing 1000g and over.

Early neonatal death rate. Early neonatal deaths of infants weighing 1000g or more at birth × 1000, *divided* by live-born infants weighing 1000g and over.

In many developed nations the extended perinatal mortality rate (extended PMR) is between 7 and 12 per 1000 births, and the standard PMR is about 9 per 1000 births. In the few developing countries which have been able to publish reasonably reliable data the standard PMR is between 35 and 55 per 1000 births.

SOCIAL FACTORS AFFECTING THE PMR

The most exact information about the effect of sociological factors on the PMR is obtained from The British Perinatal Mortality Surveys published in 1958 and 1970. All births occurring during one week and all singleton stillbirths and neonatal deaths over a 3 month period were surveyed.

The findings were that:

- The lower the social class the higher the standard perinatal mortality rate which rose from 7.5 per 1000 in social class 1 to 26.8 per 1000 in social classes IV and V.
- The mother's age affected the PMR. It was highest among the infants of mothers aged <17 and >35.
- Women who did not avail themselves of antenatal care had 5 – 10 times the mean perinatal mortality rate.
- The management of the labour affected the PMR. One-third of the perinatal deaths were due to intrapartum anoxia alone or associated with birth trauma. In some cases the intrapartum anoxia was a sequel to antepartum conditions, the fetus entering labour in poor health; in other cases mismanagement of labour or the misuse of forceps damaged the baby, which was either stillborn or died in the early neonatal period.

AN ANALYSIS OF PERINATAL MORTALITY

The precise cause of death of the fetus or neonate is not always helpful as only immediate causes of death

Standard Perinatal Mortality by Clinico-Pathological Classification Showing Mothers Likely to Have the Highest Risk	
Causes of death	**High-risk mothers**
1. Unexplained, low birth-weight (25–30 per cent of all)	Low socio-economic status Reduced height In all social classes, highest in women under 17 and over 35 Para 4 or more Cigarette smoking
2. Antepartum haemorrhage (10–15 per cent of all)	Para 4 or more Low socio-economic status
3. Fetal malformations (20–30 per cent of all) (a) CNS (b) Other	 Increase with diminishing socio-economic status; poor nutrition Primiparity, especially in primiparae under the age of 20 Increase with increasing parity and age
4. Maternal disease (3–5 per cent of all)	Increase with increasing maternal age: no effect from parity
5. Pregnancy-induced hypertension (6–10 per cent of all)	Primiparae Women over 30 History of the condition in a previous pregnancy
6. Mechanical/trauma (3–5 per cent of all)	Primiparity, especially if aged 30 or more Short stature Para 4 or more (inadequate obstetric care)
7. Unexplained, normal birth-weight (10–20 per cent of all)	Primiparae, especially aged 30 or more Para 4 or more Post term (i.e. 42 week's gestation) especially in older primigravidae
8. Iso-immunization (<1 per cent of all)	Increasing parity
9. Infections (1–4 per cent of all)	None discerned apart from? increasing age

Table 27.2 Standard perinatal mortality by clinico-pathological classification showing mothers likely to have the highest risk. (Information from Perinatal Problems, Chapter 12, by Sir Dugald Baird and A.M. Thompson; and *Perinatal Mortality Committee Reports*, The Women's Hospital, Crown Street, Sydney).

are entered. For this reason a clinico-pathological classification was devised by Professor Dugald Baird in the 1950s *(Table 27.2)*. This classification is based on why the baby became ill and died rather than the pathological cause of death. It enables health professionals to identify correctable problems. An analysis based on surveys in New South Wales and Scotland, carried out in the early 1980s is shown in *Table 27.3*. The recorded standard PMR in New South Wales was 11.03 and that in Scotland 14.0. Since that date there has been a decline of perinatal mortality in both countries, but the proportionality of the causes remains the same.

THE REDUCTION OF PERINATAL MORTALITY

Many of the measures which have been effective in reducing maternal deaths are effective in reducing perinatal deaths. In addition the provision of well-equipped, well-staffed neonatal intensive-care units (NICU) will enable a number of low birth-weight babies to survive and grow.

Comparison of the Clinico-Pathological Classification of Perinatal Deaths in New South Wales and Scotland, Proportional Percentages		
	NSW **1979**	**Scotland** **1977-81**
Environmental		
Unexplained, low birthweight	25.1	33.4
Antepartum haemorrhage	10.4	12.1
Congenital anomaly	20.6	24.1
Maternal disorder	5.5	4.1
Obstetric		
Unexplained, normal birth-weight	19.1	7.2
Pregnancy-induced hypertension	7.2	8.4
Mechanical/trauma	4.7	3.6
Iso-immunization	1.8	1.3
Infection/Miscellaneous	5.6	2.2
	n = 866	n = 3781
Standard perinatal mortality rate	11.03	14.0
Births in period	78502	270581

Table 27.3 Comparison of the clinico-pathological classification of perinatal deaths in New South Wales and Scotland, proportional percentages.

28

THE NEWBORN INFANT

Following birth the neonate undergoes several physiological changes so that it can adapt to extra-uterine life. Two main changes affect respiration and cardiovascular function.

THE FIRST BREATHS

During the last minutes of its birth the fetus becomes increasingly hypoxic from a lack of oxygen, consequent on the reduced circulation of blood through the placenta associated with the strong uterine contractions. This mild degree of hypoxia stimulates the first gasps of the neonate after it has been born. With the first gasps, the fluid which has filled the respiratory passages is driven into the expanding alveoli from where it is absorbed rapidly into the pulmonary lymphatics and circulation. Within 15 minutes of birth, the fluid has disappeared and the alveoli are distended with air, unless problems have arisen. Once breathing has been initiated, rhythmic respirations are maintained by chemoreceptors which are responsible for the ventilatory response to carbon dioxide and hypoxia.

CHANGES IN THE PATTERN OF BLOOD CIRCULATION

The second change is the redirection of the blood flow following the cessation of the high blood flow through the umbilical arteries which perfused the placental villi, and the large volume of blood returning through the umbilical vein and the vena cava. The venous pressure in the vena cava falls and the ductus venosus closes. The lungs expand with the first breath and the pulmonary vascular resistance falls abruptly. The infant's systemic blood pressure rises slightly at the same time, which results in a temporary reversal in the direction of the blood flowing through the ductus arteriosus. As the infant breathes, the oxygen tension in the blood rises and the muscular walls of the ductus contract, the passage of blood flow through it ceasing. At the same time, the pressure in the right atrium falls. There is a simultaneous increase in the blood flow through the lungs. This blood enters and increases the pressure in the left atrium. Because of the changes in pressure between the two atria, the foramen ovale closes.

With the closure of the ductus venosus, the foramen ovale and the ductus arteriosus, the adult pattern of circulation of the blood is established (Fig. 28.1; compare with Fig 5.1 page 26).

CHANGES IN LIVER FUNCTION

After the cardiovascular changes have taken place the infant's liver is perfused with a larger quantity of blood. The infant's liver can convert glucose into glycogen as efficiently as an adult liver, but some of its enzymatic functions are immature. The most important is its ability to conjugate bilirubin. In consequence a mild physiological jaundice may occur in the first 6 days of life.

Most of the glycogen stored in the liver is laid down in the last 8 weeks of intra-uterine life. This is now mobilized for the energy needs of the first few days of life. Preterm babies have smaller liver glycogen stores and may develop hypoglycaemia. After a few days of life the neonate obtains energy from food and by oxidizing fats stored in adipose tissue.

TEMPERATURE CONTROL

At birth, vasoconstriction of the skin vessels preserves body heat, but temperature maintenance is relatively difficult because of the relatively large surface area of a newborn infant. The body temperature of many newborn infants falls by 1.5°C immediately after the birth, because of rapid heat loss from the wet skin, but returns to normal within a few hours. A mature infant will have laid down fat in brown adipose tissue and can utilize this for heat production without shivering. Preterm babies have less brown fat and may become hypothermic.

Because of the instability of temperature control, neonates should be wrapped properly in cold climates, but in hot climates too much wrapping should be avoided (Chapter 22).

HYPOXIA IN PREGNANCY AND IN THE NEWBORN

Most babies establish respiration rapidly and easily. A few infants are hypoxic at birth and require resuscitation. Any condition occurring during late pregancy or labour which reduces the oxygen available to the fetus will predispose it to neonatal hypoxia. These conditions have been mentioned when discussing the 'at-risk' fetus in pregnancy and labour (page 147).

If severe fetal hypoxia develops in pregnancy, the fetus may die in utero or may be born with acidaemia and hypercapnia as well as hypoxia (asphyxia). A blood pH of <7.10 may lead to reflex pulmonary vasoconstriction which further impairs gas exchange,

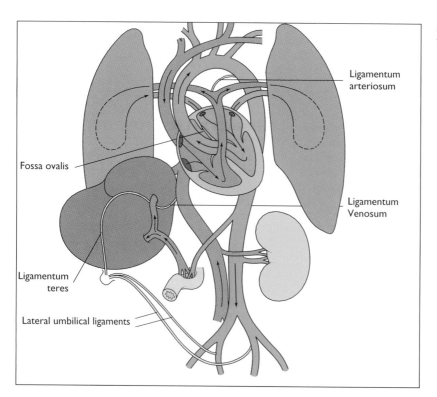

Fig 28.1 Normal circulation in the newborn.

Ligamentum arteriosum

Fossa ovalis

Ligamentum Venosum

Ligamentum teres

Lateral umbilical ligaments

Apgar Scoring Method for Evaluating the Infant			
Sign	**0**	**1**	**2**
Colour	Blue; pale	Body pink; extremities blue	Completely pink
Respiratory effort	Absent	Weak cry; hypoventilation	Good; strong cry
Muscle tone	Limp	Some flexion of extremities	Active motion; extremities well flexed
Reflex irritability (response to stimulation of sole of foot)	No response	Grimace	Cry
Heart rate	Absent	Slow (below 100)	Fast (over 100)

Table 28.1 Apgar scoring method for evaluating the infant (from Apgar and associates).

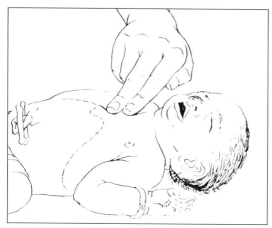

Fig 28.2 Closed cardiac massage. Intermittent pressure is applied over the middle-third of the sternum (which is pressed down about half an inch) with two fingers. The heart is compressed between the rib cage and the vertebral column and blood is expelled into the great vessel. For clarity the endotracheal tube has been omitted in the drawing (from Moya, James, Burnard and Hanks. Anaesthesiology 1961, 22, 644).

Hypoxia, on the other hand, increases the base deficit. Both of these changes increase the risk of the fetus to neurological damage. In such cases, rescuscitation is urgently needed at birth.

The severity of hypoxia around the time of birth, and its effect on the subsequent development of the infant can be measured by the Apgar scoring system *(Table 28.1)* or by the pH of umbilical artery blood. Both are useful in managing the immediate problem but are relatively poor indicators of long-term outcome.

The basic resuscitation of the newborn has been described on page 77 *Fig.10.16*. The first column of that figure equates to a 1-min Apgar score of 7–10. The second column to an Apgar score of 4–6, whilst the third column equates to an Apgar score of 0–3. The most important step in rescuscitation is administering oxygen with intermittent positive pressure respiration. If the infant does not respond and remains bradycardic the circulation should be supported by external cardiac massage *(Fig. 28.2)* and possibly endotracheal adrenalin. In addition acidosis can be corrected with sodium bicarbonate (5mmol/kg body weight) infusion via the umbilical vein.

THE RESPIRATORY DISTRESS SYNDROME (HYALINE MEMBRANE DISEASE)

Hyaline membrane disease is caused by a relative lack of surfactant in the alveoli. Surfactant determines the stability of the lung after birth, and lowers the surface tension in the alveoli, ensuring a normal residual volume of air and the capacity for gas exchange. In the absence of surfactant the alveoli become airless at the end of each breath and their ability to expand against the forces of surface tension is decreased. The consequent relative hypoxia causes pulmonary vasoconstriction and hinders the closure of the foramen ovale and the ductus arteriosus, which in turn reduces the pulmonary blood flow, with increasing respiratory and metabolic acidosis.

Hyaline membrane disease affects 0.5–1.0 per cent of all neonates. It is uncommon if the baby weighs >2500g at birth, but affects 10 per cent of low birth-weight infants, and is particularly damaging to infants weighing <1500g at birth.

Diagnosis and treatment

Within a few hours of birth the infant's respiratory rate increases, with nasal flaring, expiratory grunting and sternal or intercostal retraction. The infant may be cyanosed and limp. The diagnosis is confirmed by radiology which shows ground glass shadowing. In 80 per cent of cases the disease is only moderately severe but in 20 per cent the infant is seriously ill.

A neonatologist must be consulted and the infant admitted to a neonatal intensive care unit. The principles of treatment are:
- To keep the infant warm in an incubator adjusted to the neutral thermal range.
- To provide oxygen to obtain an arterial blood saturation of 95 per cent or a tension of 60–80mm Hg, by monitoring blood gases frequently.
- To provide assisted ventilation if needed.
- To avoid retinal damage by uncontrolled use of oxygen.
- To ensure that the baby is adequately nourished with fluid and energy, by giving an intravenous infusion of a glucose electrolyte solution, or breast milk by a nasogastric tube.
- To give either natural or synthetic surfactant in cases that require mechanical ventilation.

The mortality of hyaline membrane disease varies from 15 to 50 per cent depending on the weight of the neonate, the severity of the disease and the skill of the medical and nursing staff.

BIRTH INJURIES

With increasingly good obstetric care during child-birth, birth injuries are becoming less common and less severe. Only those injuries most likely to occur will be discussed. In all cases the injury must be explained to the parents and the treatment and prognosis discussed.

CRANIAL INJURIES
Caput succedanum

This is due to pressure on the fetal scalp when the head is being pushed deeply into the pelvis and the venous return from the scalp is impeded. The oedematous swelling covers a large area of scalp. Treatment is not required and the caput disappears within a few days.

Cephalohaematoma

Cephalohaematoma occurs following trauma by the obstetric forceps or the ventouse. The periosteum is dragged from the underlying parietal bone and subperiosteal haemorrhage occurs. The swelling is limited to the shape of the bone, is fluctuant initially, after which the rim becomes hard. The haematoma remains for 2–3 weeks and then is slowly absorbed.

Intracranial haemorrhage

Intracranial haemorrhage may be subdural or intraventricular. Both are uncommon. *Subdural haemorrhage* follows the misuse of forceps. The infant, if born alive, is shocked and shows little response to resuscitation. *Intraventricular haemorrhage* is found most often among preterm infants and is related to worsening hypoxia. Most cases are diagnosed within 72 hours of birth, when the infant's condition deteriorates suddenly. This condition is diagnosed by ultrasound examinations, which should be performed routinely on very small infants.

NERVE INJURIES

Most nerve injuries involve the face (facial palsy) or the brachial plexus and usually follow a forceps delivery or a difficult breech birth.

Facial palsy

Facial palsy is a lower motor neurone disorder with paresis or paralysis of the facial nerve and inability to close the eye on the affected side. The lesion usually resolves spontaneously within 2 to 3 weeks.

Brachial palsy

This is due to nerve damage, usually following difficulty in delivering the aftercoming head of a breech or in shoulder dystocia. In most cases the nerve sheath is torn and the nerve is compressed by haemorrhage and oedema, but its integrity is preserved. *Erb's palsy* is due to compression of the fibres of C5 and C6. The infant's arm hangs limply by the baby's side. Treatment is to put the arm into abduction with flexion of the elbow and extension of the wrist and to maintain muscle tone by moving the arm passively . Erb's palsy occurs in less than 1 in 2000 births.

Klumpke's paralysis is rare. It occurs when nerves C7 and C8 are compressed. The infant has a paralysed arm, with wrist drop and flaccid paralysis of hand muscles. The prognosis is worse than that following Erb's palsy.

BONE AND MUSCLE INJURY

These injuries may occur following a breech extraction. The clavicle, humerus or femur may be fractured. Injury to the sternomastoid muscle, due to a haematoma, may occur following a difficult delivery. It should be looked for after any difficult delivery as unless treated by stretching the muscle, permanent shortening may result.

Congenital Defects, Per 1000 Births	
Major defects	**Per 1000 births**
Chromosomal (esp. Down's syndrome)	1–3
CNS defects:	
(a) Open neural tube defects	1–1.5
1. anencephaly	0.5
(b) 2. spina bifida	0.5
Hydrocephaly	0.3–0.6
CVS defects. Heart and great vessels	2–5
Gastro-intestinal defects:	
(a) Harelip, cleft palate	1–2
(b) Alimentary tract	
(esp. pyloric stenosis)	1–3
Urogenital defects	0.5–1
Skeletal defects:	1–3
Talipes	1–3
Congenital dislocated hip	2–4
Polydactyly, etc.	0.5–1
Multiple defects	0.5–1
MAJOR DEFECTS: TOTAL	15–28
MINOR DEFECTS (skin blemishes, etc)	2–15

Table 28.2 Congenital defects, per 1000 births. (Data from Australia, UK and Sweden.

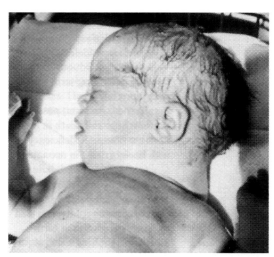

Fig 28.3 Down's syndrome.

CONGENITAL MALFORMATIONS

Congenital malformations affect between 1.5 and 3.5 per cent of all infants. These defects are major in about 2 per cent of all infants *(Table 28.2)*. More than 60 per cent of infants with congenital defects survive and benefit most growing up in a family, if this is possible. When the diagnosis has been established, the doctor should talk with the parents explaining the malformation and the prognosis, calmly and sympathetically. Most parents go though a grieving period. They may express anger and guilt, questioning if anything that they did or did not do during the pregnancy caused the fetal malformation. Most appreciate counselling sessions.

The major malformations are now described.

DOWN'S SYNDROME

Down's syndrome is the most common genetic defect. The infant has slanting eyes with epicanthic folds, short hands, small fingers, and feet with abnormal skin creases. The head is short, the cheeks fat, the back of the neck short and fat. The ears are squarish *(Fig. 28.3)*. Many Down's syndrome children have some degree of mental handicap.

The incidence of Down's syndrome increases with the age of the mother *(Fig. 28.4)*. As mentioned in Chapter 7, Down's syndrome can now be diagnosed in early pregnancy and termination offered.

Sex-linked genetic disorders can be diagnosed in early pregnancy by chorionic villus sampling .

CENTRAL NERVOUS SYSTEM DEFECTS

Anencephaly *(Fig. 28.5)* and spina bifida *(Fig. 28.6)* can be diagnosed in pregnancy as described on page 37. Hydrocephalus can be diagnosed in the second

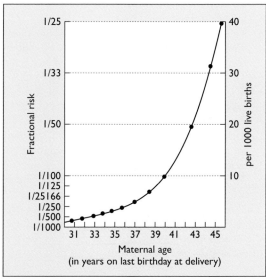

Fig 28.4 The rate of Down's syndrome in live births in relation to maternal age (from Cuckle, H.S. *et al.*, *Brit. Med. J.*, 1987; 94, 387–402).

half of pregnancy by ultrasound scanning, but may only be noticed when delivery is difficult.

CARDIOVASCULAR DEFECTS

Gross heart defects are usually demonstrated by cyanosis when the baby cries, and by marked cardiac thrills and murmurs. Care should be taken when a heart murmur is heard soon after birth as it may not be due to a congenital heart defect, because the murmur may be transient. A reassessment should be made before discharge from hospital and a paediatric consultation obtained if abnormal signs persist.

GASTROINTESTINAL DEFECTS

Harelip and *cleft palate* are obvious. *Oesophageal atresia* should be considered in the babies of women who had

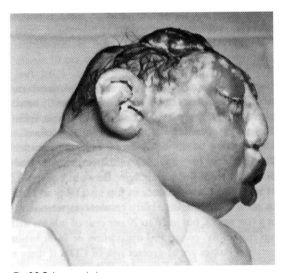

Fig 28.5 Anencephaly.

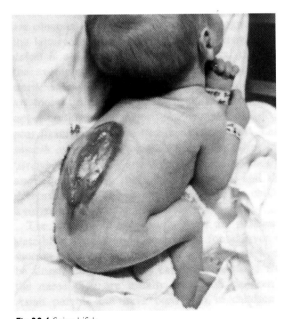

Fig 28.6 Spina bifida.

polyhydramnios. A size-9 catheter should be passed through the mouth along the oesophagus and an ultrasound examination made. Oral feeding should not be started until the condition has been excluded or treated surgically. *Duodenal stenosis* or atresia should be suspected if persistent bile-stained vomiting occurs. *Pyloric stenosis* should be suspected if the infant, usually male, has projectile vomiting in the 3rd to 6th week of life. If the infant is relaxed or feeding the hypertrophied pyloric muscle may be palpable.

UROGENITAL DEFECTS

Atresia of the kidneys

Atresia of the kidneys is rare and fatal. In 2 per cent of mature neonate males, and 20 per cent of preterm males, one or both testes will have failed to have descended into the scrotum. By the infant's first birthday less than 1 per cent of males have *undescended testes* (cryptorchidism). Surgical treatment is delayed until the child is 1.5–2.0 years old.

Circumcision

This is not required for medical reasons but some parents want it performed. Current advice is to delay circumcision until the infant is at least 10 days, and preferably 6 months, old. It should be performed under a local or a general anaesthetic.

SKELETAL DEFECTS

The most common skeletal disorders are *talipes calcaneus* (the foot is turned in and points down) and *talipes equinovarus* (the foot is turned out and points up). Usually no treatment other than gentle manipulation is needed. *Congenital dislocation* of the hip is characterized by an anteverted femoral head and neck and a shallow acetabulum from which the femoral head may be displaced partially or completely. Between 1 and 3 per cent of neonates show evidence of instability of the hip at birth but in most cases this resolves spontaneously within a week or two. In a few infants the defect persists. Examination of the newborn for congenital hip dislocation is described in Table 11.1, page 87. If congenital dislocation of the hip is confirmed, treatment should be withheld until the infant is 5 months old as 20 per cent of babies treated earlier relapse or develop dysplasia or avascular necrosis of the femoral head.

THE SKIN

Defects involving the bladder (*ectopia vesicae*) and umbilicus (*exomphalos*) are obvious at birth. The former has a poor prognosis but the latter may be treated surgically. *Angiomata* (port wine stains and strawberry marks) occur. Most defects regress spontaneously or can be treated by laser when the infant is older. *Mongolian blue spots* are patches of slate blue discoloration over the sacrum or lower spine; these occur particularly in Asian infants. They have no clinical significance.

METABOLIC DISORDERS

Cystic fibrosis affecting 1 baby in 2 000; *congenital hypothyroidism* affecting one baby in 6 000; and *phenylketonuria* affecting one baby per 10 000 can be detected by filter paper tests on blood samples taken on the 5th day of life. *Congenital adrenal hyperplasia* (1 in 10 000) can also be detected in the same way. The rare *amino-acid disorders* can be detected on a urine sample taken when an infant is 6 weeks old.

RISK OF RECURRENCE OF A CONGENITALLY AFFECTED BABY

A question of great concern to the parents of a congenitally affected baby is: 'What is the risk of our next baby being affected?'. Available data are shown in *Table 28.3*.

MATERNAL INGESTION OF DRUGS AFFECTING THE FETUS

Pregnant women should avoid taking medications as far as possible, since many pharmaceutical agents cross the placenta and may affect the fetus adversely. If a drug is required, the doctor should read the Product Information document before prescribing it. In some countries lists of drugs which should be avoided during pregnancy are obtainable from the Health Authorities.

CEREBRAL PALSY

Cerebral palsy is a descriptive term for a collection of non-progressive neuromotor disorders which are not the result of cerebral malformations. The condition affects between 1.5 and 3.5 per cent of all liveborn children. In most cases the cause of cerebral palsy is unknown, although low birth-weight infants have a greater risk of developing it. If the infant weighs less than 1500g at birth the risk is increased 25-fold. Birth trauma and hypoxia during labour (judged by a 5-minute Apgar score of 3 or less) are uncommon causes, and in many of these cases the cerebral palsy may have been due to intrinsic fetal defects rather than to events occurring during childbirth.

Clinically, cerebral palsy may not be detected in the early neonatal period, although 25 per cent of the victims have a seizure disorder at this time. The main clinical feature is a lack of motor control, usually presenting as spasticity, or less commonly as involuntary movements or muscle incoordination. Any muscle group may be affected, but quadriplegia and diplegia are seen most often. In 15 per cent of affected people, choreo-athetoid, dystonic or ataxic movements predominate. If bulbar involvement occurs, the person will have difficulty in articulating. Over half of the number of people who have cerebral palsy have normal intelligence.

The stress on the parents and on siblings is considerable, but much can be done to help them.

NEONATAL INFECTIONS

Any infant showing signs of infection should be isolated together with the mother until adequate treatment has controlled the infection. Infection may occur during pregnancy, as discussed in Chapter 19. During labour, infection may occur, particularly if the membranes have been ruptured for a long time; or from vaginal infection by group B streptococci (see page 134).

The common infections occurring after birth are:
- *Candida* spp which infects the infant's mouth, where it forms white patches.
- Staphylococcal infections which present as skin pustules, periumbilical infection, or blepharoconjunctivitis.
- *Chlamydia trachomatis* which may cause conjunctivitis, 1–3 weeks after birth, or pneumonia 3 weeks later.
- *E. coli* infections causing gastroenteritis or urinary tract infection (which is difficult to diagnose).

Any ill infant with unexplained fever should have a urine specimen, obtained by suprapubic puncture, examined, and if the diagnosis remains unclear, a chest x-ray and a lumbar puncture should be made to exclude meningitis.

Treatment is to give the appropriate antibiotic depending on local bacterial sensitivities and experience.

Risks of Recurrence of Some Congenital Defects			
Disorder	**Incidence** (per 100 births)	**Risk (per cent)** Normal parent having a second affected child	**Affected parent having an affected child**
Down's syndrome	0.2	1	–
Anencephaly	0.2	2	
Spina bifida	0.3	4	4
Cleft palate	0.04	2	7
Cleft lip and palate	0.1	4	4
Congenital heart disease	0.6	2	2

Table 28.3 Recurrence of congenital defects.

29

THE LOW BIRTH-WEIGHT INFANT

The intra-uterine growth and birth-weight of the fetus depends on its inherited growth potential and the effectiveness of the support to its growth provided by the uteroplacental environment. The latter is affected, in a general sense, by the health of the mother and the presence or absence of maternal disease.

Provided the growth support exceeds the growth potential, fetal intra-uterine growth will continue; but when the fetal growth potential is limited, as in the case of many malformed fetuses, or maternal growth support diminishes, as in cases of multiple pregnancy and maternal diseases, a deviation from the normal growth curve occurs. The deviations usually arise after the 30th gestational week and are most marked after the 35th week of pregnancy (Fig. 29.1).

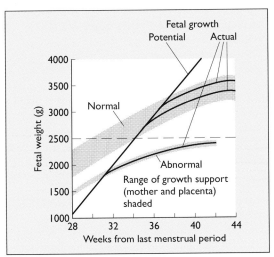

Fig 29.1 Fetal growth potential and maternal growth support.

Fetal growth retardation is identified if the estimated weight of the infant is >2 standard deviations below the mean; a low birth-weight baby is arbitrarily defined as weighing < 2500g at birth. This definition presents some problems, as the mean birth-weight of babies in many developing countries is less than for those in developed countries. For example, the mean birth-weight of a baby born to a poor woman in Tamil Nadu, India, is about 2800g compared with a mean birth-weight of 3400g in most developed countries. Defining low birth-weight as less than 2500g in southern India would place over 15 per cent of healthy infants in the low birth-weight category. The mean birth-weight of babies born to mothers living in developed countries at various gestational periods is shown in *Fig. 29.2*. The figure shows that the birth-weight of 2 500g is achieved at the end of the 35th week of pregnancy, and hospital statistics show that between 5 and 6 per cent of the infants weigh less than 2500g at birth, in other words have a low birth-weight.

Data are available from several developed countries which show the proportion of babies who are of low birth-weight, their perinatal mortality and the survival of those babies born alive *(Table 29.1)*. These data obscure the fact that low birth-weight babies comprise two populations: preterm (premature) babies; and small for gestational age babies.

Preterm babies have grown normally in the uterus but are born preterm, that is by definition, before the 37th week of gestation.

Small for gestational age (SGA) babies are also referred to as small-for-dates babies. This population of infants weighs less that their expected weight for a given gestational age, and comprise two groups. The growth potential of the first group has been low

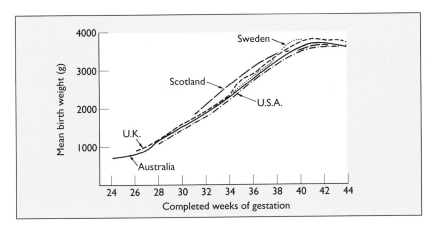

Fig 29.2 The mean birth-weight at various gestational ages in several developed nations. Note that the mean birth-weight at the end of the 35th gestational week is approximately 2500g.

Perinatal Mortality Related to Weight and Period of Gestation (UK, Australia 1975–85)				
Weight (g)	Gestation (in weeks)	Percentage of all births	Perinatal mortality (per 1000)	Live birth per cent survival
<500	All		990	<1
501–750	All	0.5	750	25
751–1000	All		500	50
1001–1500	All	0.5	250	75
1501–2000	less than 36		200	90
	more than 36	1.0	150	95
2001–2500	less than 36		100	95
	more than 36	5.0	50	98
2501–3000	All	18.0		
3001–3500	All	39.0	30	98
3501–4000	All	28.0		
>4000	All	8.0	50	95

Table 29.1 Perinatal mortality related to weight and period of gestation (UK, Ireland, Australia 1980–90).

at all gestational ages and they are light-for-dates, but otherwise healthy. The growth of the second group has faltered in utero, as detected by at least two measurements (usually by ultrasound scanning). These babies have suffered intra-uterine growth retardation and are at greater risk of dying, either in the uterus or in the neonatal period. The baby is wasted with little subcutaneous fat.

Risk Factors in the Incidence of Low Birth Weight Babies
Socioeconomic
Maternal age <17 or >35 Socioeconomic class IV or V Prepregnancy weight <50kg or >75kg Cigarette smoking Excessive alcohol consumption
Obstetric history
Previous low birth weight baby Maternal anaemia
Present pregnancy
Hypertensive disease (especially if severe) Antepartum haemorrhage Multiple pregnancy
Fetal
Congenital defects Intra-uterine infection

Table 29.2 Risk factors in the incidence of low birth weight babies.

Combinations of the two main populations may occur: a preterm baby may be small for dates.

AETIOLOGICAL FACTORS IN LOW BIRTH-WEIGHT

The common aetiological factors are shown in *Table 29.2*. It has to be said that in many cases no precise factor has been identified. The socioeconomic factors are the most amenable to change with a possible reduction in the proportion of low birth-weight babies born. However trials of supplemental nutrients, the frequency of antenatal visits, or antenatal education have not significantly reduced the proportion of low birth-weight infants born.

MANAGEMENT OF THE LOW BIRTH-WEIGHT INFANT

The birth-weight and gestational age of the infant predict its morbidity and mortality to a large extent. A special category of high-risk babies are those whose birth-weight is less than 1 500g – the Very Low Birth-Weight Baby.

The care of a low birth-weight baby should be conducted by a neonatologist, with the resources available in an intensive neonatal care unit. As mentioned in Chapter 21, a woman who goes into labour before the 35th week of pregnancy should, if possible, be transferred to a hospital with a level 3 nursery.

The objectives of management are:
- To provide an environment as close to the intra-uterine environment as possible.
- To prevent infection.
- To provide adequate nourishment.
- To detect and treat possible metabolic and other complications.

The best environment for a small baby is in a nursery maintained at a temperature of no less than 24°C, or if the infant is very small in an incubator maintained at a temperature of 26–32°C and a humidity of 65–75 per cent. Oxygen is provided via a head box or enters the incubator in a controlled manner.

Infection is controlled by careful attention to avoid overcrowding and medical attendants and others introducing infection into the nursery. Hand washing before handling a baby is the most important preventive measure.

Feeding is started about 6 hours after birth and breast milk is used as soon as possible. The baby is fed by gavage or spoon, and is put to the breast as soon as it suckles strongly. Vitamin supplements are given with or after feeding. Recommended daily doses are: vitamin D 400U; ascorbic acid 50mg; niacin 6mg; riboflavin 1mg; and vitamin A 5000U.

Complications may occur and can be listed:

- Hyaline membrane disease (see page 201).
- Cyanotic attacks, which may be due to inadequate ventilation of the lungs or cerebral damage.
- Jaundice (see page 87).
- Hypoglycaemia. This affects about 15 per cent of low birth-weight babies. For this reason regular checks of the infant's blood glucose are made until feeding has been established. If detected, glucose is given via intravenous infusion (6–9mg/kg/min).
- Hypocalcaemia may occur in very low birth-weight babies, usually in the first 24 hours of life. If the plasma calcium level is <2mmol/L, calcium gluconate is slowly given intravenously.
- Intracranial haemorrhage. Periventricular haemorrhage (intraventricular and/or parenchymal haemorrhage) occurs mainly in babies weighing 1500g or less, when about 20 per cent are affected. It is detected by real-time ultrasonography.

RETINOPATHY OF PREMATURITY

This disease of immature retinal vessels increases in incidence the lower the birth-weight of the infant, affecting over 40 per cent of infants weighing <1 500g at birth. In most cases, the disease is mild, but one infant in five who has retinopathy is severely affected. Excessive doses and prolonged exposure to oxygen is thought to be the main cause, but other factors are probably involved. Continuous monitoring of oxygen supply has helped to reduce the incidence of the disease, but cases continue to occur. Treatment of established severe cases is by cryotherapy or laser, applied transscleratally.

THE MORTALITY AND MORBIDITY OF LOW BIRTH-WEIGHT INFANTS

Low birth-weight infants contribute 70 per cent of early neonatal deaths; the smaller the infant the less is its chance of survival. With the development of special neonatal intensive care units, the mortality of these small babies has decreased. Few infants weighing 500g or less survive; 25 per cent of infants weighing 501–750g survive, as do 50 per cent of infants weighing 751-1000g. Babies weighing 1001–1500g have a 75 per cent chance of surviving and those weighing 1501–2499g have a 90–95 per cent survival rate.

The morbidity of the surviving infants has also decreased in recent years, the highest morbidity among infants whose birth-weight is less than 1000g. Examined at the age of 1 year, 20 per cent of these infants are severely disabled with cerebral palsy, blindness or deafness, and another 5–15 per cent have minor physical defects. By age 3, one in three of these children show a serious defect or are developmentally delayed or 'uncooperative'.

An ultrasound scan of the infant's brain, if normal, is highly predictive of a normal neurological development. However, considerable problems remain. For example, the disability rate of survivors who weighed <700g at birth is over 60 per cent. This raises an ethical question. Should the medical attendants persist with complex, expensive, traumatic procedures or, with the agreement of the parents, permit the infant to die peacefully?

30

DISORDERS OF MENSTRUATION

Menstruation is normal if it occurs at intervals of 22–35 days (from day 1 of menstruation to the onset of the next menstrual period) as mentioned in Chapter 2; if the duration of the bleeding is less than 7 days; and if the menstrual blood loss is less than 80ml. It was also noted that menstrual discharge consists of tissue fluid (20–40 per cent of the total discharge), blood (50–80 per cent) and fragments of the endometrium. However, to the woman menstrual discharge looks like blood and is so reported.

By convention the notation of menstruation and its disturbances is written as, for example, 5/28. This indicates that the woman bled for 5 days and that menstruation occurred at an interval of 28 days. The quantity of menstrual loss is entered as slight, normal or heavy.

Disorders of menstruation occur most commonly at each extreme of the reproductive years, that is under the age of 19 and over the age of 39. The disorder may relate to the length of the menstrual cycle, or to the amount and duration of the menstrual loss. A woman may have both disturbances.

CHANGES IN THE LENGTH OF THE MENSTRUAL CYCLE

Menstruation may occur at intervals longer than 35 days, when it is termed *oligomenorrhoea*; if menstruation does not occur for more than 70 days (in the absence of pregnancy) a diagnosis of *secondary amenorrhoea* is made. *Primary amenorrhoea* is diagnosed if menstruation has not commenced by the age of 16 years. Menstruation may also occur at intervals of less than 21 days when it is given the term *epimenorrhoea or polymenorrhoea*.

CHANGES IN THE AMOUNT OF MENSTRUAL LOSS

The quantity of menstrual discharge may vary, without altering the cyclicity of menstruation. Scanty or light menstrual discharge is termed *hypomenorrhoea*. Heavy 'bleeding' is termed *menorrhagia*. In menorrhagia there may be an excessive amount of blood lost, or the apparently heavy bleeding may be due to an increased loss of tissue fluid.

Menorrhagia may occur in association with an organic condition in the uterus, or may occur in the absence of any detectable uterine abnormality. In this case it is termed *dysfunctional uterine bleeding*.

DISTURBANCES IN CYCLICITY AND AMOUNT OF MENSTRUAL LOSS

In this disturbance the cyclicity of menstruation is lost, bleeding occurring at irregular intervals, the quantity of menstrual loss varying considerably. This pattern is termed *metrorrhagia*. Generally it indicates a local condition in the uterus.

AMENORRHOEA AND OLIGOMENORRHOEA

PRIMARY AMENORRHOEA

Primary amenorrhoea (affecting 5 per cent of amenorrhoeic women) may be due to a genetic defect such as gonadal dysgenesis in which case the secondary sexual characteristics will not have developed. It may be due to a Mullerian duct abnormality, such as an absent uterus, vaginal agenesis, a transverse vaginal septum, or an imperforate hymen. In the last three causes, menstruation may occur but the menstrual discharge cannot escape from the genital tract. The condition is *cryptomenorrhoea* rather than amenorrhoea. Rarely is testicular feminization the cause.

In many cases, however, no abnormality is found and the young woman may be expected to menstruate on time. Some of these women have an eating disorder or exercise compulsively.

SECONDARY AMENORRHOEA

The most common cause of **secondary amenorrhoea** is pregnancy but the condition may occur during the reproductive years from a variety of causes. In *Fig. 30.1* and *Table 30.1* the most common causes of amenorrhoea and their frequency are shown. Only these causes will be discussed in this chapter.

As noted in Chapter 2, normal menstruation depends on a normal uterus and vagina, and on the reciprocal interaction between hormones released from the hypothalamus (gonadotrophic releasing hormones), the pituitary (the gonadotrophins – follicle stimulating hormone (FSH) and luteinizing hormone (LH) and the ovaries (oestrogen and progesterone).

The investigation of secondary amenorrhoea

Unless organic disease is suspected or the woman is desperately seeking relief of infertility, most experts would not investigate amenorrhoea until it has lasted for 6–12 months, as most women start menstruating during this time.

When investigation is indicated, a careful history is essential, in which the doctor inquires about the woman's general health, seeks to determine if she has an eating disorder or exercises excessively, or if any medical or psychiatric condition is present. A physical examination, including a vaginal examination follows,

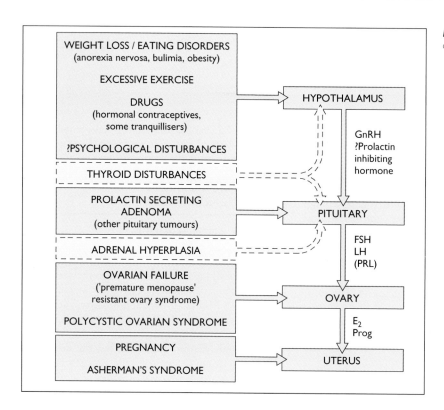

Fig 30.1 The aetiology of secondary amenorrhoea.

and a pelvic ultrasound examination may be made in certain cases. If these examinations reveal no definite diagnosis, the following tests are ordered.

- Hormone assays:
  (i) *FSH and LH.* An FSH level outside the normal range of the laboratory, confirmed by repeating the measurement indicates primary ovarian failure.
  (ii) *Prolactin (hPr).* A raised HPr level on two or more occasions indicates hyperprolactinaemia and makes a CAT scan of the pituitary obligatory.
  (iii) *TSH* (and serum T_4).
  (iv) *Oestradiol 17-beta.* This may be measured or a 'progestogen stimulation test' made.
- *Progestogen stimulation test.* The test seeks to determine if the uterus responds to progestogen withdrawal. Progesterone and progestogens will only provoke bleeding if there is sufficient circulating oestradiol (>150pmol\l). The test determines if the endometrium will respond and indirectly determines that the oestradiol is above a critical level. Medroxyprogesterone acetate 5mg is given daily for 5 days. If menstrual bleeding occurs within 7 days the test is positive, and clomiphene is likely to induce ovulation.
- X-ray of the pituitary fossa or a CT scan if the hPr level is raised, to exclude the presence of a pituitary tumour.

The purpose of the investigations is to exclude organic disease (for example, a prolactin-secreting microadenoma or hypothyroidism) and to treat anovulation as a cause of infertility. If organic disease is not detected and infertility is not a problem, amenorrhoea does not represent a danger to the woman, but because low oestrogen levels may lead to bone loss, after 6 months amenorrhoea hormone replacement treatment (see page 307) should be advised.

The sequence of investigations is shown in *Fig. 30.2.*

THE MORE COMMON CAUSES OF AMENORRHOEA
Weight loss

Women who have an eating disorder, particularly anorexia nervosa, cease to menstruate as do some women who are compulsive exercisers. The cause of the amenorrhoea is a failure of the hypothalamus to release sufficient gonadotrophic releasing hormone to initiate the release of gonadotrophins and in consequence, only a small quantity of oestrogen is secreted by the ovaries. If this persists for more than 6 months,

The Causes of Secondary Amenorrhoea (per cent)	
Weight loss	20–40
Polycystic ovaries	15–30
Pituitary insensitivity (post pill)	10–20
Hyperprolactinaemia	10–20
Primary ovarian failure	5–10
Asherman's syndrome	1–2
Hypothyroidism	1–2

Table 30.1 The causes of secondary amenorrhoea (per cent).

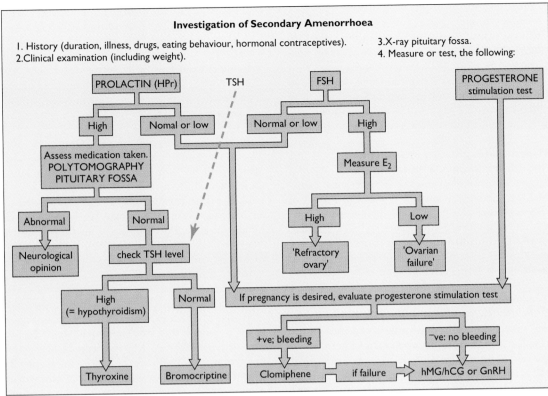

Fig 30.2 The investigation and treatment of secondary amenorrhoea.

bone loss may occur at a time when bone formation is reaching its peak. A consequence of this is a greater risk of osteoporosis in later life. Even during the recovery phase, menstruation may not occur for several months, which may aggravate the problem.

Hyperprolactinaemia and prolactin-secreting tumours

Prolactin secretion by the pituitary gland is inhibited, under normal conditions, by dopamine released from the hypothalamus. In certain circumstances, this control is diminished. Examples are: hypothyroidism, and the administration of dopamine depleting agents or dopamine receptor blocking agents. A more common cause of hyperprolactinaemia is a potential or actual microadenoma of the pituitary gland. In these cases, the increased circulating levels of prolactin act directly on the hypothalamus to reduce the secretion of gonadotrophic-releasing hormone (GnRH) which in turn prevents the FSH and LH rises needed for follicle development and ovulation.

In most cases of hyperprolactinaemia the only symptom is amenorrhoea, but occasionally oligomenorrhoea or hypomenorrhoea is present. In 30 per cent of women inappropriate milk secretion (galactorrhoea) occurs. In addition, some women show signs of hypoestrogenemia, complaining of vaginal dryness and reduced libido.

As hyperprolactinaemia accounts for about 20 per cent of cases of amenorrhoea, investigation is important. The diagnosis is made if a raised blood level of prolactin is found. If this is noted during investigation, a high-resolution CT scan of the pituitary is made to detect a prolactin secreting tumour, although in most cases none is found.

If a tumour is detected, a microadenoma (<10mm in diameter) is more common than a macroadenoma.

Treatment is needed if a macroadenoma is detected or if the woman desires to become pregnant, but in *all* cases of hyperprolactinaemia careful follow-up is needed as some women with this condition but no tumour eventually develop one. Women who have functional hyperprolactinaemia require assessment at 1–3 year intervals, when the level of prolactin in a blood sample is measured and a CT scan made. Women who have a microadenoma need to be assessed annually, but treatment is not required unless they are infertile or have marked symptoms of low circulating levels of oestradiol. In both these groups if amenorrhoea persists for more than 6 months, as is likely, hormone replacement treatment should be offered to prevent bone loss and the development of osteoporosis.

If a macroadenoma is detected, treatment is to prescribe a dopamine agonist such as bromocriptine in a dose which reduces the prolactin levels to the normal range and maintains them in these.

Surgery is only indicated if bromocriptine treatment fails. During treatment and after ceasing to take the drug, regular measurements of serum prolactin and an annual CT scan are mandatory.

A patient who has a macroadenoma should avoid becoming pregnant until the tumour has shrunk to lie completely within the pituitary fossa as shown by a CT scan, as the tumour may grow during pregnancy.

Hypothalamic pituitary insensitivity: 'hypothalamic amenorrhoea'

In about one-third of cases of amenorrhoea, hypothalamic–pituitary insensitivity is postulated. Many of these cases coincidentally follow the use of oral contraceptives, but eating disorders may also be involved, as may psychosomatic factors; for example, change of work, marital disharmony or separation. Severe depression or acute or chronic illness may be factors.

Treatment of hypothalamic amenorrhoea

If the amenorrhoea has persisted for 9–12 months and anovulation is the only or the main cause of the couple's infertility, ovulation may be induced in 80 per cent of women by using clomiphene, especially if the progestogen test is positive. Clomiphene is an antioestrogen (which may sometimes act as a weak oestrogen). It acts by binding on to oestrogen receptors in target cells, thus preventing oestradiol binding to them. Transferred to the cell nucleus, it renders the cells relatively insensitive to the effects of endogenous oestradiol. This inhibits the negative feedback with the release of GnRH and subsequently FSH and LH. The regimen for clomiphene use is shown in *Table 30.2*.

Should anovulation persist in spite of the clomiphene regimen, the patient should be referred to an infertility specialist, as laboratory control is needed if other drugs regimens are used.
The regimens are:
- Human menopausal gonadotrophin (hMG, Humegon, Pergonal) and human chorionic gonadotrophin (hCG, Pregnyl, Profasi).
- Gonadotrophic releasing hormone (GnRH) or one of its analogues.

The details of the treatments can be found in books about infertility as shown in the Bibliography.

Using these treatments about 90 per cent of women with amenorrhoea and 40 per cent of women with oligomenorrhoea will ovulate, and 70 per cent and 25 per cent will conceive. A number of women continue to ovulate after the treatments have ceased and become pregnant.

Polycystic ovarian syndrome (PCO)

The ovary contains multiple (>4) immature and atretic follicles (not cysts in spite of the name), which are aligned near the surface, often in a necklace-like formation. Oligomenorrhoea or amenorrhoea is usual and may be associated with hirsutism, acne, infertility and sometimes obesity. The aetiology of PCO is unknown, but an increase in insulin resistance and inappropriate gonadotrophin stimulation of the ovaries has been postulated.

A diagnostic problem has arisen with the increased use of transvaginal ultrasound to image pelvic organs. Using this technique, about 20 per cent of normally menstruating women have been found to have >15 subcapsular follicles, measuring 2-10mm in diameter). In addition, three-quarters of women who have bulimia nervosa have been found to have either multiple small ovarian follicles (MFO) or PCO. It is possible that chaotic eating, particularly of carbohydrates, leads to insulin resistance, which in turn indirectly causes PCO.

A key feature of PCO is that there is an increased level of luteinizing hormone. This may lead to hypertrophy of the theca interna with an increased secretion by the ovaries of androstenedione and to a lesser extent testosterone. The high level of LH may also prevent the proper maturation of oocytes when they complete the first meiotic division. This may account for the infertility of some women who have PCO.

The diagnosis of PCO is made on the case history and confirmed by transvaginal ultrasound and the finding of a raised LH:FSH ratio.

Therapeutic Regimen Using Clomiphene to Induce Ovulation		
Stage	Month	Dose
1	1	Clomiphene 50mg daily for 5 days
2	2	Clomiphene 100mg daily for 5 days
3	3	Clomiphene 150mg daily for 5 days
4	4	Clomiphene 200mg daily for 5 days
5	6-8	No treatment
6	9	Clomiphene 100mg daily for 5 days + HCG 5000 IU 7 days later
7	10	Clomiphene 150mg daily for 5 days + HCG 5000 IU 7 days later

Table 30.2 Therapeutic regimen using clomiphene to induce ovulation.

Treatment depends on the presenting symptom and on the wishes of the woman. If there are no symptoms no treatment is indicated. If hirsutism is a problem this is treated appropriately (see page 228), as is obesity. In most cases the reason for visiting a doctor is infertility, and the treatment is that described for hypothalamic–pituitary dysfunction.

Uterine abnormalities

Surgical removal of the uterus, endometrial ablation or radiation results in amenorrhoea. Excessive curettage (particularly following an abortion or postpartum) may act in the same way as endometrial ablation, producing amenorrhoea by removing the basal endometrial layer and permitting synechiae to form (Asherman's syndrome). The diagnosis is made by hysteroscopy, transvaginal ultrasound scanning or from a hysterogram. Treatment is considered later.

Primary gonadal (ovarian) failure

The cause of primary ovarian failure in most cases is unknown. In this condition the ovarian follicles disappear before the age of 40, and the woman reaches a premature menopause. In other women the follicles persist but the woman develops autoantibodies which mask the gonadotrophin receptors in the ovaries so that the gonadotrophins can no longer bind to them. These women may have a premature menopause, but some months or years later inexplicably, the woman ovulates and menstruates – the 'resistant ovarian syndrome'. Treatment is to provide hormone replacement to control menopausal symptoms and to prevent bone loss and cardiovascular sequelae (see page 306). If the woman wishes to have a child, she may enter an assisted conception programme and receive a donor ovum.

MENORRHAGIA

Menorrhagia may be due to an organic cause, but in most cases is dysfunctional, in other words due to an alteration in the endocrine or local endometrial control of menstruation (see page 11). Organic causes include: uterine myomata, particularly if the myoma is intramural or submucous and distorts the endometrial cavity; diffuse internal endometriosis (adenomyosis); endometrial polyps and rarely, chronic pelvic infection (pelvic inflammatory disease); a blood dyscrasia; and hypothyroidism. If the clinician thinks hypothyroidism is a possible diagnosis TSH and free T_4 levels should be measured. Treatment in these cases is directed to the cause.

INVESTIGATION

A careful history and a physical examination should be made and from this specific laboratory tests be ordered. These include a full blood picture, including a coagulation screen if indicated and possibly tests for thyroid function.

These tests may be sufficient to reach a diagnosis, but if the woman is over the age of 35 it is usual to investigate further.

The additional tests are:hysteroscopy and endometrial biopsy, endometrial sampling, transvaginal ultrasound scanning and diagnostic curettage.

Hysteroscopy

Using a hysteroscope the uterine cavity can be inspected and abnormalities such as endometrial polyps, or submucous myomata can be detected and often removed; in addition an endometrial sample can be taken for histological examination. Hysteroscopy is an office procedure which can be performed either with or without a local anaesthetic.

Endometrial sampling (biopsy)

Endometrial sampling (biopsy) is made by introducing a narrow biopsy curette through the uterine cervix and obtaining a representative sample of the endometrium. The procedure can take place in the doctor's office.

Transvaginal ultrasound

This procedure has been suggested as a non-invasive method of imaging the uterine cavity. The presence of submucous myomata can be detected and the width of the endometrium measured. An endometrium more than 5mm wide in a postmenopausal woman indicates the need for a curettage to exclude endometrial pathology.

Diagnostic curettage

The procedure is invasive and is performed under general anaesthesia. It requires admission to hospital as a day case. It is performed between bleeding episodes. The entire endometrium is curetted and sent for histological examination. It is being replaced by hysteroscopy and endometrial sampling.

DIAGNOSIS

If no organic cause for menorrhagia is found, a diagnosis of **dysfunctional uterine bleeding (DUB)** is made. In these cases the immediate cause of the menorrhagia is thought to be that there is reduced vasoconstriction and a lack of platelet aggregation, hence the haemostatic plugs occluding the endometrial blood vessels are less effective in achieving haemostasis. These changes may reflect increased prostacyclin and prostaglandin E_2 secretion by the endometrium. Studies have shown that DUB is more common under the age of 19 and after the age of 39.

DYSFUNCTIONAL UTERINE BLEEDING

The importance of an accurate menstrual history cannot be overstated. If the patient is agreeable, and the bleeding is not too severe, or if she has not recorded a menstrual history herself, it is helpful if she records the duration of, the interval between, and the perceived amount of menstrual discharge for a 3-month period. This last is difficult for a woman to measure as it is usually overestimated. Ideally the actual blood loss should be determined (by collecting all pads and tampons and measuring the haemoglobin content by the alkaline haematin method) but this is not practical except in a research programme. Certain clinical pointers help. These are: the occurrence of 'flooding'; saturation of tampons or pads or changing pads every 1/2 to 2 hours; the presence of large blood clots; and a prolonged duration of the menstrual period.

Although dysfunctional uterine bleeding is usually regular, the duration of the menstrual cycle may be increased so that the menorrhagia occurs less frequently. In this group of cases, which are usually found at the extremes of the reproductive period, oestrogen secretion may be less than usual and is not opposed by progesterone. In other words the bleeding is *anovulatory*. In other cases the unopposed oestrogen levels are high, resulting in an increased thickness of the endometrium, causing *cystic hyperplasia (Fig. 30.3)*.

Fluctuations in the circulating levels of oestrogen tend to occur, resulting in lack of 'support' for the endometrium leading to cyclical, profuse bleeding. In other cases, the heavy bleeding occurs at shorter intervals, the cycle length being reduced. This is referred to as *polymenorrhagia*. The treatment of these variants is the same as that of dysfunctional uterine bleeding.

TREATMENT OF DYSFUNCTIONAL UTERINE BLEEDING

Patients seen during a severe bleeding episode

In this situation treatment may be required urgently. Two methods are available: to perform a curettage; and to administer hormones. The hormones usually chosen are combined equine oestrogens (CEE), 25mg given intravenously and repeated 4-hourly for 6 doses. CEE in this dosage may cause marked nausea in some women. Once CEE has stopped the bleeding, a progestogen must be given for 14 days to induce secretory change and then endometrial shedding. An alternative to CEEE is to give 17-hydroxyprogesterone acetate 125–250 mg intramuscularly, or oral norethisterone 20–30 mg each day in divided doses, for 4 days. If a progestogen is used, a withdrawal bleed may be expected 3–6 days later. This can be avoided if norethisterone (5–10 mg daily) is continued for 20 days.

Patients seen between bleeding episodes

In this situation several choices are available. They should be discussed with the woman as her wishes

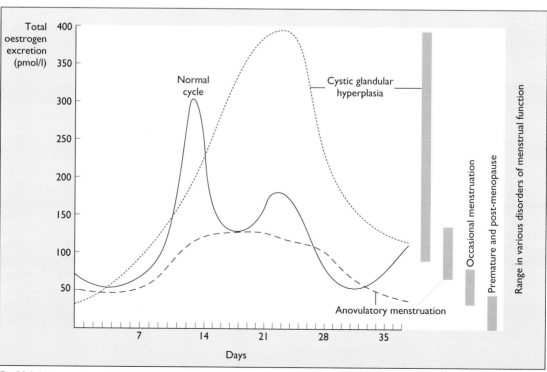

Fig 30.3 Urinary oestrogen excretion (in ug/24 hours) in certain gynaecological conditions related to the menstrual cycle.

and concerns should be addressed before treatment is instituted. The choices fall into two main groups: (1) hormonal treatment and (2) surgical treatment.

Hormonal treatment

This consists of:

- *Progestogens.* Either norethisterone (5–15mg daily) or medroxyprogesterone acetate (10mg twice or three times daily) is given from day 5 to day 25 of the menstrual cycle. A new progestogen, gestrinone 2.5mg twice weekly is also being used. The treatment should be continued for 4–6 menstrual cycles.
- *Oral contraceptives.* If the bleeding is not too severe, a monophasic, progestogen dominant hormonal contraceptive may be chosen.
- *Danazol.* This hormone in a dose of 200mg a day may be chosen. If this dose does not control the bleeding it is increased to 400mg a day. At these doses side effects such as lassitude, weight gain, muscle pains and acne are uncommon but may occur. Danazol is expensive, but is highly effective in courses of no more than 6 months.
- *A levonorgestrel intrauterine device* is being trialled. This device releases 20μg of levonorgestrel a day and is effective for 5 years. As well as regulating the menorrhagia it is an effective contraceptive. The menorrhagia is cured within 3 months in 90 per cent of women.

Surgical treatment

Curettage. Before the availability of hormones or the newer surgical treatments, curettage was the only treatment of menorrhagia, apart from hysterectomy. Curettage controlled heavy bleeding for a short time but it usually recurred in 4 to 6 months.

Endometrial ablation. The concept of this procedure is that by ablating the basal layer of the endometrium, endometrial regeneration is prevented or reduced and the menorrhagia is cured. Endometrial ablation should only be performed by a gynaecologist experienced in the technique, or the results will be poor and the women may be at risk of severe complications. Before endometrial ablation is performed the cavity of the uterus is inspected with a hysteroscope. Many gynaecologists prescribe danazol 200mg two or three times a day for 4 weeks before the operation or a GnRH analogue; for example, depot leuprolide 7.5mg, 4 weeks before the procedure to reduce endometrial thickness. Endometrial ablation may be performed using 'roller ball' electrocoagulation, loop resection or by laser, after distending and flushing the uterine cavity with a glycine mixture. If laser is chosen the uterine cavity is continuously flushed with a sodium chloride infusion system. An alternative is to use radiofrequency induced thermal endometrial ablation. In this method the uterine cavity is not distended with fluid.

The procedures are not without problems. In 1 per cent of cases the uterine wall is perforated. Glycine and sodium chloride are absorbed into the vascular system and may cause fluid overload, pulmonary oedema, and hyponatraemia.

The different methods produce similar results: 30–60 per cent of women become amenorrhoeic; 35–60 per cent become hypomenorrhoeic and the remaining 5–15 per cent require a repeat of the procedure or a hysterectomy. Interviewed up to 2 years after the procedure, three-quarters of women express satisfaction, the remainder complaining of persistent menstruation, dysmenorrhoea or pelvic pain.

The benefits of endometrial ablation are that it is less invasive and painful than hysterectomy; the woman is in hospital for 1–2 days rather than 7–10 days and it is less expensive. The woman should be convalescent for 3–7 days. The procedures must still be considered experimental and the patient informed of this.

Hysterectomy. Whilst there is no argument that hysterectomy is an appropriate operation in many cases of uterine myomata, advanced endometriosis, uterine malignancy and in some cases of pelvic infection, its position in the treatment of dysfunctional uterine bleeding is not so clear. Although many women welcome hysterectomy for the relief of a distressing symptom, others believe that hysterectomy diminishes their femininity. The importance of this observation is that a woman must have the opportunity to discuss the choices for the treatment of menorrhagia, and be given time to reflect, if hysterectomy is recommended to her. There is rarely any need for an 'urgent' hysterectomy, and once the operation has been recommended by a gynaecologist, it may be helpful for the woman to talk with her general practitioner about the benefits of and problems related to the operation. These matters are discussed further on page 220.

METRORRHAGIA

In metrorrhagia. the bleeding is irregular in quantity, acyclical in character and often prolonged in duration. The condition is usually due to a pathological condition in the uterus or other internal genital organs. It presence demands that the doctor investigate further. The investigations include either a hysteroscopy and endometrial biopsy or a diagnostic curettage. Treatment is directed to the underlying cause. Hysterectomy is often appropriate.

OTHER DISTURBANCES OF MENSTRUATION

In some women the duration of the cycle is shortened to less than 21 days (*polymenorrhoea*). Most women have no concern about this, but if the change is annoying, the menstrual period can be regulated by prescribing an oral contraceptive.

Some women complain of *slight menstrual staining* occurring either two or three days before or following the end of a normal menstrual period. Apart from being annoying, the condition has no sinister consequences, although some doctors believe that premenstrual staining is a sign of endometriosis. The woman should be reassured, but if she requests treatment menstruation is usually regulated by prescribing oral contraceptives or norethisterone 2.5mg from day 20–25 of the menstrual cycle for a few months.

Another concern of some women is that the amount of menstrual discharge has decreased. The condition, known as *hypomenorrhoea*, occurs most commonly in women taking oral contraceptives. The woman should be reassured that it has no abnormal consequences.

31

PSYCHOSOMATIC AND PHYSICAL DISORDERS OF THE MENSTRUAL CYCLE

In the proliferative phase of the menstrual cycle few problems occur. Some women experience pain in the lower abdomen which is unilateral and occurs at the time of ovulation. The pain is usually not severe and lasts for about 12 hours or less. The condition is called *mittleschmerz*. It indicates that ovulation has occurred, but investigations show no intra abdominal pathology. If mittleschmerz is recurrent and distressing, relief can be obtained if the woman takes a hormonal contraceptive.

MOOD AND PHYSICAL SYMPTOMS IN THE MENSTRUAL CYCLE

Most women in the reproductive years experience some psychological (negative mood) or physical symptoms in the luteal phase of the menstrual cycle. The symptoms vary in character and tend to become worse as menstruation approaches. They do not occur in every cycle and may vary in intensity in different cycles. A few women have severe mood and physical symptoms; a diagnosis of premenstrual syndrome may be made in these cases.

PREDOMINANTLY PSYCHOSOMATIC DISORDERS

PREMENSTRUAL SYNDROME (LATE LUTEAL PHASE DYSPHORIC DISORDER, DSM-III-R)

In 5–15 per cent of women, who are usually aged in their late twenties or early thirties (range 20–40 years) the negative mood and physical changes occurring in the luteal phase are of sufficient severity to affect a woman's day-to-day living and her social and personal relationships, particularly with her partner or children, most or all months. With the onset of menstruation or during it, the symptoms disappear. During the postmenstrual period, for at least a week, the woman feels well, often euphoric. With or soon after ovulation the symptoms reappear. The condition is the *premenstrual syndrome (PMS)*.

The symptoms vary in character and in severity in different menstrual cycles, but are always cyclic, a symptom-free interval occurring. The most common symptoms are shown in *Table 31.1*. The mood changes tend to cluster together and can be grouped into one defined factor – general negative mood. The physical symptoms cluster into two groups. First: breast symptoms, abdominal fullness, increased appetite and food cravings; and a second group which starts during the one to two days before menstruation. The symptoms include: abdominal discomfort or pain, headache, backache, lassitude, decreased appetite and menstrual cramps. This second group may be identified as the *perimenstrual syndrome*.

The diagnosis of PMS

The diagnosis of PMS is made after evaluating the periodicity of the physical and mood symptoms, ascertaining that there is a symptom-free period after menstruation and ensuring that the symptoms cannot be explained by some other illness.

The suspected diagnosis should be confirmed by asking the woman to complete a daily record of symptoms over three menstrual cycles (see Fig. 31.1). As well as establishing a firm diagnosis, the value of the daily record is that the woman develops an insight into her symptoms and is encouraged by the fact that the medical practitioner has an interest in her problems.

The aetiology of PMS

The aetiology of PMS is unknown. There may be a genetic component, but the current theory is that PMS is multifactorial. One underlying abnormality may be a fluctuation in the levels of oestradiol in the luteal phase which may cause the symptoms directly or by decreasing brain serotonin activity. A problem in accepting this theory is that no consistent fluctuations have been detected with daily monitoring.

The management of PMS

The importance of obtaining an ongoing therapeutic relationship with the woman cannot be underestimated. Once this has been established, explanation

Symptoms Associated With PMS	
Symptoms	
Mood (Emotional)	**Physical**
Irritability	Abdominal bloating
Anxiety	Abdominal discomfort, tenderness or pain
Nervous tension	Breast swelling, tenderness or pain
Depression (feeling sad or blue)	Feeling of weight gain
Lethargy, exhaustion, mood swings, aggression, panic	Oedema
Confusion	Headache
Craving for sweet foods	Backache
	Nausea

Table 31.1 Symptoms associated with PMS.

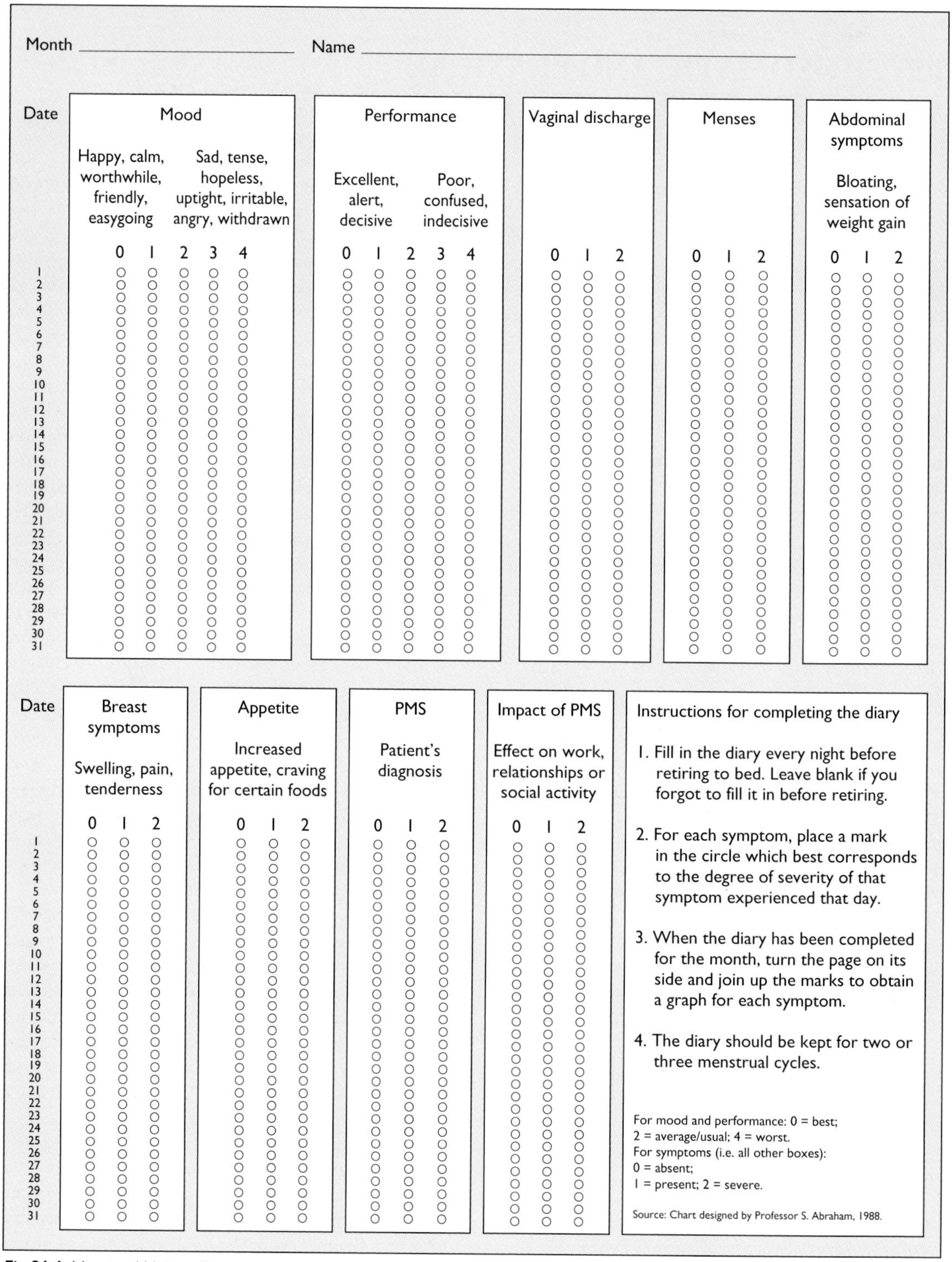

Month _____ Name _____

Mood

Happy, calm, worthwhile, friendly, easygoing — Sad, tense, hopeless, uptight, irritable, angry, withdrawn

0 1 2 3 4

Performance

Excellent, alert, decisive — Poor, confused, indecisive

0 1 2 3 4

Vaginal discharge

0 1 2

Menses

0 1 2

Abdominal symptoms

Bloating, sensation of weight gain

0 1 2

Date: 1–31 (rows of circles for marking)

Breast symptoms

Swelling, pain, tenderness

0 1 2

Appetite

Increased appetite, craving for certain foods

0 1 2

PMS

Patient's diagnosis

0 1 2

Impact of PMS

Effect on work, relationships or social activity

0 1 2

Date: 1–31 (rows of circles for marking)

Instructions for completing the diary

1. Fill in the diary every night before retiring to bed. Leave blank if you forgot to fill it in before retiring.

2. For each symptom, place a mark in the circle which best corresponds to the degree of severity of that symptom experienced that day.

3. When the diary has been completed for the month, turn the page on its side and join up the marks to obtain a graph for each symptom.

4. The diary should be kept for two or three menstrual cycles.

For mood and performance: 0 = best; 2 = average/usual; 4 = worst.
For symptoms (i.e. all other boxes):
0 = absent;
1 = present; 2 = severe.

Source: Chart designed by Professor S. Abraham, 1988.

Fig 31.1 Menstrual history diary.

and counselling will be accepted. The woman's lifestyle should be explored and suggestions made to reduce 'stress'. The predominant symptoms should be identified from the completed charts and treatment directed to specific problems.

Several medications have been tried *(Table 31.2)*, but in spite of enthusiastic reports none has proved better than placebo. If altered serotonin levels are relevant, the use of fluoxetine, a selective serotonin uptake inhibitor, may relieve the

Medications Used to Treat PMS	
Bromocriptine	2.5mg twice daily (This may relieve breast symptoms but has no other benefit)
Diuretics	Including spironolactone
Dydrogesterone	10mg twice daily
Evening primrose oil	
Fluoxetine	
Mefenamic acid	250mg 4 times daily (this may relieve the symptoms of the perimenstrual syndrome)
Progesterone	(vaginal suppositories) 200–800mg daily
Pyridoxine	(vitamin B6) up to 300 mg a day, a dose which may produce peripheral neuropathy.

* These drugs are prescribed from 2 days before symptoms are expected until the onset of menstruation

Table 31.2 Medications used to treat PMS.

symptoms in some women. A recent pilot study shows that the drug may be effective.

The concept that PMS is associated with diurnal fluctuations of oestradiol is also being investigated. Three approaches for women who have severe intractable PMS have been suggested. The first is to prescribe a hormonal contraceptive. The Pill (not a triphasic pill) has been prescribed for some years with varying rates of success in relieving PMS. More recently transdermal oestrogen patches, or an oestrogen implant have been prescribed. In these cases the woman has to be protected from the development of endometrial carcinoma from unopposed oestrogen and a progestogen is prescribed cyclically. During the period when the progestogen is taken, symptoms of PMS may recur. The third approach is radical. It is either to suppress ovarian activity with GnRH agonists or to perform a bilateral oophorectomy (and total hysterectomy).

THE PERIMENSTRUAL SYNDROME

Women with this syndrome complain of symptoms which occur within 2 days of the onset of menstruation, the earlier part of the menstrual cycle being symptom-free or may exhibit symptoms of PMS.

The most common mood symptoms are lassitude and headache. The most common physical symptoms are abdominal discomfort and bloating, pelvic pressure and dysmenorrhoea. A few women may develop severe premenstrual migraine. The symptoms may vary in character and intensity in different menstrual cycles. They cease within 48 hours of the onset of menstruation.

Treatment when requested is to prescribe one of the non-steroidal anti-inflammatory drugs.

IRRITABLE BOWEL SYNDROME

A number of PMS sufferers also have irritable bowel symptoms. The irritable bowel syndrome affects 15 per cent of women aged 20–60, although only 1–2 per cent seek medical help.

Normally, bursts of regular, powerful, propulsive contractions move the faeces along the bowel. Patients with the irritable bowel syndrome have exaggerated patterns of bowel motility, the bursts of activity occurring at shorter or longer intervals. The cause of the bowel motility dysfunction is unknown, but as there is a strong psychosomatic element, the medical practitioner should explore if the woman is depressed, anxious or has a sexual problem. The patient complains of abdominal pain, usually left-sided, which is relieved by defaecation, gaseous abdominal distention, an alteration in bowel habit and episodes of diarrhoea alternating with constipation. Investigations should be made to exclude organic disease, and the faeces should be examined for occult blood, giardiasis and other parasites.

Treatment

Treatment is unsatisfactory, unless a clear cause (for example giardiasis) has been detected. Patients should review their diet to find if any foods cause 'gas'. If the predominant symptom is pain and diarrhoea, loperidine or codeine phosphate may help. Support and explanation are required.

CHRONIC PELVIC PAIN

A few women complain of chronic pain in the lower abdomen and pelvis which fluctuates in intensity and tends to increase in the premenstruum. It may occur on either side of the abdomen and may be felt on different sides at different times. The woman may also complain of deep dyspareunia or a postcoital pelvic ache which may last for 24 hours. The woman may have a history of several episodes of 'pelvic inflammatory disease' which have been diagnosed on clinical findings rather than by laparoscopy and she may have had episodes of pelvic surgery.

The diagnosis is made after excluding organic causes of chronic pelvic pain such as adenomyosis, endometriosis and pelvic inflammatory disease, which are present in about one-third of cases. This fact indicates that laparoscopy is mandatory to make a diagnosis. The procedure should be made during menstruation to disclose endometriotic lesions deep in the cul de sac when the lesion is most likely to be seen. At laparoscopy although the pelvis shows no evidence of disease a venogram via the uterus may occasionally show varicosities in the broad ligament.

Treatment

The investigations themselves may constitute a form of treatment, as in one study of 60 women, in whom laparoscopy showed no pathology, 90 per cent of the patients assessed 6 months later said that since the laparoscopy they had no pelvic pain or that there was much less pain.

The woman's psychological, marital and psychosexual problems need to be explored and supportive psychotherapy offered. If the woman asks for medications, medroxyprogesterone in a dose of 30mg a day may be prescribed. An alternative is to prescribe danazol 200mg three times daily for 2 or 3 months, although the side effects may deter the woman from taking this treatment.

PREDOMINANTLY PHYSICAL DISORDERS

DYSMENORRHOEA

Dysmenorrhoea means painful menstruation. Two types are described: primary or spasmodic dysmenorrhoea; and secondary dysmenorrhoea.

Primary dysmenorrhoea

This form usually starts 2 or 3 years after the menarche and is maximal between the ages of 15 and 25. It decreases with age and usually ceases after childbirth. The crampy pains start during the 24 hours before menstruation, and may last 24–36 hours, although they are only severe for the first 24 hours. The cramps are felt in the lower abdomen, but may radiate to the back or down the inner surface of the thighs. In severe cases vomiting or diarrhoea may accompany the cramps.

Spasmodic dysmenorrhoea is experienced by 60–75 per cent of young women. In three-quarters of affected women the cramps are of minor or moderate severity, but in 25 per cent they are severe and incapacitating.

The aetiology of spasmodic dysmenorrhoea has now been clarified. When progesterone is secreted following ovulation, the luteinized endometrium is able to synthesize prostaglandins. If the balance between prostacyclin, which causes vasodilatation and myometrial relaxation, prostaglandin $F_{2\alpha}$, which causes vasoconstriction and myometrial contraction, and prostaglandin E_2 which causes myometrial contraction and vasodilatation is disturbed, so that $PGF_{2\alpha}$ predominates, myometrial ischaemia (uterine angina) and uterine hypercontractility occur. In addition, vasopressin is involved in dysmenorrhoea. Vasopressin increases prostaglandin synthesis and may act on the uterine arteries directly.

Treatment. Treatment is either to suppress ovulation by prescribing an oral contraceptive or to prescribe one of the prostaglandin synthetase inhibitors (NSAIDS), such as mefenamic acid, ibubrufen, diclofenac sodium or naproxen. There appears to be little difference in their effectiveness.

Oral contraceptives. These may be preferred by a woman who is sexually active as the pill will protect her against an unwanted pregnancy as well as relieving the dysmenorrhoea.

NSAIDS. NSAIDS may be preferred by women who do not wish to use hormones and prefer to take medication for as short a time as possible. The chosen medication is taken at the first sign of pain and continued for up to 5 days.

Dysmenorrhoea is relieved in 95 per cent of cases, whether oral contraceptives or NSAIDS are chosen. If the chosen treatment fails to relieve the dysmenorrhoea, an alternative can be tried.

Secondary dysmenorrhoea

Secondary or acquired dysmenorrhoea is unusual before the age of 25 and uncommon before the age of 30. In most cases the underlying cause is either endometriosis or pelvic inflammatory disease. Typically the cramps start 2 or more days prior to menstruation, and the pain increases in severity until late menstruation when it peaks, taking 2 or more days to cease. The management is that of the primary condition.

TOXIC SHOCK SYNDROME

This syndrome which is due to an endotoxin released by *Staphylococcus aureus* may occur in women who use tampons for menstrual protection. The reported annual incidence is <1:25000 tampon users. Toxic shock may also occur in males and in children when it follows infected surgical wounds, furuncles or other skin infections. It is characterized by the acute onset of fever >38.9°C, sore throat, headache, aching muscles, dizziness and, sometimes, watery diarrhoea. The woman may develop shock. A rash develops on the skin 3 days after the onset of the disease; later dandruff-like desquamation of the skin occurs, which is followed a week later by epidermal sloughing of skin from the hands and feet. Treatment is to restore blood volume and to prescribe penicillinase-resistant antibiotics such as flucloxacillin. As the syndrome is associated, although rarely, with tampon use, tampons should be changed 4-hourly, and a pad used at night.

PSYCHOSOMATIC PROBLEMS AFTER HYSTERECTOMY

In recent years the frequency of hysterectomy has fallen as other methods of treatment for conditions previously treated by hysterectomy have been developed. The psychosomatic effects of the operation depend on the condition which led to the hysterectomy, and the woman's knowledge of and attitude to hysterectomy. Some women recover quickly (after the first 24–48 hours when pain may be severe).

Other women are mildly or moderately incapacitated for up to 3 months. One-third of women take three months to recover fully from the operation, and 20 per cent take longer. Five to ten per cent of women feel well generally but have bowel or bladder symptoms, particularly genuine stress incontinence, which may persist for months.

Some women feel mutilated after hysterectomy and develop an anxiety state. This is more likely to occur if the woman believes that her body image, her femininity and sexual atttactiveness are reduced after the operation. The anxiety that her sexual attractiveness will be decreased follows misconceptions about hysterectomy. These include that:

- a woman will be unable to have or enjoy sexual intercourse because her vagina is shorter.
- she will become obese.
- she will be severely depressed after the operation.
- she will become postmenopausal.

The patient should be reassured about the first two misconceptions before the operation takes place. The third misconception is untrue. There is no evidence that hysterectomy increases clinical depression, unless the woman had psychiatric morbidity prior to surgery. The fourth misconception is only likely to be true if she has her ovaries removed at the operation, or if the surgeon has damaged the ovarian blood supply. There is information that up to 20 per cent of women aged 40–45 experience ovarian failure within 3 years of hysterectomy. However, this and menopausal symptoms following bilateral oophorectomy at the time of hysterectomy can be eliminated if the woman is offered hormone replacement treatment (see p 307).

The question of bilateral oophorectomy of normal ovaries at the time of hysterectomy is contentious. Ovarian extirpation is not usually carried out in women aged less than 45 but some gynaecologists perform it in older women. Their reasons for oophorectomy are first, that if the ovaries are left 1 in 1000 women will develop ovarian cancer, and second, the ovaries have no function after the menopause. The woman should make her own decision, after discussion with her doctors and after she has had time to think it over and seek other advice if she wishes.

Hysterectomy is safe today, but it is not without mortality. A nationwide epidemiological study in Denmark in 1990 of hysterectomy for non-cancerous conditions, where no major 'co-surgery' took place, showed that the 30-day mortality rate, although only 16 per 10 000 cases, was four times as high as for a reference group. This finding suggests that if an alternative to hysterectomy is available (as it is in cases of dysfunctional uterine bleeding) this should be tried first.

To reduce the psychological and physical problems which may occur after hysterectomy, the attending doctors, whether specialist or GPs, have an obligation to talk with the woman and her partner. The reason for the operation should be explained, its extent described, alternative treatments discussed and problems which may arise mentioned. In most cases the woman should be given time to think about the discussion and to ask further questions, if she has any, before the operation is performed.

32

HUMAN SEXUALITY AND PSYCHOSEXUAL PROBLEMS

In the past three decades more people than ever before have been able to learn about human sexuality and the human sexual response. Discussion about human sexuality has become more open.

Sexual problems within a relationship are not uncommon and more women and men now feel able to seek advice about them. Often the first reference point is the person's general practitioner. General practitioners, like other people, have inhibitions about sexuality and a variety of values about sexual behaviour. These inhibitions and values are based on the person's religious beliefs, upbringing and on values obtained from parents. Some medical practitioners are uncomfortable about discussing sexual problems with their patients; others are able to listen and give advice in a nonjudgemental manner. If a medical practitioner is unable to do this he or she should refer the patient to a colleague and not impose her or his own sexual values on the patient. If the medical practitioner feels able to treat sexual dysfunctions, he or she should try to determine the patient's sexual values and try to solve the problems within that value system.

Sexual advice can only be given if the practitioner has some knowledge of sexuality and sexual behaviours.

SEXUALITY

Sexuality may be defined as the sum of a person's inherited characteristics, knowledge, experience, attitudes and behaviour as they relate to being a woman or a man. It includes those ways of behaving which enrich the personality and increase love between people. Human sexuality is as much psychological as physical, involving feelings as well as physicality. It involves communication with the other person, not talking at him or her or remaining silent, but listening and interpreting. It involves touching and exploring each other's bodies to learn the textures and surfaces, and the sight and smell of another person.

Sexuality includes the sexual drive which is the sum of the desire to have sex and the ability to accomplish the act. Sexual drive varies considerably between different people. In some a low drive is due to constitutional factors such as ill health or advanced age. In others the low drive is due to a traumatic sexual experience in childhood or adolescence. Recently more women are reporting that they have been sexually assaulted in childhood or early adolescence and this may be the basis of a fear of sex and a low sexual drive.

During adult life the intensity of the sexual drive is maximal in the years up to the age of 40 and tends to lessen after this time, but there are considerable variations. Problems arise if the sexual drive of two partners is markedly different.

THE HUMAN SEXUAL RESPONSE

The physiology of the human sexual response was not described until 40 years ago, in the studies of Masters and Johnson. For descriptive purposes they divided the sexual response in women and men into five phases, although the distinction between each phase is often blurred and one phase tends to merge into the next provided the appropriate stimulation occurs.

The phases are:
- Sexual desire.
- Sexual arousal or excitement.
- Plateau.
- Orgasm.
- Resolution.

Sexual desire is stimulated by the thought, sight, touch or smell of another person. It may be suppressed or merge into the arousal phase.

In the *arousal phase*, a man's penis becomes erect and a woman's vagina becomes lubricated. In this phase sexual enjoyment is increased if the couple pleasure each other sexually by cuddling, stroking and exploring each other's body with fingers, tongue, lips and thighs. Arousal is increased further if the erogenous zones of the body, a woman's clitoral area, breasts and vulva and a man's penis and scrotum are stimulated. A woman's breasts become bigger due to engorgement with blood and her nipples become erect. Her clitoris increases in width and becomes more sensitive to touch. Her labia and the lower part of her vagina become congested and softer and thicker. The sub-vaginal tissues become increasingly congested and fluid transudes between the vaginal cells to increase vaginal lubrication.

The *plateau phase* follows. During this phase, the sexual pleasure is intensified, and the partners desire to have penile–vaginal, penile–oral or penile–anal penetration. The thrusting movement of the penis in the vagina or its oral stimulation causes an *orgasm* in a man with the ejaculation of seminal fluid. In 90 per cent of women, the thrusting of the man's penis in her vagina indirectly, or the digital or oral stimulation of her clitoral area directly, leads to *orgasm*. Fifty per cent of sexually active women reach orgasm when the clitoral area is stimulated by finger or tongue; 25 per cent reach orgasm during penile thrusting in the the vagina; 15 per cent of women can achieve multiple orgasms; and the remaining 10 per cent are unable to achieve orgasm although they may enjoy their partner's pleasure.

Orgasm provides an intense feeling of pleasure. During orgasm the perineal muscles,the medial fibres of the levator ani and the sphincter ani muscles contract rhythmically and involuntarily as do the muscles surrounding the vagina. Many other muscle groups, particularly those of the back, contract at the height of the orgasm and a deep feeling of ecstasy (in its original sense) and relaxation follows.

In the *resolution phase* both sexual partners are relaxed. In the initial moments the clitoris and the penis are exquisitely sensitive to touch, but this passes rapidly and the tissues of the lower genital tract in both sexes decongest, the penis becoming flaccid, the clitoris small and the woman's external genitals and vagina decongested.

The physiological basis of the observed changes during sexual response occurs in two parts. Both are mediated by psychic or physical sexual stimulation, or more usually by both. Both parts can be inhibited by subconscious influences to a greater or lesser degree.

The phases of the sexual response up to orgasm are mediated by the parasympathetic nerves, which lead to vasodilatation and vasocongestion of the genital organs. In a man this leads to an inflow of blood into the cavernous spaces of the penile cylinders and an inhibition of outflow from the cylinders. The result is an erection. In a woman the changes leads to the development of congestive 'cushions' around the lower part of the vagina and to vaginal lubrication.

Failure of sexual arousal prevents these changes with resulting erectile failure in a man, and general sexual dysfunction in a woman.

The second, orgasmic phase is mediated by the sympathetic nerves, the stimulation of which leads to the clonic muscle contractions of the pelvic and other muscles. In a man these contractions lead to ejaculation and in both sexes to the more general muscle contractions. The feeling of pleasure experienced by both sexes appears to have its origin in a 'sex centre' in the thalamic and limbic areas of the old cortex which are closely related anatomically to the pleasure centres in the paleocortex. The messages which stimulate these centres are initiated from clitoral and vaginal stimulation in females and penile stimulation in males. Failure of the sympathetic element to proceed in an orderly fashion results in premature or retarded ejaculation in a man. Failure of the sensations invoked in the clitoris and vagina to be transmitted to the brain and interpreted as pleasurable is the reason for orgasm failing to occur in women.

SEXUAL DYSFUNCTIONS

Most sexual dysfunctions arise from a poor relationship with the partner, ignorance about sexuality and sexual technique, a low sexual drive, or performance anxiety. In addition physical illness or the fear that sex will aggravate an existing illness, excessive alcohol use, or clinical depression are factors.

As men and women age changes occur in their sexual desire and sexual response. These are considered on p 306.

Women have three main sexual dysfunctions:
- Inhibited sexual desire.
- Failure to achieve orgasm.
- Dyspareunia (including vaginismus).

In *Table 32.1* the sexual dysfunctions which occur in men and women are listed.

Table 32.1 Sexual dysfunction.

Sexual Dysfunction		
	Clinical syndrome	
	Male	**Female**
1. Inhibited sexual desire	No arousal	No arousal
2. Fear of sexual (genital) activity	Primary erectile failure (impotence)	Vaginismus
3. Impairment of sexual arousal. Absence or inadequate vaso-congestion* due to failure to respond to erotic stimulation because of anxiety, guilt or fear of injury	Reduced libido and secondary erectile failure (impotence)	Reduced libido
4. Impairment or failure of orgasm. Extremely rapid, or absence of clonic rhythmic contractions of pelvic musculature due to inhibition of genital tactile or psychic erotic stimulation	Premature ejaculation Retarded ejaculation	Orgastic dysfunction

*In the male, penile erection; in the female, vaginal lubrication and perivaginal swelling.

INHIBITED SEXUAL DESIRE (HYPOACTIVE SEXUAL DESIRE DISORDER)

Women with this disorder do not have sexual fantasies and have no desire for sexual activity. Its prevalence in society is not known but may be as high as 10 per cent. Allied to this disorder is a failure to become sexually aroused either by sexual fantasies or when sexually teased by her partner, and she may find the teasing distasteful. This may not mean that the woman will reject sexual advances by a husband or partner, but that she will obtain little or no enjoyment from the contact.

Inhibited sexual desire or inhibited sexual arousal may have been present since puberty or may occur after some months or years of sexual activity. In the latter case it may be the manifestation of a deteriorating relationship or a sign of depression. If two partners have inhibited sexual desire, problems are not perceived, but if one has inhibited sexual desire and the other has a normal or raised desire the problem becomes manifest. The condition appears to affect more women than men.

FAILURE TO ACHIEVE ORGASM (ANORGASMIA)

Orgasm may be achieved during penile thrusting, but not usually simultaneously with the man's orgasm, or it may only be achieved if the woman's clitoral area is stimulated by finger or tongue. In both cases orgasm is reached and the woman cannot be considered to be anorgasmic. However, some women (and men) believe that unless a woman reaches orgasm during penile thrusting, preferably simultaneously with the man, she is sexually dysfunctional.

APAREUNIA (VAGINISMUS) AND DYSPAREUNIA

In apareunia the woman is unable to accept a penis penetrating her vagina. The condition may be due to vaginal atresia or to vulvovaginal infection. In some cases the problem lies with the male who is unable to acquire or to sustain an erection, although this condition would be classified as erectile failure.

In most cases the problem is psychosomatic, the woman involuntarily tightening the muscles which surround the vaginal introitus and the lower one-third of the vagina. This is termed *vaginismus*. In severe cases of vaginismus the woman is unable to accept an examiner's finger into her vagina, so marked is the muscle spasm. Vaginismus may be transient or permanent, and affects between 1 and 3 per cent of women aged 15 to 50.

Although the woman is unable to have sexual intercourse she may be able to enjoy masturbating her partner, but avoids any contact with her own external genitals.

The cause of vaginismus lies in inadequate or faulty sex education, particularly in a belief that sex is 'dirty', or a fear based on ignorance that the penis may painfully damage the woman's body. Occasionally vaginismus can be traced to a sexual assault during childhood, or to a painful, brutal initial experience of sexual intercourse.

Dyspareunia, or painful intercourse, is shown as recurrent and persistent pain during or after sexual intercourse. It usually has an organic component. Examples are vulvovaginal infections, a painful episiotomy scar, atrophic vulvovaginitis, endometriosis, pelvic inflammatory disease, and ovarian cysts or tumours. Organic disorders must be excluded before the condition is ascribed to psychosomatic factors. These are usually found in cases of prolonged dyspareunia. The aetiology of psychogenic dyspareunia is unclear, but lack of sexual knowledge, guilt about sexuality, or a childhood sexual assault have been postulated. The problem is aggravated when the woman fails to be aroused sexually and fails to lubricate.

GENERAL MANAGEMENT STRATEGIES

The objectives of treatment are to alter an existing destructive attitude to sexuality; to reduce or resolve any underlying interpersonal sexual conflict, anxiety or fear; and to help a couple create an environment in which sexuality is perceived as a mutually pleasurable experience.

To achieve these objectives the counsellor seeks to help the woman examine her attitudes to her sexuality and to discover what stimulates her sexually; to correct any false ideas or myths about sexuality; and to help her make her partner aware of her sexual feelings, needs, and desires so that they can better express their needs to each other.

The management of sexual dysfunctions in women begins by the medical practitioner obtaining a comprehensive general and sexual history. The general history should pay particular attention to physical illness and psychiatric problems such as depression. The sexual history must be obtained with great sensitivity. During the history the medical practitioner explores the relationship and seeks to find out the woman's attitudes to her body, to menstruation and to her feelings about her sexuality.

This can be difficult and it may help to use the acronym LEPERS:

Listen for hidden signals

Explore the patient's attitudes to her sexuality, sexual activities and responses

Provide information about the female and male body

Examine relationships

Reduce the patient's anxiety

Suggest strategies for helping her, such as giving permission and prescribing specific treatment, which may differ for different problems as discussed later.

The question of whether the partner should be involved depends on the sexual problem elucidated and, more particularly, on the patient's wishes.

THE MANAGEMENT OF SPECIFIC SEXUAL PROBLEMS (FIG. 32.1)

Although the general management of sexual problems is the same for all the sexual dysfunctions, the different categories of female sexual dysfunction require different strategies.

INHIBITED SEXUAL DESIRE

The most used approach is to involve both partners when possible. The partners attend together and are

helped to communicate better with each other, though words and actions. If they are poorly informed the therapist helps them learn the anatomy and physiology of sexual intercourse. The main part of treatment is for the couple to perform a series of graded 'tasks' at short intervals over a period of weeks. The tasks are undertaken at home in a relaxed atmosphere. In the first stage, lasting one week, the couple set aside at least 30 minutes each day for non-genital pleasuring. The man fondles, caresses and massages his partner at her direction, avoiding her breasts and genitals, and responding if

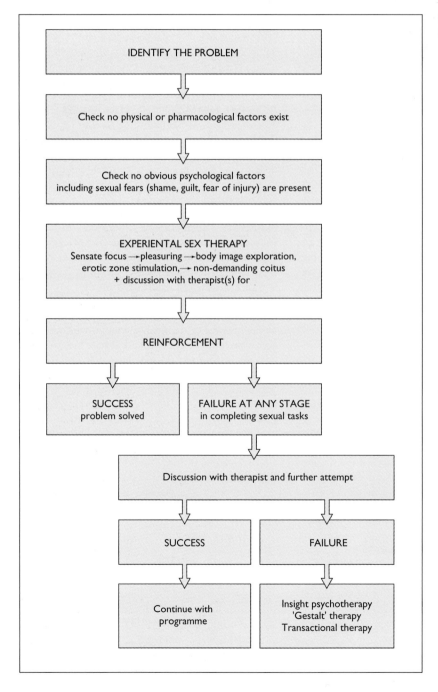

Fig 32.1 The Management of sexual problems.

she says that she doesn't like a particular area being touched. The couple then change roles.

At the end of the seven days, if the couple have made steady progress, they move to the second phase of genital pleasuring. In this phase the couple can touch, massage, kiss or lick each other's bodies and genitals. During the touching the active participant inquires 'Do you like me touching you like this?' 'Does it feel good?' 'How would you like me to do it?'. After about 15 minutes the couple exchange roles.

The couple reach the third phase when they feel that they are confident that they have enjoyed the second phase. In the third phase they proceed through the first phases fairly quickly and then attempt sexual intercourse, preferably with the woman astride the man facing him so that she can introduce his penis into her vagina at her speed.

The couple see the therapist at intervals so that their progress can be reviewed and any problems discussed.

Anorgasmia

If a woman wishes to increase her ability to achieve orgasm or has never achieved orgasm several techniques are available. Of these masturbation has produced the most successes. Many young women have masturbated but have felt guilty about it and have not reached orgasm. Others have never masturbated. Learning to achieve orgasm by masturbation often cures anorgasmia, but the woman needs to supplement this with discussion and counselling with a trained practitioner. For masturbation to be effective in reaching orgasm, the woman has to give herself time and privacy and be able to fantasize or view or read erotic literature as she masturbates either using her fingers or a vibrator.

Apareunia and dyspareunia

Any physical cause of these sexual dysfunctions must be identified, discussed with the woman, and treated if treatment is possible. If it is not, suggestions may be made about techniques in with which the woman may better enjoy her sexuality. For example, if she has a chronic pelvic infection she may find a different position for sexual intercourse is more pleasurable. If sexual intercourse is painful whatever position the couple adopt, she may obtain sensual pleasure by body caressing and clitoral stimulation, whilst giving her partner pleasure by oral sex or by masturbating him.

If the woman has vaginismus, the therapist reinforces the general strategies discussed earlier by stressing that she is not 'small made' and that she can learn to relax her perineal muscles. She may be asked to try to insert a lubricated finger in her vagina, and given instructions to continue with the exercise at home. If her relationship with her partner is good, she may choose for him to insert his finger. Once one finger is accepted, she progresses to insert two and then three fingers, or if she prefers, a series of graded metal dilators. These steps require reinforcement and encouragement by the therapist who should be visited weekly. Once she has introduced three fingers with comfort and without muscle spasm occurring, she may be ready to sit above her partner and to control his penis so that it touches the entrance to her vagina. In progressive steps on different days she inserts his penis into the entrance, then deeper into her vagina. When this is comfortable and accepted, she may move rhythmically with his penis deep in her vagina, and then permit him to thrust. Finally, having become confident that intercourse is painless, she will be able to have sexual intercourse with the man on top.

THE EVALUATION OF TREATMENT OUTCOMES

There is much confusion about treatment outcomes as many of the patients seen were selected and the data collection uncontrolled. A literature survey suggests that 50–60 per cent of women who have inhibited sexual desire or arousal are cured; 60–70 per cent of women who have anorgasmia are cured; and over 75 per cent of women who have vaginismus or psychosomatic dyspareunia enjoy normal sexual intercourse.

OTHER SEXUAL PROBLEMS

SEXUAL ASSAULT

Sexual assault includes incest and rape, which is defined as 'unlawful carnal knowledge of a woman without her consent by force, fear or fraud'. In over three quarters of cases of rape the offender is known to the woman. Statistics about the prevalence of rape are difficult to obtain as fewer than one-third of rapes are reported, but about one woman in 200 has been raped or suffered attempted rape in a year.

A woman who has been raped needs to be treated with great care and consideration when she presents to a medical practitioner. In most cases the woman attends a hospital or a 'rape crisis centre' where staff are trained to handle the woman's emotional and physical problems.

The woman should be listened to sympathetically and nonjudgementally as she tells her story. She should then be examined. It is important to explain, during the examination, what is being done and why it is being done. The presence of scratches or bruises on the woman's arms or body should be looked for and the vulva inspected to look for blood, bruising or seminal staining. A vaginal inspection is made and a vaginal smear taken to detect spermatozoa. The woman should be asked to return later so that she can be tested to exclude gonorrhoea and so that serological tests can be made to exclude infection, particularly syphilis and HIV infection. If the rape took place at the time of ovulation the woman should be given the choice of taking postcoital contraception the 'morning after pill' or asked to return if she fails to menstruate.

It is important to record carefully all findings.

HIRSUTISM

The development of body hair is to a large extent genetic. Chinese people, for example, tend to have little body hair, whilst southern Europeans tend to have much more body hair. Hirsutism is defined as a woman having increased, or excessive body hair particularly on her face, breasts or legs compared with other women of her ethnic group. Current fashion in most of the developed countries of the world has decreed that to be attractive a woman should have no hair in her armpits, or on her body. Hirsutism is perceived as diminishing a woman's attractiveness and her femininity.

In most cases hirsutism is due to the 'benign androgen excess syndrome', which shows as raised levels of free testosterone and of the final degradation product, androstenedione glucuronide.

The diagnosis is reached after excluding other, uncommon, causes of hirsutism, such as Cushing's syndrome, congenital adrenal hyperplasia and virilism. It is important to exclude virilism as this condition is usually due to virilizing ovarian or adrenal tumours. In affected women as well as hirsutism, the clitoris is enlarged, the breasts are atrophic, the hairline recedes, the voice deepens and the muscle mass increases.

In the absence of virilism, few laboratory tests are needed. Blood should be taken to measure free testosterone, and androstenedione glucuronide. A transvaginal ultrasound test may be made, as some hirsute women also have polycystic ovaries.

The management of hirsutism

The management of benign androgen excess is broad. The medical practitioner should enquire about any psychosexual problems and explore the woman's concerns about her appearance. Information should be offered about cosmetic aids, such as bleaching, shaving (which contrary to popular belief does not accelerate hair growth), waxing and the use of depilatory creams or electrolysis.

Treatment

If the woman does not wish to use these methods or they have been used and have not relieved her, several drugs are available to treat hirsutism:

- *Oral contraceptives*, particularly those containing one of the 'new generation' progestogens (such as Marvelon) often reduce the hirsutism. A new oral contraceptive containing 35 µg ethinyl oestradiol and 2 mg cyproterone (Diane) is now available which may prove an advance in treatment.

- *Cyproterone acetate* in a dose of 100 mg from day 5 to 14 of the menstrual cycle with ethinyl oestradiol 30 µg from day 5 to 25 of the cycle to maintain a regular menstrual cycle. An alternative is to give cyproterone 300 mg as a single intramuscular injection on day 5 of the menstrual cycle. Cyproterone is a competitive inhibitor of androgens at peripheral receptors and may reduce androgen synthesis. It takes about 3 months' use of cyproterone before any reduction of hirsutism is noted and the drug should be continued for 9 months to achieve the maximal effect. About 20 per cent of women fail to respond, and a similar proportion develop side effects, if the larger dose regimens are chosen. The side effects include lassitude, increase in body weight, loss of libido (10 per cent) and breast discomfort. Fewer side effects occur if the oral contraceptive pill containing cyproterone is chosen.

- *Spironolactone*. Given in a dose of 200 mg a day in divided doses, this drug reduces the amount of hirsutism over a three month period, and if continued maintains the reduction. Spironolactone works in the same way as cyproterone. There is some concern that spironolactone given for prolonged periods may induce tumour formation. In the short term, it causes polymenorrhoea (a shorter menstrual cycle) in some women. If the woman becomes pregnant and the fetus is male, he may be feminized. For both these reasons a woman taking spironolactone should also take an oral contraceptive.

33

CONCEPTION CONTROL

The availability of safe modern contraceptives has enabled women to avoid having an unwanted pregnancy, and couples to space their children. Spacing children to intervals of 2 or more years, improves a woman's health.

Contraceptive choices now available permit the woman or the couple to choose the most appropriate contraceptive for their particular circumstances. Younger women usually prefer oral contraceptives or expect their male partners to use condoms, whilst older women are more inclined to choose the intrauterine device or a permanent method of birth control such as tubal ligation or her husband a vasectomy *(Fig. 33.1)*.

Before choosing a particular contraceptive most people want to know its effectiveness in preventing pregnancy, its safety and the side effects associated with its use.

A method of evaluating the effectiveness of the various contraceptive methods is the *Pearl Index*, which calculates the unintended pregnancy rate from the formula:

$$\frac{\text{The number of unintended pregnancies}}{\text{Total months of exposure to pregnancy}} \times 1200$$

The result is expressed as the *failure rate per 100 woman years (HWY)*.

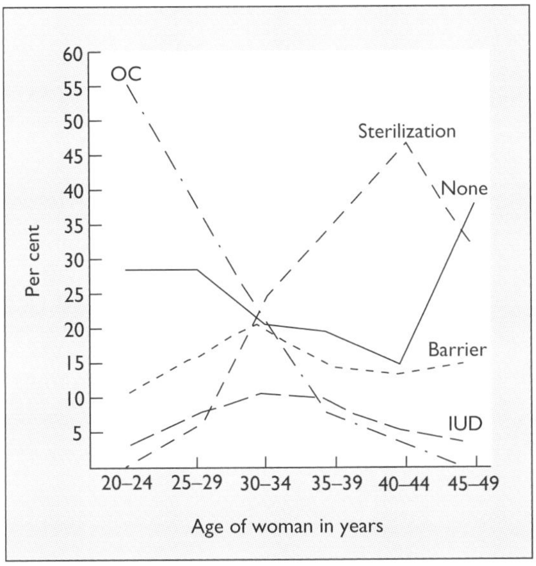

In *Table 33.1* the reliability of various available contraceptive methods in preventing pregnancy is shown.

Some women find it embarrassing to consult a medical practitioner about contraception and a sensitive doctor will do everything possible to diminish that embarrassment. The ability to listen to and to talk with the woman is of great importance.

The doctor should take a general history, a menstrual history and a sexual history in a nonjudgemental way. With this information the doctor will be better able to help the woman decide which method of contraception she would prefer.

A gynaecological examination should be made, although if the woman is teenaged and has not previously had a vaginal examination it can be deferred to a subsequent visit, when the woman may be less embarrassed. If she has not had a pap smear taken in the previous year, the doctor should suggest that this is done, explaining how the smear is taken and the reason for it.

Fig 33.1 Methods of fertility control in Britain 1986.

Ranking of Contraceptive Methods by Rate of Effectiveness		Failure rates per 100HWY
Group A	**Most effective**	
	Tubal ligation/vasectomy	0.005–0.04
	Combined oral	0.005–0.30
	Sequential oral	0.20–0.56
Group B	**Highly effective**	
	IUD	0.5–3.5
	Continuous progestogen	1.5–2.3
	Diaphragm or condom + cream	
	All users	4.0–7.0
	Highly motivated	1.5–3.0
	Periodic abstinence	
	All users	10.0–30.0
	Highly motivated	2.5–5.0
Group C	**Less effective**	
	Coitus interruptus	30.0–40.0
	Vaginal foam or cream	30.0–40.0
Group D	**Least effective**	
	Post-coital douche	45.0
	Prolonged breast feeding	45.0

Table 33.1 Ranking of contraceptive methods by rate of effectiveness (as calculated from unexpected pregnancies per 100 woman-years).

REVERSIBLE METHODS OF CONTRACEPTION USED BY THE COUPLE

✓ PERIODIC ABSTINENCE

The knowledge that ovulation occurs about 14 (±3) days before the next menstrual period and that the sperm can only fertilize the ovum over a 48-hour period, led to the development of the several methods of contraception. One of these which has largely superseded the older methods is the Periodic Abstinence Method, which is also called the Mucus Method.

The woman is taught to detect the presence of mucus at the vaginal entrance each morning (before any sexual arousal). Three types of mucus can be detected and from this the days on which sexual intercourse can take place whilst avoiding to some extent the chance of an unwanted pregnancy occurring can be calculated (Fig. 33.2). The compliance of the man is essential if pregnancy is to be avoided.

Because of the difficulties in interpreting the mucus and the need for the man to cooperate fully, the pregnancy rate varies from 10 to 30 per HWY for all couples other than motivated couples is 2.5–5.0 per HWY.

✓ COITUS INTERRUPTUS

Withdrawal or coitus interruptus is the oldest form of birth control, apart from induced abortion. With the development of more modern contraceptives its frequency has declined, but it is still the favoured method among some sections of society. Its reliability for preventing pregnancy depends on the ability of the man to recognize the pre-ejaculatory phase and his agility in withdrawing his penis from the woman's vagina before ejaculation. Because of these constraints, the efficacy of coitus interruptus in preventing an unwanted pregnancy is rather low (Table 33.1). 30 – 40 perHWY

REVERSIBLE METHODS OF CONTRACEPTION USED BY THE MALE PARTNER

✓THE CONDOM

Modern condoms which are made of latex, prelubricated by adding silicone, and supplied in hermetically sealed aluminium sachets are cheap, efficient and hardly noticeable to either partner. Their advantages are that they can be obtained from a variety of outlets without a doctor's prescription, and that they offer some protection against the transmission of sexually transmitted diseases, including the human papillomavirus, chlamydia and the human immuno-deficiency virus (HIV). The disadvantages of condoms is that many younger men refuse to use them as they believe that they reduce sexual pleasure and may burst during use.

The pregnancy rate following condom use relates to their usage, to the way the condom is put on the penis and how it is held on after penile detumescence. The doctor should explain how a condom should be used if consulted by a woman or her partner (Fig. 33.3).

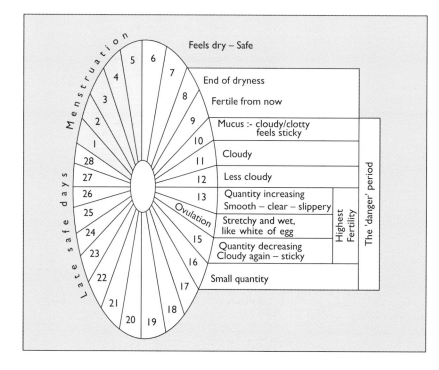

Fig 33.2 Periodic abstinence: the mucus (ovulation) method.

REVERSIBLE METHODS OF CONTRACEPTION USED BY WOMEN

Women have more choices of reversible or temporary contraception than have men. Women may choose:

- *Barrier methods* – the vaginal diaphragm, the cervical cap, the vaginal sponge and the female condom.
- *Hormonal contraceptives* – the Pill, injectables and implants.
- *The intrauterine device (IUD)*.

BARRIER METHODS
The vaginal diaphragm and cervical cap

The vaginal diaphragm and the cervical cap consist of a thin plastic or latex dome attached to a circular flat, coiled or arching spring rim. The vaginal diaphragm is easier to use than the cervical cap. As the diaphragm fits diagonally across the vagina, the correct size is determined by a medical practitioner examining the woman vaginally and inserting the index and middle fingers as far as they will go into the posterior vaginal fornix and noting how far the index finger reaches behind the symphysis pubis.

The diaphragm is made in sizes from 50mm to 100mm, in 5mm steps. After measuring the vagina the doctor inserts a series of diaphragms or fitting rings until the most appropriate size is found.

Using a diaphragm or a cervical cap requires practise, and after teaching the woman how to use it, *(Fig. 33.4)* many doctors ask the woman to learn the technique at home and return with the diaphragm or cap in her vagina for checking.

When the woman is confident about the technique, she inserts the diaphragm each day or at any convenient time before sexual intercourse is anticipated. It should not be removed for cleaning until at least 6 hours after the last ejaculation. Some women

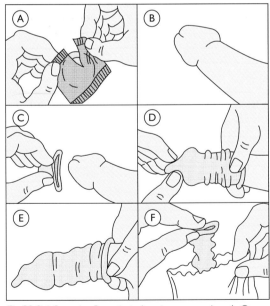

Fig 33.3 *Information for patients: how to use a condom.* A. Open the packet carefully, and do not unroll the condom before putting it on. B. Semen can leak out soon after the penis becomes erect, prior to ejaculation. To prevent pregnancy or infection, the condom must be put on before any sexual contact takes place. C. Ensure that the condom is the right way up. Squeeze the teat on the tip of the condom and hold it against the tip of the penis. D. Unroll the condom all the way to the base of the penis. E. After ejaculation, the penis should be withdrawn before the erection is totally lost. When withdrawing, hold onto the condom. F. Do not allow the condom or penis to come into contact with the female's genital area, and carefully dispose of the condom.

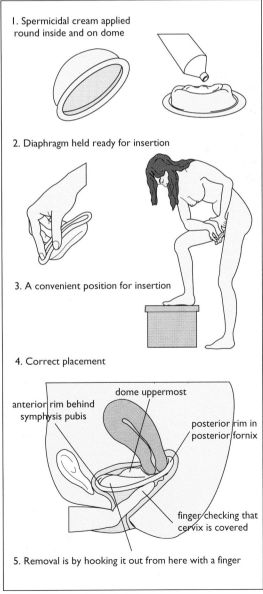

1. Spermicidal cream applied round inside and on dome

2. Diaphragm held ready for insertion

3. A convenient position for insertion

4. Correct placement

anterior rim behind symphysis pubis

dome uppermost

posterior rim in posterior fornix

finger checking that cervix is covered

5. Removal is by hooking it out from here with a finger

Fig 33.4 The use of vaginal diaphragm.

choose to smear a nonoxynol-9 spermicidal cream around the rim, but whether this adds to the effectiveness of the diaphragm in preventing pregnancy is uncertain. It is known to destroy the HIV, to some extent, which is a benefit.

If a woman chooses a cervical cap, she must have a healthy, short cervix. Fitting is made by a medical practitioner. The technique of insertion and removal is that of the vaginal diaphragm.

Vaginal sponges

These devices incorporate an active spermicide in a polyurethane mushroom shaped sponge. The sponge is inserted before sexual intercourse and is not removed until 6 hours after the last ejaculation.

The female condom — NOT EFFECTIVE

This device is a tube of polyurethane plastic about 15 cm long and 7cm in diameter. It is closed at one end (Fig. 33.5). The lower open end is surrounded by a soft ring which holds it against the vulva. A problem is that the female condom may be pushed into the vagina during intercourse or slip out together with the penis.

HORMONAL CONTRACEPTIVES ✳

Hormonal contraceptives contain oestrogen and a progestogen (combined oral contraceptives – COCs); or progestogen alone. Oestrogen suppresses FSH secretion and reduces LH secretion and in this way prevents ovulation. The progestogen further suppresses LH release, alters the quality of the cervical mucus rendering it less penetrable to sperm and produces endometrial changes culminating in glandular exhaustion. Importantly, the progestogen also permits a withdrawal bleed which is regular in onset, short in duration and light in amount.

COMBINED ORAL CONTRACEPTIVE (COCS)

These formulations are chosen by most contraceptive users as they are effective in preventing pregnancy and are easy to take. Most currently available COCs contain less than 50μg of ethinyl oestradiol (one contains mestranol, which is rapidly converted into ethinyl oestradiol), and one of several progestogens. These COCs are called 'low-dose COCs'.

Most of the COCs prescribed are monophasic or triphasic. In the monophasic formulations the amount of oestrogen and progestogen is constant in each tablet throughout the cycle. The triphasic formulation tablets contain varying doses of both oestrogen and progestogen. The total progestogen in a cycle is less and the total oestrogen is more than in the monophasic formulations. The two sequential (biphasic) formulations and a formulation containing cyproterone acetate have a limited use; they are prescribed for women who have acne or are markedly hirsute.

The concept behind the development of the triphasic formulations was to reduce the effects of the Pill on lipid metabolism. Oestrogen increases high density lipoprotein cholesterol (HDL-c) and reduces low density lipoprotein (LDL-c); whilst the first generation progestogens decrease the level of HDL-c. Combined as in the Pill, total cholesterol is not increased, but that of HDL-c is reduced slightly (compared with oestrogen alone), the decrease being related to the total dose of progestogen. The triphasic formulations reduce the total quantity of progestogen given in a cycle and thus reduce the decrease in the circulating levels of HDL-c.

Oral contraceptives containing the newer (second generation) progestogens, such as desogestrel and gestodene, do not reduce HDL-c and thus can be given in a monophasic preparation. They are replacing the older COCs.

Contra-indications to the prescription of COCs

The International Planned Parenthood Federation recommends that the following groups of women should not choose COCs if they have:

- A past or present history of venous or arterial thrombosis, ischaemic heart disease, or a severe hypertension.
- Familial hyperlipidaemia.
- Any condition favouring cerebral ischaemia, particularly severe focal migraine.
- Acute liver disease and some forms of chronic liver disease.
- Oestrogen dependent cancer.
- Undiagnosed per vaginam bleeding.

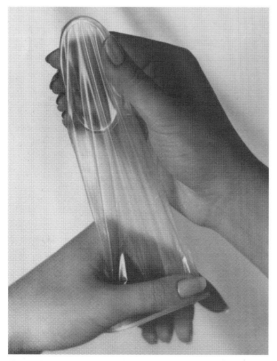

Fig 33.5 The female condom (illustration courtesy of Chartex, U.K.).

Noncontraceptive benefits of COCs

As COCs are the most used form of contraception in the world, it is important to note the noncontraceptive benefits of the preparations:

- Most menstrual cycle disorders are reduced including menstrual blood loss, menorrhagia, dysmenorrhoea (by <80 per cent) and the premenstrual syndrome. However, about 1 per cent of COC users develop amenorrhoea.
- Pelvic infection (pelvic inflammatory disease) is reduced among women who have several sexual partners or whose partner has or has had several sexual partners.
- Benign breast disease and benign breast tumours are reduced by up to 50 per cent; breast carcinoma is not increased.
- Functional ovarian cysts are less common.
- Uterine myomata are less common as is endometriosis.
- Endometrial and ovarian cancers are reduced.
- Rheumatoid arthritis appears to be reduced among COC users who have taken the medication for <5 years.

Clinical side effects of COCs

Two main areas of concern are: circulatory disease and certain cancers. Other clinical conditions may also occur.

Circulatory disease. *Thromboembolism* is slightly more common among COC users, although the risk is small (<0.5 per 1000 users per year). The increase is due to an increase in fibrinogen concentration and of factors II, VII, IX, X and XII and a decrease in antithrombin III. There is a concomitant increase in fibrinolysis but it does not equal the coagulation changes. The risk is increased in smokers and in obese women. If these two variables are excluded the relative risk of developing thromboembolism in a woman taking low-dose COCs is not increased.

As major surgery adds to the risk of thromboembolism, women taking COCs should change to another form of contraception for 4 weeks before the surgery. Thrombotic stroke is increased six-fold (compared with women using no, or other forms of contraception) but is very uncommon in this age group.

The use of COCs leads to a small increase in the systolic blood pressure, which is reversible. *Hypertension* of greater magnitude occurs in about 2 per cent of women, particularly women who have a family history of hypertension, are overweight and over the age of 35. Women who have had pregnancy-induced hypertension are more likely to be affected. The cause is an increased sensitivity to the progestogen content of the Pill, but oestrogen may be involved, so that a low-dose oestrogen Pill is to be preferred.

The use of low-dose COCs does not increase the risk of *myocardial infarction*, unless the woman is a smoker, overweight and is over the age of 35, when a small increased risk occurs.

Cancers. The use of COCs reduces the risk of developing ovarian cancer (by 40 per cent) and endometrial cancer (by 50 per cent). The prolonged use of COCs increases the risk of developing cervical cancer slightly, but this may be due to the sexual behaviour of the women rather than to the use of COCs. The overall incidence of breast cancer does not increase, except perhaps for a small subgroup of women presenting with breast cancer in their 30s, who have taken the Pill for at least 5 years before their first pregnancy.

Other clinical conditions occurring in women using COCs

Acne. The oestrogen content of the COCs tends to improve acne, whilst the progestogen tends to aggravate it. Monophasic COCs, especially containing a 'second generation' progestogen (e.g. Marvelon), sequential COCs or an OC containing cyproterone (e.g. Diane) should be chosen.

Break-through bleeding (BTB) and spotting. Many women starting to use hormonal contraceptives have episodes of break-through bleeding or spotting in the early months of use. In the first cycle 20 per cent of women experience BTB; by the sixth month less than 3 per cent have the symptom. BTB is less likely if the woman takes the Pill *at the same time each day*. BTB causes considerable concern to many women, and doctors should advise women starting to use the Pill or 'switching' Pills, that BTB may occur. The doctor should explain that in most cases it settles within a few months and that it is not dangerous. If BTB continues for longer than six months, the woman should be prescribed a COC with a higher content of oestrogen.

Chloasma. Hyperpigmentation of the skin may occur in susceptible women exposed to sunlight, but is uncommon. It is thought to be due to oestrogen. Treatment is to change to a progesterone only pill (POP) or to use another form of contraception, to avoid direct sunlight, and if the woman is very concerned, to apply 2% hydroquinone ointment. Even with these measures the chloasma takes up to 9 months to fade.

Drugs and COCs. Women who need to take antibiotics should take extra precautions during the time they take the antibiotic and for seven days after, as absorption of the Pill is reduced and pregnancy may occur. Women who require to take carbamazepine, griseofulvin, phenytoin or rifampicin, should use another form of contraception, as these drugs increase hepatic enzyme activity which increases the metabolism of contraceptive steroids and reduces their efficacy.

233

✓ **Eye problems.** A few women who use contact lenses may experience discomfort due to a change in the topography of the cornea.

✓ **Gall bladder disease.** The development of gall bladder disease is accelerated among women taking a higher oestrogen dose COC (>50µg).

✓ **Headaches and migraine.** The prevalence of headaches among women taking COCs is variable and headaches may occur on days when no hormones are taken. If the headaches are severe and occur on days when the Pill is not taken (or a non-active Pill is taken in a 28-day pack), the frequency of headaches can be reduced by taking the Pill continuously for 3 months. The woman will not have a withdrawal bleed until the end of the three-month cycle, but will have fewer headaches each year.

A few women develop migraine when taking COCs. If the migraine is focal or persists severely for 3 days or more, the woman should change to another form of contraception.

✓ **Mood changes, including depression.** Some women who have premenstrual mood changes find that the symptoms decrease when taking a monophasic COC, particularly if it contains a second generation progestogen. Clinical depression is not increased among Pill users.

✓ **Nausea and vomiting.** These symptoms may occur in the first few months of taking COCs as the body adjusts to the hormonal milieu.

✓ **Sexual desire.** A few women report a decrease in libido when taking COCs; others report an increase.

✓ **Vaginal discharges.** An increased amount of vaginal secretions is usual, but candidosis does not occur more frequently among women taking modern COCs.

✓ **Weight gain.** Transient weight gain occurs in the premenstrual week in most women, and may be increased among women taking COCs; it is lost when menstruation starts. A few women gain weight after a few months' use of COCs. Whether this is due to the progestogen content of the COC or to an increased appetite is unclear.

NON-OESTROGEN HORMONAL CONTRACEPTIVES

Progesterone-only pill (POP) – the mini-Pill. This oral contraceptive is a good choice for women who have contra-indications for COCs or who are breast feeding. It is an alternative for some diabetic women or women who have risk factors for cardiovascular disease, women who have hypertension related to COCs or needing control by antihypertensives, and some migraine sufferers. The POP is associated with break-through bleeding and unpredictable menstruation in about one in four users. The failure rate (pregnancy rate) is shown in *Table 39.1* on page 229.

Long-acting injectable progestogens. This formulation contains medroxyprogesterone acetate (DMPA) 150mg, injected 3-monthly or northisterone oenanthate (NET-OEN) 200 mg injected every 2 months. A new monthly injectable is currently under trial by the WHO. The advantage of the injectables is that they remove the need to take a Pill every day. Their disadvantage is that during the first 4–6 months of use, menstruation tends to be irregular. Concern that the injectable might provoke breast cancer has been removed.

Subdermal Implants. Six Silastic capsules, measuring 30mm by 2.5mm and each containing 36mg of levonorgestrel are introduced subdermally into the anterior aspect of the forearm through a cannula, after making a 2mm incision through the skin. As with other progestogen formulations they may provoke irregular episodes of uterine bleeding, which may be prolonged, in the first year of use, in about 20 per cent of women. The woman's fertility is not reduced once the implants have been removed.

The vaginal ring. This novel contraceptive, currently under study, has been developed in two forms (1) a ring containing an oestrogen and a progestogen mimicking the COCs (2) a ring containing levonorgestrel. The ring fits in the upper vagina around the cervix. The advantage of the vaginal ring is that it is the only long-acting method under the woman's control. The woman removes the ring at will but generally replaces it at once after washing it. The disadvantage of the vaginal ring is that it may be associated with irregular bleeding in the first months of use and may be expelled from the vagina.

PRESCRIBING HORMONAL CONTRACEPTIVES

The history is taken and the woman is examined as described in Chapter 2. The choices of hormonal contraceptives available may be discussed with the woman, although often she had a good idea of the one she would prefer. She should be advised to read and to follow the instructions in the packet. Some doctors provide a pamphlet which reinforces these instructions.

POSTCOITAL CONTRACEPTION

If a woman has unprotected sexual intercourse at ovulation time she has two choices. The first is to wait and see if she misses a menstrual period and then have an immunological pregnancy test. If this is positive she can then choose to continue with the pregnancy or to have an induced abortion (see p 105). The second choice is to use a form of postcoital contraception, provided she seeks help within 72 hours. Three methods are available:

- The woman may be prescribed a COC containing ethinyl oestradiol 50μg and levonorgestrel 250μg (the 'morning after' pill). Two of these tablets are taken together with an antiemetic, because of the side effects of nausea and vomiting. The dose is repeated after 12 hours.
- The woman is prescribed mifepristone (RU 486) in a dose of 600mg (at present), in countries where the drug is available. The advantage of mifepristone over the 'morning after' pill is that nausea and vomiting are less frequent.
- The woman may choose to have an IUD inserted within 5 days of the unprotected intercourse. This method is inadvisable if the woman is nulliparous.

Pregnancy is prevented in over 95 per cent of cases, but the woman should return a week after the time of her expected period for a pregnancy test if she fails to menstruate.

THE INTRAUTERINE DEVICE (IUD)

Intrauterine devices were used in humans in the last years of the 19th century, but had so many adverse side effects that they were abandoned. The development of a polyethylene IUD in 1950, which had a memory for its shape, revived interest.

A satisfactory IUD should be easy to introduce, easy to remove, have few side effects and a high degree of efficiency in preventing pregnancy. In the 1980s a series of legal actions against IUD manufacturers led to the removal from the market of most

IUDs, and today only three types remain. Two of the devices have fine copper wire surrounding the stem, which permits a smaller device to be used and reduces some of the side effects (Fig. 33.6). The third IUD contains levonorgestrel in its stem (Fig. 33.7). In the first 4 months of use some women have unpredictable episodes of spotting or bleeding. After this time the levonorgestrel IUD reduces menstrual flow, controlling menorrhagia in women who have this menstrual disturbance and may cause amenorrhoea. It may be chosen by women in their 40s who would otherwise consider tubal ligation.

Copper IUDs prevent pregnancy by incapacitating the sperms making them dysfunctional for fertilization. The progestogen IUD releases 20mcg of levonorgestrel a day and acts in the same manner as the progesterone-only Pill.

The Advantages of the IUD

The IUD requires only a single decision to have the device introduced into the uterus, and unless problems arise, will prevent pregnancy for 3–7 years (depending on the device). It is highly effective in preventing pregnancy (see Table 33.1).

The Adverse Effects of IUDs

During insertion: Perforation of the uterine wall occurs in about 1 per 1000 insertions and is directly proportional to the skill of the individual performing the insertion. Perforation may cause bleeding and pain, but is often silent. If perforation is suspected,

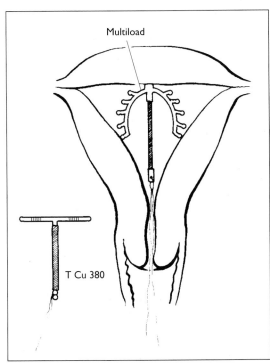

Fig 33.6 Currently used IUDs.

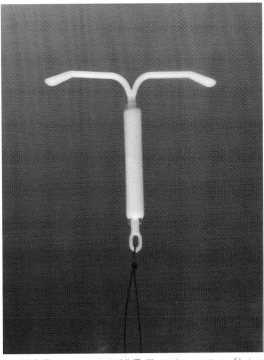

Fig 33.7 The Levonorgestrel IUD (illustration courtesy of Leiras Oy, Finland).

the location of the IUD is determined using an ultrasound scan. If this indicates that the IUD has perforated the uterus and is wholly or partly in the abdominal pelvic cavity, it should be removed because the copper may cause a tissue reaction leading to intraperitoneal adhesions. The removal is effected by finding the IUD by using a laparoscope or by making a laparotomy.

Expulsion: The uterus tends to expel 'foreign bodies' and the IUD is no exception; between 1 and 10 women in every hundred who have an IUD inserted expel the device. Expulsion may occur at any time after insertion, but usually occurs in the first 6–8 weeks, often during a menstrual period. Younger women and women who have never been pregnant are more likely to expel the device than other women.

Cramping and bleeding: Over a two-year period these complications have been shown to occur with a frequency varying from 4 per 100 women to 10 per 100 women in the case of the copper-containing IUDs. The problem usually occurs in the first month after the insertion and diminishes as time passes. One half of the number of medical removals of an IUD is for this cause.

Pregnancy and the IUD

Although the IUD is highly effective (>98 per cent) in protecting a woman against an unwanted pregnancy, occasionally a pregnancy occurs with the IUD in situ. The continued presence of the IUD increases the risk of miscarriage to 25 per cent (compared with a 10 per cent risk in a woman who has no IUD in situ), so that if the woman agrees, an attempt should be made to remove it from the uterine cavity. The procedure does not increase the miscarriage rate above that in the population. If the IUD cannot be removed and the woman chooses to continue with the pregnancy, a miscarriage occurring in the second quarter of pregnancy may be associated with infection (septic abortion), although the frequency of this complication is not known. Should infection occur, antibiotics should be given promptly and an attempt made to remove the IUD, if feasible. These problems should be discussed with the woman. Given the information she may choose to have an induced abortion.

Pelvic Inflammatory Disease. Pelvic inflammatory disease (pelvic infection) is discussed in detail in Chapter 35. The background incidence of PID in the community is 1 per 100 women per year, aged 15–45. It has been claimed that the IUD increases the chance of PID. A recent meta-analysis has shown that this only applies if the infection occurs within the first month of the IUD insertion in women who have symptomless cervical infection due to *chlamydia trachomatis*, *N. gonorrhoeae* (or, rarely, *polymicrobial infection*) at the time of the IUD insertion.

These findings suggest that sexual activity rather than the IUD is the cause of PID, and that the introduction of an IUD through the infected cervix of a woman may increase slightly the chance that she will develop PID.

Tubal infertility. The relative risk of a woman who has never been pregnant developing tubal infertility (primary infertility) associated with the use of a copper IUD is 1.6. Women who have only one sexual partner have no increased risk of primary infertility.

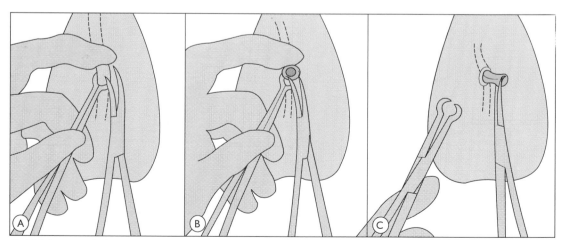

Fig 33.8 In a no-scalpel vasectomy the vas (dotted line) is grasped by special ring forceps and the skin and the vas sheath are pierced by sharp-tipped dissecting forceps (A). The forceps then stretch an opening (B) and the vas is lifted out (C).

INFERTILITY

A couple who have had regular unprotected intercourse for a period of 12 months without a pregnancy occurring is considered to be infertile and may seek help from a medical practitioner. Infertility affects about 10 per cent of couples.

FACTORS IN INFERTILITY

The factors which may be involved in the couple's infertility vary depending on local conditions, the population investigated and the referral procedures. Analyses reported by several clinics of large numbers of patients in the past two decades are as follows:

Male factors (defective sperm production, insemination difficulties).	30–40 %
Ovulation factors.	5–25 %
Tubal or uterine factors.	15–25 %
Cervical/immunological factors.	5–10 %
Unexplained after investigations.	10–25 %

In a quarter of cases more than one of the factors is believed to be involved in the infertility.

INVESTIGATION OF INFERTILITY

Of the many investigations suggested over the years, most have been found to be of little value and today there is relative agreement about what tests should be made to reach a diagnosis.

In most cases the woman makes the first contact with a health professional. During this visit the doctor should obtain information about the history of past illnesses and operations; the woman's menstrual history; and the couple's sexual behaviour, including frequency of sexual intercourse. Some women are concerned that they do not have an orgasm and that semen runs out of the vagina. The doctor should reassure the woman that neither of these affects the woman's fertility.

A general physical examination, including a pelvic examination, is made to exclude any current disease. The pelvic examination is made to detect any gross abnormalities of the genital tract, such as uterine myomata, ovarian tumours and endometriosis (see later). If a cervical smear (pap smear) has not been made in the previous year this should be taken. Laboratory tests should be ordered. These should include: a full blood examination, including tests for syphilis and HIV infection, and a urine analysis. If the woman has attended during the luteal phase of her menstrual cycle blood may be taken to measure the progesterone level, to establish if she is ovulating.

Having completed these initial investigations the medical practitioner should outline the investigations which will be made and their sequence. It is customary to start the investigations with a seminal analysis, as the man may have azoospermia or severe oligospermia. This finding would make unjustified further investigations of the woman.

SEMINAL ANALYSIS

Ideally a man should accompany his partner at the first visit so that the investigation plan can be discussed with both and so that a history can be obtained from the man and he can be examined. However, it is unusual for a man to accompany his partner. Because of this and because a woman knows if penetration and ejaculation occur during sexual intercourse, the first step is to arrange for a semen analysis, and only if this is abnormal need the man be seen.

The seminal specimen can be obtained in two ways. In the first the man attends the laboratory and masturbates there providing a fresh seminal specimen. The second way is for the man to masturbate at home (or have his partner masturbate him) and to ejaculate into a clean, dry glass container. This is then taken to the laboratory within 1 hour of the test, and the analysis made.

Standards for a 'normal' seminal specimen have been developed by the World Health Organization and are shown in *Table 34.1*. If the first seminal appraisal is abnormal, two further specimens should be evaluated before a prognosis is made.

Evaluation of the samples permits the specimens to be graded as:

Normal Seminal Analysis	
Volume	>2ml
Sperm concentration	>20 million per mL
Total sperm concentration	>40 million
Motility 60min after ejaculation	>50% with forward progression
Morphology	>50% with normal morphology
When the sperm count is less than 20 million per ml, abnormal morphology and motility is often found.	

Table 34.1 Normal seminal analysis.

- Normal.
- Oligospermia (a count <20 million per ml)
  (i) with normally motile sperm
  (i) with asthenospermia.
- Severe oligospermia (>5 million in total specimen).
- Azoospermia.
- Asthenospermia with a normal sperm count.

Abnormal results indicate that the man should be examined and a history taken. The history may show that he is exposed to high heat, certain chemicals, or is taking anti-cancer drugs. The examination of the man's genitals is important. The size of his testicles is evaluated, and his scrotum is palpated, with the man standing, to detect if he has a varicocele, although the importance of this as a factor in infertility is disputed. If azoospermia or severe oligospermia is diagnosed, blood is drawn to measure the level of FSH. A raised level (×3 the normal upper limit) indicates testicular failure. If severe oligospermia is diagnosed, and the testicular volume and the FSH levels are normal, a testicular biopsy is sometimes made.

Absolute infertility is diagnosed if azoospermia and raised FSH levels are found. Severe infertility is diagnosed if severe oligospermia is found. Relative infertility is diagnosed if the sperm count is between 5 million and 20 million per ml. Treatment may be offered to men with relative infertility, although it has to be said that none has proved more effective than placebo.

The technique of microinjection of a spermatozoon into the vitelline space between the zona pellucida and the ovum or into the substance of the ovum has produced a few pregnancies recently in cases of severe male infertility.

INVESTIGATING THE WOMAN

The factors which may delay or prevent fertility in women are:

- Anovulation or infrequent ovulation.
- Tubal damage which prevents the passage of the sperm.
- Uterine factors such as intra-uterine adhesions (Asherman's syndrome).
- Cervical mucus 'hostility', which is an immunological defect in most cases.

These factors require to be investigated in the work-up of infertility.

Ovulation

The most effective way of determining if the woman is ovulating is to measure the serum progesterone level in the midluteal phase of the menstrual cycle. The older method of daily temperature charting is now obsolete. In past years many gynaecologists performed a diagnostic curettage to obtain a specimen which could be examined to determine if endometrial luteinization had occurred, indicating ovulation. This invasive procedure is no longer justifiable except in countries where genital tuberculosis is common.

Anovulation is obvious if the woman is amenorrhoeic and may occur in women who have normal menstrual periods. The investigation of anovulation has been discussed in Chapter 30.

Tubal factors

The patency of the Fallopian tubes can be evaulated in two ways.

The first, a hysterosalpingogram, is performed by inserting a cannula attached to a syringe into the cervix and injecting a radio opaque substance into the uterus under direct imaging. The passage of the dye is observed as it fills the uterine cavity and passes along the Fallopian tubes to spill into the peritoneal cavity. The advantages of the hysterosalpingogram are that it is a minor operation and the patient does not need to be admitted as a day-case, and that it will detect any intra-uterine abnormalities *(Fig. 34.1)*.

The second method is to perform a laparoscopy and then to inject a water-soluble dye into the uterine cavity and to observe it as it spills through the fimbrial ends of the Fallopian tubes. The advantage of laparoscopy is that as well as ascertaining that the Fallopian tubes are patent, peritubal adhesions and endometrial deposits can be detected if they are present. Endometriosis is the only abnormality found in about 10 per cent of infertile women, and 40 per cent of women who have endometriosis are involuntarily infertile, but the relationship between the two conditions is unclear. The topic is discussed further in Chapter 37.

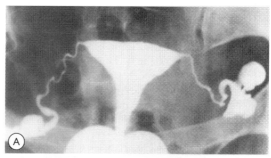

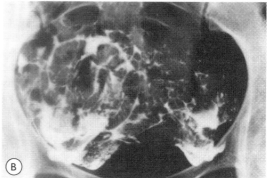

Fig 34.1 (A) Hysterosalpingogram showing a normal uterus and tubes. (B) A film taken some hours later confirmed that oil was present in the peritoneal cavity and the tubes were patent.

Currently the use of colour Doppler ultrasonography is being investigated, as is tuboscopy.

Cervical 'hostility'

Although this term is usually used to indicate that the sperm fail to penetrate the cervical mucus at ovulation time, it is more likely that the failure is due to defective sperm function, probably immunological.

Many gynaecologists continue to believe in 'cervical hostility' and test this by means of the *postcoital test*. The test has been in use for over 100 years and was originally made to detect sperm in the cervix. The test is made in the following way: The couple have intercourse on one of the two days before ovulation or on the day of ovulation. After the man has ejaculated, the woman remains on her back for 20 minutes, and attends the doctor 8–12 hours later so that a sample of cervical mucus can be removed from her cervix, using a plastic tube attached to a syringe. The specimen is smeared on a slide and is examined to determine the degree of penetration of the mucus by actively moving sperm and their numbers per field. A positive test (>5 actively moving sperm per field) indicates that there is unlikely to be an immunological problem causing the infertility; a negative test provides no useful information. Because of this, more specific sperm-mucus tests have been developed *(Table 34.2)*.

UNEXPLAINED INFERTILITY

After adequate investigation a group of about 15 per cent of infertile couples remain in whom no cause for their infertility can be found. Unexplained infertility is frustrating both for the couple and the team of health professionals.

THE TREATMENT OF INFERTILITY

MALE INFERTILITY

Azoospermia is an absolute barrier to conception, and it is unusual for a pregnancy to occur in a couple if the man has severe oligospermia. For these couples, donor semen insemination (DI) is a choice. Using DI monthly for 12 months, if necessary, will enable over 65 per cent of women to become pregnant. (An alternative is to microinject a spermatozoon into the space under the zona pellucida or into the ovum. This is still experimental.)

Improvement in the sperm count of men with non-severe oligospermia has been attempted using an oral form of testosterone (mestrolone) and more recently clomiphene prescribed for at least 12 weeks, but it is doubtful if any real improvement has occurred or that the pregnancy rate is higher than that obtained by chance.

An attractive alternative is to concentrate a seminal sample and fertilize several ova using the In-Vitro Fertilization (IVF) technique.

FEMALE INFERTILITY
Anovulation (usually associated with amenorrhoea)

The treatment is that discussed in the treatment of amenorrhoea on p 212.

Tubal damage

Two choices are available and the one chosen depends on the severity of the tubal damage and on the wishes of the patient. The first approach is to attempt to make the Fallopian tubes patent, using microsurgery. If only the fimbrial ends of the tubes are blocked, a salpingostomy or fimbriolysis is made. This results in a 40 per cent chance of the woman conceiving in a 2-year period following the operation. Greater tubal damage necessitates a tubal anastomosis, with a success rate of no more than 20 per cent, whilst reversal of a tubal ligation is followed by a pregnancy rate of 60 per cent.

Given these relatively poor results (except in the case of reversal of a tubal ligation), the alternative approach, that of IVF, has been recommended by some gynaecologists. They claim that the procedure is less invasive, the risk of ectopic gestation is less and the chance of giving birth to a healthy baby greater.

Sperm-Cervical Mucus Crossed Hostility Test				
Penetration of wife's cervical mucus with donor's sperm	+	–	+	–
Penetration of donor's cervical mucus with husband's sperm	+	+	–	–
Diagnosis	Specific immunological problem in couple	Cervical mucus of wife abnormal	Specific immunological problem in male	Problem in husband *and* wife
Treatment	Donor insemination Intra-uterine insemination husband's semen ?IVF	?Ethinyl oestradiol 0.01mg b.d. day 5–12	Donor insemination or corticosteroids to male	?

Table 34.2 Sperm-cervical mucus crossed hostility test.

The new assisted reproductive technologies

These technologies, that is IVF and its variants, have added a new dimension to the treatment of the infertile couple. In the past decade considerable advances have been made in reducing the pain involved, the invasiveness of the procedure and the cost. The procedure is as follows:

- The woman is given ovulatory drugs to produce superovulation.
- The eggs are retrieved from the ovaries by the transvaginal route under ultrasonic guidance.
- The eggs are prepared for fertilization and only 'good' ova are selected.
- Sperm is added in vitro to the selected eggs.
- Two (occasionally three) fertilized eggs are transferred into the uterus; or into the Fallopian tubes using a technique called gamete intrafallopian transfer (GIFT).

The success rate of a single IVF procedure in terms of a live healthy baby is about 10 per cent, whilst that of a single GIFT procedure is about 20 per cent. If either procedure is repeated 5 times, the cumulative 'take home baby rate' using IVF is 40 per cent and that using GIFT about 50 per cent.

Cervical hostility (immunological infertility)

The oldest method of treatment is for the man to use condoms for 6 months in the hope that the antisperm antibodies will be eliminated. Other treatments are for the man to take low dose corticosteroids (prednisone 20mg twice a day for the first 10 days of the woman's menstrual cycle) for 3 months; to use washed sperm introduced into the uterine cavity; or to use IVF or GIFT techniques. None of these treatments has been properly evaluated and it appears that as many pregnancies occur if no treatment is given.

Unexplained infertility

Current opinion about the treatment of couples who have been diagnosed as having unexplained infertility is confused. If no treatment is given, beyond reassurance that no cause for the infertility has been found, over 40 per cent of the women will become pregnant within 3 years. However, if the couple wish, or if the woman is over the age of 35, IVF or GIFT may be chosen soon after diagnosis, rather than delaying for 3 years.

THE SUCCESS RATE OF TREATMENT

Four couples in every ten treated for infertility will have a 'take home baby'. In most cases the pregnancy occurs because of treatment but in about 20 per cent it can not be attributed to the treatment. The success rate for the treatment of various infertility factors is shown in *Table 34.3*.

PSYCHOSOCIAL PROBLEMS ASSOCIATED WITH INFERTILITY

The conception and later the birth of a healthy child is a significant life event. To most women, motherhood is the expression of her nurturing gender role and of her femininity. To most men the siring of a child is a visible demonstration of their masculinity and potency. To most couples parenthood is an expression of their love for each other. To society infertility is still regarded as an illness.

The psychological impact of being infertile can be considerable and the necessary investigations psychologically disturbing, particularly to the woman, who has more investigations performed than her partner. She may perceive these investigations as invasive and intimate, involving a loss of control over her body.

Pregnancy Rates in Infertility*			
	Proportion of all cases of infertility (%)	Pregnancy rate** (%)	Proportion of all pregnancies (%)
Male:			
Azoospermia	7	65 (using DI)	4.5
Oligospermia	25	30	7.5
Female:			
Amenorrhea	7	90	6.3
Other ovulatory	14	60	7.4
Tubal damage	16	20	3.2
Endometriosis (severe)	2	30	0.6
Uterine abnormalities	1	70	0.7
Male-female (immunological)	5	15	0.7
Unexplained	23	60	13.8
			44.7

*'Take home' baby rates are about 7 per cent lower.
**Within 2 years of diagnosis with or without treatment.

Table 34.3 Factors influencing fertility in several large studies.

If a bar to fertility is detected in either partner, or if after investigation and treatment a pregnancy does not occur, the couple may be subjected to considerable psychological strain and may develop psychosexual problems.

The possibility of problems developing can be reduced in several ways, which involve the infertility specialist and the couple's general practitioner, who should have a key role, as he knows the couple better than does the specialist. This implies that there must be good communication between specialist and G.P.

- As early as possible in the infertility 'work-up' the medical practitioner should provide the patients with a clear detail of the investigations proposed, the reasons for them, and the sequence in which they will be performed. As the patients may be so anxious that they may listen to but not hear what is being said, it is helpful to suggest that they read a book about infertility or are provided with pamphlets.
- The investigations should be kept to a minimum, and only those which produce reliable information should be made. Once information is obtained the couple should be told the results and have the opportunity to ask questions.
- The attitude and behaviour of the doctor should be supportive, communicative and empathetic.
- If an absolute or severe barrier to conception is found, appropriate counselling should be offered. Inability to have a child represents a real loss, and mourning is an appropriate response. In counselling, the approach is to consider the findings as causing the couple's unhappiness, so that neither partner blames the other.
- Couples who are in an IVF or a GIFT programme need special care, as in most cases these technologies are a 'last resort' in their attempt to have a child. The egg retrieval may be painful and the whole process psychologically traumatic, particularly if the woman perceives parenthood as a prerequisite for personal fulfilment. Most couples cope well but one-third of women experience anxiety or depression and one woman in 7 becomes severely distressed.

35

INFECTIONS OF THE GENITAL TRACT

VULVOVAGINAL INFECTIONS

The skin of the vulva, in common with other parts of the skin which are liable to friction and chafing may be infected by common skin pathogens. Boils may occur on the vulval skin, particularly when the standard of hygiene is low. Multiple vulval ulcers occur occasionally, particularly in dehabilitated women, and are due to staphylococcal infection. The ulcers are shallow with a grey, discharging base and surrounding oedema. The vulva is extremely tender. Treatment is to prescribe antibiotics and apply 1 per cent chlorhexidine cream if this can be done without causing much pain.

GENITAL HERPES

Herpetic infection of the vulva is becoming increasingly common. The virus, herpes simplex virus (HSV) exists in two forms, HSV1 and HSV2. HSV1 usually causes cold sores on the lips, but is the cause of genital herpes in 15 per cent of cases. HSV2 causes genital herpes in 85 per cent of cases.

The first attack of genital herpes is the worst. It follows sexual contact with an infected person who at the time was recovering from an attack of genital herpes. The inner surfaces of the labia majora are most likely to be infected. After a short period of itching or burning, small crops of painful, reddish lumps appear which become blisters within 24 hours. The blisters ulcerate rapidly to form multiple shallow painful ulcers *(Fig. 35.1)*. The surrounding tissues become oedematous and secondary infection may occur, aggravating the oedema and pain, and in some cases making micturition painful and difficult. Over 5 days the ulcers crust over and heal slowly, the healing being complete in 7 – 12 days after the appearance of the blisters. During this time and for 7 days after healing, virus is shed from the infected area. The virus also enters the myelin sheath of the sensory nerves supplying the affected area, and tracks to lie in the dorsal root ganglion. It may lie dormant for the rest of the person's life or may be reactivated and track back along the nerves to cause a new attack of herpes. Second and subsequent attacks are less severe but can cause considerable discomfort and affect relationships.

A single recurrence occurs in 30 per cent of infected women, and between 2 and 5 per cent have recurrent attacks, sometimes more than 6 times a year. As time passes the attacks become less frequent and may cease. In most cases the cause of the recurrence is not known, but recurrences are more common in the luteal phase of the menstrual cycle; if the woman has other sexually transmitted infections; or if she is emotionally stressed.

Diagnosis

The appearance of the ulcers leads to a provisional diagnosis of genital herpes, which should be confirmed by pricking the blisters to obtain vesicular fluid or by rubbing the ulcers with a cotton tipped bud (after applying 2% topical lignocaine a few minutes before) to obtain epithelial cells and sending the swab in a virus transport medium for culture.

Treatment

During an attack a woman should wear panties at all times as she may inadvertently scratch the infected area when sleeping and transfer the virus to her eyes. She should wash her hands after touching the infected area or applying medications. If the woman is unable to pass urine because of pain, a catheter may need to be inserted. Local applications of ice or anaesthetic jelly provide some relief.

The only effective medication is acyclovir. This drug is expensive. Acyclovir reduces the duration and severity of the initial and recurrent attacks, and shortens the time of viral shedding if given early in the attack. It is given orally in a dose of 200mg five times daily for 5 days. Given prophylactically it

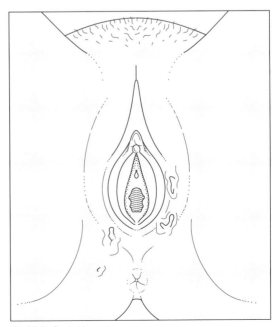

Fig 35.1 Genital herpes.

reduces the frequency of recurrent attacks. The need for prophylactic acyclovir should be reviewed annually.

GENITAL WARTS (CONDYLOMATA ACUMINATA)

Genital warts are caused by one or more types of the human papilloma virus (HPV), most commonly types 4 and 11, but sometimes types 16 and 18. The virus is usually (but not necessarily) transmitted sexually. Vulval infections are the most common, and the virus may spread to infect the vagina or the cervix; these areas may be infected initially.

Vulval warts usually present as cauliflower growths of varying sizes, but may be clinically undetectable. It has been estimated that 5–10 per cent of sexually active adults are infected annually, and that 30 per cent have evidence of previous infection (based on DNA hybridization).

The growths may occur on any part of the vulva and may involve the anal area *(Fig. 35.2)*. In most cases the warts are symptomless but some women complain of vulval itching or burning. If the warts involve the vaginal entrance or the vagina, the woman may complain of dyspareunia.

The importance of HPV infection is that types 16 and 18 are involved, in some way, with the development of cervical carcinoma. The risk of this occurring from vulval warts is small (Relative Risk 1.5: 0.9–2.5). This is discussed further in Chapter 39.

Treatment

Genital warts, if not too exuberant, may be treated with podophyllotoxin (twice daily for 3 days, repeated if needed after 4 days) applied by the woman herself, after trimming away any vulval hair around the wart; or the medical practitioner may apply 20 per cent podophyllin in benzoin tincture to the wart without touching the surrounding skin, to avoid skin burns and ulceration. The mixture is allowed to dry and the woman washes it off 4 hours later. This is repeated twice weekly if necessary. Larger condylomata on the cervix may respond to the application of tricholoracetic acid.

Large warts or warts which fail to respond to medical treatment, are treated by diathermy or by laser. The procedure is painful and anaesthesia is needed. Post operatively, pain requires analgesics. A problem which has recently been reported is that neither diathermy nor laser may cure the woman, as the virus may have infected neighbouring normal cells and warts may recur. Because of the concern that HPV infection with types 16 and 18 may be involved with the development of cervical carcinoma, a woman who has vulval warts should have an annual pap smear made.

SYPHILITIC VULVAL ULCER

Syphilis is caused by the invasion of the tissues by *Treponema pallidum* and is sexually transmitted. The initial lesion is a small papule which appears at the site of inoculation, usually 14 – 28 days after the person is infected. In women the usual site of infection is one of the labia majora, but the cervix may be infected instead. The papule rapidly enlarges to form an oval lesion of variable size, the centre of which becomes eroded and granulomatous. The edges of the eroded area are sharp, and outside this a thickened, indurated zone occurs, hence the name for the lesion – hard chancre *(Fig. 35.3)*. The chancre is

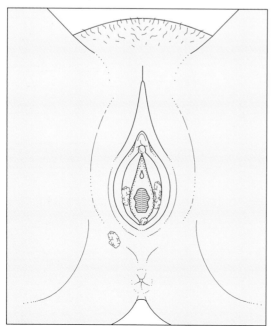

Fig 35.2 Genital warts.

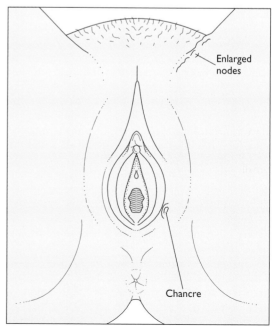

Fig 35.3 The primary lesion of syphyilis

painless and may be ignored by the woman or considered a small sore of no consequence, but as it is teeming with Treponema it is highly infectious. The primary lesion disappears in 21 days or so.

Diagnosis

The diagnosis is confirmed by examining a swab taken from the ulcer through a microscopic under dark ground illumination. To obtain an accurate diagnosis the chancre is first cleaned with a swab, and then, if necessary, its edge and base is scarified using a scalpel so that exudate appears before the specimen is taken. Six weeks after the primary infection serological tests for syphilis (VDRL or Rapid Plasma Reagin) become positive.

Treatment

Treatment is to give antibiotics, for example, procaine penicillin 1.0 megaunits for 10 days; or a long-acting benzathine penicillin 2.4 megaunits; or erythromycin 500mg orally 4 times a day for 10 days. Meticulous follow-up is essential.

INFECTION OF BARTHOLIN'S GLAND (BARTHOLINITIS)

The infection is usually due to *E.coli* or *staphylococci* but may follow gonorrhoeal infection. In the acute stage both the duct and gland are involved. If it is not treated the infection may subside or a Bartholin's abscess may form. Occasionally the gland becomes chronically enlarged following an inflammatory conglutination of the duct epithelium, to form a Bartholin's cyst.

Diagnosis

In acute Bartholinitis the woman complains of acute discomfort in the region of the gland, and a reddened tender swelling appears beneath the posterior part of the labium majus.

Treatment

Treatment is to prescribe analgesics and a broad spectrum antibiotic. If an abscess has formed, marsupialization of the abscess should be performed. An elliptical piece of the vagina and abscess wall just inside the hymen is removed. The vaginal and abscess walls are sutured to maintain patency and a small drain is inserted.

VAGINAL DISCHARGES AND INFECTIONS

The vagina of a woman in the reproductive years is lined by a layer of stratified epithelium, 10 to 30 cells thick. As is described on page 313, the superficial cells of the vagina are shed constantly into the vaginal cavity and release glycogen which is acted on by Doderlein's bacilli (lactobacilli) to produce lactic acid and hydrogen peroxide, natural defences against vaginal infection, and to maintain the vaginal pH between 3.5 and 4.5.

The vagina harbours large numbers of bacteria, which constitute its normal flora *(Table 35.1)*. However, a significant number of women harbour potential pathogens in the vagina. The pathogens are *Trichomonads*, *Candida spp.*, and *Gardnerella*. These organisms produce symptoms in only a few women.

The vagina is normally kept moist by transudation of fluid through the vaginal walls, which mixes with the exfoliated vaginal cells, aliphatic acids and the microorganisms mentioned earlier. The quantity of vaginal secretions varies through the menstrual cycle, peaking at ovulation time. The quantity is also increased by emotional stress. If an increased quantity of vaginal secretion is present, it may form a white coagulum, which may cause concern to the woman when she notices a whitish discharge which may cause itching. The discharge is termed leucorrhoea which is defined as a non-infective, non-bloodstained physiological vaginal discharge.

LEUCORRHOEA

When a woman presents to a doctor with leucorrhoea, infection by pathogenic organisms must be excluded by obtaining a vaginal smear which is examined and/or cultured.

Treatment

Treatment is to reassure the woman that the discharge is not pathogenic, that its fishy smell is undetectable to others, and to explore reasons for the woman's concern. A few women have recurrent vaginal discharges which show no pathogens on repeated laboratory investigations. These cases are difficult to treat. Many of these women have abnormal scores on psychometric tests, or have the somatizing syndrome, so that the woman's life-style including her sexuality should be investigated, rather than concentrating on the vaginal discharge. Some women repeatedly douche themselves for 'vaginal hygiene', a practice which may increase the chance of vaginal infection by reducing the number of vaginal lactobacilli.

Normal Vaginal Flora	
	Per cent
Lactobacilli	80–90
Staphlococci, micrococci	50–70
Ureaplasma	40–50
Anaerobes	20–50
Streptococci	20–30
Gardnerella	10–30
E. coli	5–15
Candida sp	5–15
Bacteroides	5–10
Trichomonads	3–7

Table 35.1 Normal vaginal flora.

If the woman wants medication, a vaginal acidifying jelly (Acijel) may be prescribed. Antibiotics should be avoided as they may aggravate the discharge rather than relieve it.

PATHOLOGICAL VAGINAL DISCHARGES

The three common pathological irritating vulvovaginal discharges are caused by:

- Trichomoniasis.
- Candidosis.
- Amine vaginosis.

In many cases they can be differentiated in the doctor's office or outpatient clinic by taking a sample of the discharge and looking at a smear under a microscope. Part of the swab is mixed with a drop of saline and part is mixed on a second slide with two drops of 10% potassium hydroxide (KOH). The saline preparation may reveal *trichomonal flagellates*, which can be observed moving and thrashing their tails *(Fig. 35.4)*. This slide may also show vaginal epithelial cells with serrated borders 'Clue cells' which suggest that the woman has *amine vaginosis (Fig. 35.5)*. Clue cells are more readily apparent on a Gram stained slide. Amine vaginosis is also suggested by a strong fishy smell from the KOH preparation (the amine test). The KOH preparation is examined under a microscope when hyphae of *Candida albicans* can be seen if this is the cause of the discharge *(Fig. 35.6)*.

The alternative is to take the vaginal swab and place it in a culture medium, such as Transgrow, and send it to a laboratory for tests.

TRICHOMONIASIS

The *trichomonas vaginalis* parasite is a 20µm long flagellate. It is a little larger than a leucocyte *(Fig. 35.4)*. Once introduced into the vagina it shelters at the bottom of the crypts of the velvet-like vaginal epithelium. As it is found in the vagina of symptomless women it appears only to become a pathogen in certain conditions, which raise the pH to 5.5 or more. The conditions are not known. It is readily sexually transmitted. It infects the man's urethra and is symptomless. It may also infect women who have not had sexual intercourse.

Clinical aspects

The main complaint is a moderate to profuse vaginal discharge which produces itching and irritation inside the vagina and around the vaginal introitus. In long-standing cases the discharge is greenish in colour and frothy.

Treatment

The patient is given a single oral dose of tinidazole 3g or metronidazole 2g. Alternatively, oral metronidazole may be prescribed in a dose of 200mg three times a day for 7 days. The woman's sexual partner should be invited to take the same treatment. These regimens cure 90 per cent of infected women. A vaginal swab is taken 7 days after completing treatment and if the flagellates are still present, a second course of treatment is given. All patients are asked to have a further vaginal swab made 2 months after the completion of treatment but few do. Side effects of treatment are minimal: a few women feel nauseated. Alcohol should be avoided whilst taking the tablets as it may lead to headaches and flushing.

CANDIDOSIS

Candida spp infect the vaginal epithelial cells, particularly if in the fungal germinating stage, when they develop spores and long threads (hyphae) *(Fig. 35.5)*. Inside the vaginal epithelial cells they may lie dormant until environmental conditions encourage germination. *Candida spp* may also infect the vulval skin, the anogenital region, the mouth and the intestinal tract. If the vaginal acidity falls, its growth is encouraged, as it is in diabetic women and women taking antibiotics or corticosteroids.

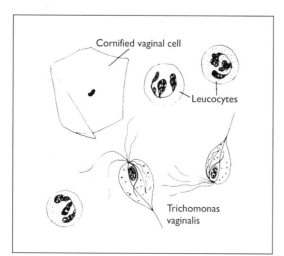

Fig 35.4 *Trichomonas vaginalis.*

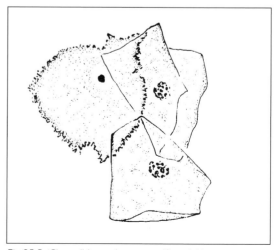

Fig 35.5 'Clue cells', seen in non-specific vaginitis.

Clinical aspects

The woman complains of severe vulvo-vaginal irritation which is associated with a vaginal discharge. Her sexual partner may complain of itching of his glans and foreskin in some cases.

Typically the discharge is thick and 'cheesy' and adheres to the vaginal wall in plaques, but these findings often are not present.

Diagnosis

Diabetes mellitus should be excluded, and a vaginal swab should be taken and processed as mentioned earlier.

Treatment

One of the imidazole group of drugs (clotrimazole; econazole; isoconazole, or miconazole) is prescribed as a vaginal tablet, either as a single dose or daily for 3 days. If vaginal treatment fails or oral treatment is preferred, fluconazole or ketoconazole may be prescribed. Vulval irritation may be intense, and an imidazole cream may be applied at intervals. A course of treatment cures 85 per cent of patients.

RECURRENT CANDIDOSIS

Between 5 and 15 per cent of women with vaginal candidosis have recurrent attacks, sometimes 4 times a year. Most are relapses of the initial infection, possibly because of a reduced local host defence against *Candida spp.* Recurrent attacks can cause a considerable disruption to the woman's personal and sexual life, and she may resort to alternative medicine.

Treatment

It is difficult to treat this condition. In women who have frequent recurrences, prophylactic ketoconazole 100mg by mouth daily for 6 months or fluconazole 150mg weekly may offer protection. Some women complain of nausea. Ketonazole causes liver damage in 1 in 15 000 users, and the woman should have liver function tests at the start of treatment and after 3 months. The woman is usually told not to wear nylon pantihose or tight jeans, but the value of this has not been established.

AMINE VAGINOSIS (NON-SPECIFIC VAGINITIS)

This condition is believed to be caused by an interaction between the normal vaginal inhabitant, *Gardernella vaginalis* and *Vaginal anaerobes*.

Clinical aspects

The woman complains of a thin greyish discharge which has a strong fishy odour.

Diagnosis and treatment

The diagnosis is established as mentioned earlier. Treatment is that suggested for trichomoniasis.

INFECTIONS OF THE INTERNAL GENITAL ORGANS

The fact that the genital tract, apart from the lowest third, derives from the Mullerian duct and has anastomosing systems of arteries, veins and lymphatics, means that infections of individual organs, are less frequent than sequential ascending infection of the organs.

Ascending vaginal infection is controlled to some extent by the following mechanisms. First, the vaginal walls lie in apposition and the vaginal secretions are acidic, which inhibits bacterial growth; second, the cervical mucus forms a meshwork, except at the time of ovulation, which limits upward spread; third, the endometrium is shed each month during menstruation. However, if the cervix is infected directly, the above mechanisms are less effective.

Most cervical infections occur in sexually active women and usually follow a sexually transmitted organism acquired from an infected man, who has gonorrhoea or non-gonococcal genital infection (in most cases *Chlamydia trachomatis*). In a few cases, microbial agents which are normal vaginal inhabitants may spread upwards and cause infection of the internal genital organs. These 'polymicrobial' infections are usually found in long-standing cases of pelvic infection and may be secondary contaminants.

As it may be difficult clinically to determine which organ is infected, and as more than one organ is usually infected, the condition is usually diagnosed as acute pelvic infection or *pelvic inflammatory disease (PID)*. It is currently thought that chlamydial infection causes 50 – 65 per cent of all cases of PID, and gonorrhoea 15 – 30 per cent; in the remaining cases the aetiology is unclear, but may be polymicrobial. The women in this last group tend to be older and to have had PID for a longer time.

Infection of the internal genital organs also may occur following an abortion or after childbirth. In

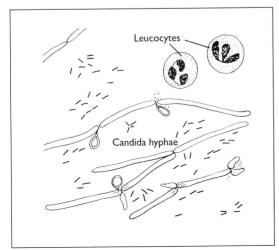

Fig 35.6 Candida albicans.

these cases the infective agents, which are usually staphylococci, streptococci, *E. coli* or anaerobes, enter the tissues through cervical lacerations, or more frequently, through the placental bed. Infections following pregnancy or childbirth are discussed in Chapter 25.

In a few cases pelvic infections occur either from haematogenous spread, as in tuberculosis, or from pelvic peritonitis.

NON-GONOCOCCAL (NGGI) AND GONOCOCCAL GENITAL INFECTIONS

As mentioned, most cases of PID follow sexual intercourse with a man who has gonorrhoea or non-gonococcal urethritis. In many cases the man has no symptoms and may be unaware that he is infected. The microorganisms invade the columnar cells lining the crypts of the cervical canal. They may be eliminated by the body's immune system, spread rapidly to cause an acute infection or remain quiescent in the columnar cells, with the potential to spread to other pelvic organs. Spread occurs via the lymphatics or the veins or possibly by 'riding on the back of spermatozoa'. In a few instances the infection is carried into the uterus during the insertion of an intrauterine device (see page 236).

The endometrium is first infected, causing endometritis. From here the infection may spread to the myometrium causing myometritis, or through the uterine cavity to the Fallopian tubes causing acute or subacute salpingitis. In some cases the ovaries and the pelvic peritoneum may be involved *(Fig. 35.7)*.

The two principal infecting agents are *Chlamydia Trachomatis* and *Neisseria gonorrhoeae*. They require further discussion.

CHLAMYDIAL INFECTION

Infection with *Chlamydia trachomatis* is usually symptomless, but a few women (<20 per cent) may complain of a mucopurulent discharge from the cervix, or of dysuria. Community studies have shown that between 15 and 30 per cent of healthy women have circulating antichlamydial antibodies, indicating previous subclinical infection, and that 1 – 4 per cent have symptomless infection of the endocervical cells. Symptomatic chlamydial genital infection affects less than 1 per cent of sexually active women aged 15 – 50 each year. A higher incidence occurs in women under the age of 25 who have a history of a sexually transmitted disease and who have had several sexual partners or whose sexual partners have had several partners.

GONOCOCCAL GENITAL INFECTION

Gonococcal genital infection may be symptomless or produce early symptoms of dysuria, urinary frequency and a purulent discharge per vaginam. The discharge originates from infected endocervical cells

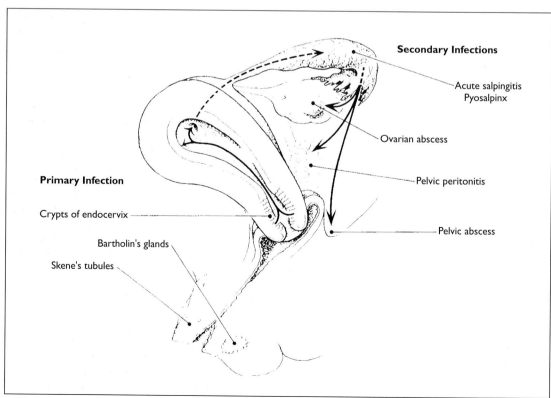

Fig 35.7 Diagram of route of spread of non-gonococcal and gonococcal infection.

and from Bartholin's glands, but not from the vaginal mucosa as the gonococcus is unable to penetrate vaginal stratified epithelium. The severity of the initial infection varies and in 50 – 80 per cent of infected women symptoms are so mild that they are ignored. Spread, if it occurs, is upwards to the endometrium and Fallopian tubes, or downwards to infect Bartholin's glands.

CLINICAL PRESENTATIONS OF PID

Cervical infection has been discussed and endometritis is usually symptomless except when it follows a bacterial infection after abortion or childbirth.

Salpingitis may be symptomless or symptomatic. In acute symptomatic cases, the growth of organisms of the cells lining the oviduct produces the acute phase of primary infection. A large amount of mucus is secreted, together with a fibrinous exudate which produces agglutination of the mucosal folds of the endosalpinx. The Fallopian tubes become inflamed and oedematous, producing recognizable symptoms. These are:

- Severe bilateral lower abdominal tenderness and pain.
- Abdominal muscle spasm.
- Fever (>38.0 °C), often with rigors.
- Leukocytosis.

On examination, the lower abdomen is tender and on pelvic examination bimanual palpation of the lateral vaginal fornices is excruciatingly painful.

In particularly virulent infections, pus may collect in the Fallopian tube, producing a pyosalpinx, or the infection may spread to the ovaries.

Diagnosis

The diagnosis may be established clinically but confirmation by laparoscopy is required in most cases, as the symptoms are non-specific and may occur in tubal pregnancy, accompany an infected ovarian cyst, or have a psychosomatic basis. Recently, it has been suggested that an endometrial sample (using a Vabra or similar biopsy curette) which is sent to a laboratory to detect plasma cells and transvaginal pelvic ultrasound scanning are as accurate as laparoscopy and less invasive. The transvaginal ultrasound looks for:

- Multiple ovarian cysts.
- Thickened fluid-filled Fallopian tubes.
- Free fluid in the pelvis.

Laboratory tests should be made. Urethral and cervical swabs should be taken and sent in appropriate transport media for examination. Screening for chlamydia is made by an immunofluorescence test or an ELISA test using a monoclonal antibody.

Treatment

In most cases treatment should be started before the exact infective agent has been identified. In severely ill patients antibiotics should be started intravenously. In less severe cases intramuscular or oral antibiotics should be given. Because of the frequent association of chlamydia and gonococcal infection, and the increasing prevalence of penicillin-resistant N gonococci, the Centre for Disease Control in the USA recommends that the current treatment of doxycycline and metronidazole should be replaced with a single dose of probenecid 1g and ceftriaxone 250mg IM (one dose), or cefixime 400–800mg orally, followed by doxycycline 100mg orally twice daily for 14–21 days. Other authorities recommend clindamycin 450mg four times a day for 10 days or ciprofloxacin 750mg twice daily for 12 days.

In severe infections, including tubovarian abscess, intravenous treatment should be started with cefoxitin 2g IV four times daily plus doxycycline 100mg IV twice daily. This regimen is continued for 4 days and is followed by doxycycline 100mg twice daily for a further 10 days.

Surgery is indicated if the drug treatment fails, or in the presence of obvious abscesses, which do not respond to antibiotic treatment. The surgery should be as conservative as possible, draining being preferred. A 'total clearance' of the genital organs is rarely indicated.

Prevention

Both chlamydia and gonorrhoea are sexually transmitted. Prevention is therefore best obtained if people are prepared to use 'safer sex', that is, limiting the number of sexual partners and insisting on the use of a condom if the couple choose vaginal or anal penetration and either partner cannot be relied on to disclose his or her previous sexual behaviour. This advice is idealistic, and usually is ignored. An alternative is to suggest that a person who has several sexual partners or whose partner has several sexual partners is 'screened' for chlamydia and gonorrhoea every 6 months or so.

Long-term effects of PID

A first chlamydial genital infection, unless treated, causes damage to the Fallopian tubes in 10 per cent of cases. If a second infection occurs the proportion of women who develop tubal damage increases to 25 per cent and after a third infection to over 50 per cent. Gonococcal infection unless treated is associated with an even higher chance of tubal damage. As many infections, particularly chlamydial infections, are symptomless it is not surprising that evidence of previous tubal infection often is first detected during investigations for infertility. If a previously infected woman, who has had tubal damage, does succeed in getting pregnant she has 5 – 7 times the risk of having an ectopic pregnancy compared with a woman who has not had PID.

SUBACUTE SALPINGITIS

This is often symptomless or the woman may feel unwell. A vaginal examination may show a tubal mass. This is found in half the number of women infected with gonorrhoea, but in only a quarter of those infected with chlamydia.

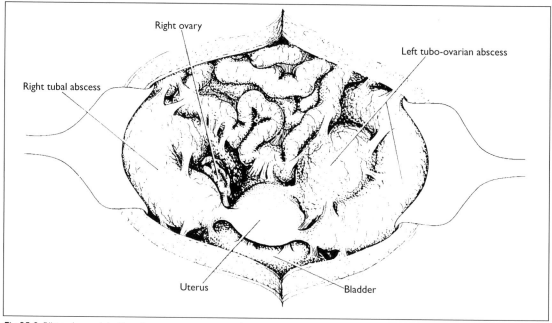

Fig 35.8 Bilateral pyosalpingitis – the appearance at operation.

CHRONIC GENITAL INFECTION (CHRONIC PID)

Chronic genital infection is a long-term sequel of acute or subacute infection and may follow post abortion or puerperal infection. It may present as a pyosalpinx, a hydrosalpinx or a chronic tuboovarian abscess *(Fig. 35.8)*. In other cases the infection involves the connective tissues of the pelvis, causing chronic pelvic cellulitis.

PYOSALPINX

Pyosalpinx, or 'chronic pus tube' forms as a result of blockage of the lumen of the oviduct at the fimbrial end and at one or more points along the Fallopian tube. This occurs in the acute phase of the infection, and exudate accumulates distending the oviduct to a greater or lesser degree *(Fig. 35.9)*. The distension of the oviduct flattens the endosalpinx and the wall of the oviduct is thickened by the inflammatory

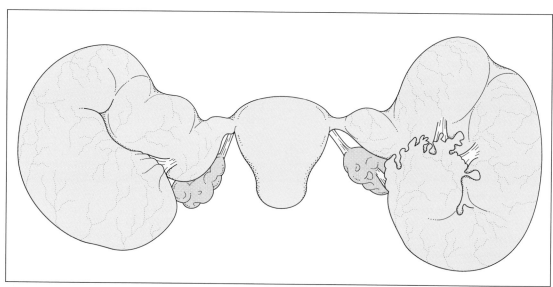

Fig 35.9 Bilateral chronic salpingitis.

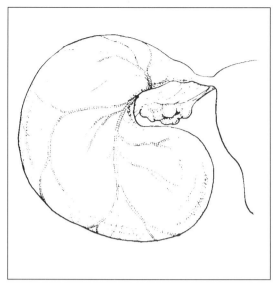

Fig 35.10 Hydrosalpinx. Note the 'retort'-shaped distension of the oviduct.

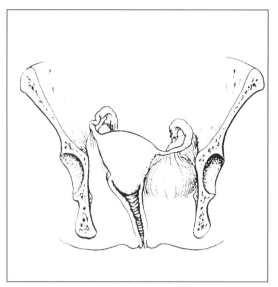

Fig 35.11 Diagram of chronic pelvic cellulitis.

process. Since the inflammatory process extends through the thickness of the wall of the oviduct, adhesions to surrounding structures are usual. The ovary may be involved to form a chronic tubo-ovarian abscess.

There may be no symptoms, or vague pelvic pain may occur which is intermittent or constant. It is often worse in the premenstrual phase of the menstrual cycle. Some women complain of deep dyspareunia. These symptoms are not specific for chronic pelvic infection and may be due to psychosomatic conditions. The symptoms may vary in severity, possibly because of an exacerbation of the infective process. This may occur months or years after the first infection. Laparoscopy may be needed to establish the diagnosis. In some cases the woman becomes acutely ill.

Treatment of chronic pyosalpinx which is causing symptoms is surgical. The extent of the surgery depends on the severity of the condition, and in general requires bilateral salpingectomy and often oophorectomy, although some ovarian tissue may be saved. Hysterectomy is also usually performed in case residual infection is present.

HYDROSALPINX

Hydrosalpinx is the end result of burnt-out pyogenic salpingitis, which was of low virulence but highly irritating, producing large quantities of clear exudate within the closed portion of the oviduct. The distended oviduct has a thin wall, which is translucent and is usually retort shaped *(Fig. 35.10)*. Adhesions to contiguous structures may be present.

Hydrosalpinx may be symptomless but if symptoms are present they are many and variable.

They include general ill-health, lassitude, disturbances of menstruation and chronic aching in the lower abdomen, which is worse premenstrually. Abdominal examination often shows no abnormality. Vaginal examination may reveal generalized tenderness or a smooth cystic enlargement. Because of these nonspecific complaints, laparoscopy is often required to make a diagnosis. Treatment is surgical. The extent of the surgery is determined by the condition of the other Fallopian tube and the woman's desire to have children.

CHRONIC PELVIC CELLULITIS

Chronic pelvic cellulitis is less common today than in the past but still occurs. It is usually the sequel of acute pelvic cellulitis and results in thickening and fibrosis of the connective tissues of the parametrium, so that the position of the uterus is distorted and it is relatively or absolutely immobilized *(Fig. 35.11)*. The symptoms of chronic pelvic cellulitis are variable. The most common complaint is a chronic deep pelvic ache, often localized to one side, and backache. Deep dyspareunia is frequent and may be so severe as to prevent sexual intercourse. Vaginal examination shows a tender uterus drawn to one side and relatively fixed in position.

Treatment is unsatisfactory, some patients responding to pelvic short-wave diathermy. Hysterectomy is another option. Unfortunately, in spite of treatment, in many women the pain persists.

TUBERCULOUS INFECTION OF THE GENITAL TRACT

In the developed countries genital tract tuberculosis is very uncommon, accounting for less than 0.5 per cent of all pelvic infections. In the developing countries the incidence is much higher. The disease is spread in the post-primary haematogenous phase of tuberculosis. If this happens to coincide with puberty when an increased growth of and blood supply to the internal genital organs occurs, infection may occur.

The disease may be limited to the oviducts, but spread to the endometrium is common. Symptoms are minimal, and the condition is detected when investigations for infertility are made. Treatment is that for pulmonary tuberculosis, surgery only being used if there are large adnexal masses and only after medical treatment has been tried.

36

ATROPHIC AND DYSTROPHIC CONDITIONS

In the years after the menopause, the internal genital organs become smaller and atrophic. The changes occur, because the amount of circulating oestrogen falls to a very low level.

THE INTERNAL GENITAL ORGANS

By the age of 75 years, the uterus, the Fallopian tubes and the ovaries have shrunk considerably.*(Fig. 36.1)*. In the uterus, the endometrium has become atrophic and the muscle fibres of the myometrium have been replaced progressively by fibrous tissue. The cervix has atrophied and the cervical canal may become obliterated. If the woman develops uterine infection, the pus may not escape, leading to a *pyometra*. This may also occur if the woman develops an endometrial or cervical carcinoma. The woman may complain of lower abdominal pain. Examination shows that the uterus is larger than expected for her age. The diagnosis is confirmed by ultrasound scanning which shows that the uterine cavity is enlarged and filled with fluid. If carcinoma is detected it is treated appropriately; if it is not present, the cervix is dilated and a drain inserted for a few days.

THE VAGINA

The changes in the vagina depend on the amount of oestrogen which continues to be synthesized in peripheral tissues, but in most women the vaginal epithelium becomes atrophic. The superficial cells diminish in number and intermediate and parabasal cells predominate. These changes show clinically as vaginal discomfort and burning, and painful intercourse.

THE PELVIC FLOOR

Deprived of oestrogen the blood supply to the muscles of the pelvic floor diminishes. The pelvic floor muscles lose their tone and the connective tissue its elasticity, so that relaxation of pelvic floor tissues damaged during childbirth is likely to occur with varying degrees of prolapse (see Chapter 40).

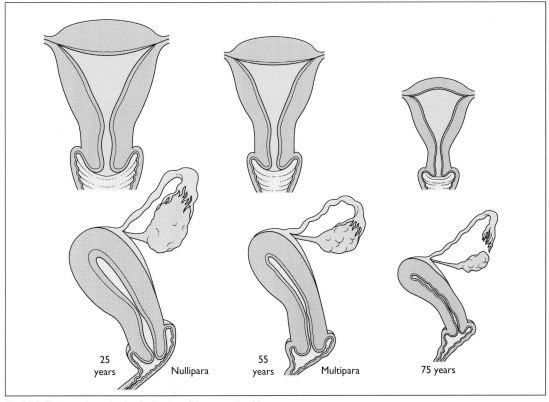

25 years · Nullipara 55 years · Multipara 75 years

Fig 36.1 To show the reduction in the size of the uterus in old age.

THE VULVA

As a woman's age increases the labia majora lose their fat and elastic tissue content, becoming smaller, and the vaginal introitus is exposed. In very old women only a narrow cleft indicates the presence of the vaginal introitus.

The vulval epithelium becomes thin, with loss of elastic and collagen fibres. These changes may lead to vulval irritation, although this may occur at earlier ages.

THE ITCHY VULVA (PRURITUS VULVAE)

One woman in 10 who attends a medical practitioner for genital tract complaints, will say, among other complaints, that she has an itchy vulva. The reason may be infection, general skin or medical disease or emotional problems. Emotional problems are thought to cause vulval itch in some women because the skin covering the vulva, and its underlying capillaries are 'unstable'. Thus sexual or marital problems, anxiety and depression may manifest somatically as vulval itch.

Whatever the cause, the itch, mediated by a release of histamines, leads to scratching, which aggravates the itch. Over a period of months the itch–scratch cycle may initiate a variety of histological changes in the vulval skin – chronic vulval epithelial dystrophies. Dermatologists prefer the term 'non-neoplastic epithelial disorders of the skin and mucosa'.

HISTOPATHOLOGY OF CHRONIC VULVAL DYSTROPHIES

The changes to be described usually only occur if the itchy vulva has persisted for 6 months or more. Biopsies taken before this time will usually show a normal vulval skin *(Fig. 36.2)*.

Atrophic dystrophy

In young women this histological change is termed by dermatologists as lichen sclerosus et atrophicus. In older women it is termed senile vulvitis.

Clinically the skin is pale red and shiny. A skin biopsy will show that the horny layer is unchanged or hyperkeratinized with marked thinning of the epidermis and disappearance of rete pegs. The sub epidermis is oedematous, some degree of hyalinization is present, collections of round cells are also present *(Fig. 36.3)*.

Hypertrophic dystrophy (squamous cell hyperplasia)

Dermatologists used to call this condition chronic dermatitis or neurodermatitis but now call it squamous cell hyperplasia. The skin looks red and is thickened with exaggerated skin folds. In moist areas, where maceration of the horny layer occurs, white patches may be seen. On histological examination, the epithelium is thickened and the papillae are elongated, but the rete pegs retain a finger-like shape. The dermis is oedematous and contains numbers of plasma cells and sometimes collagen fibres, but elastic fibres are usually absent *(Fig. 36.4)*.

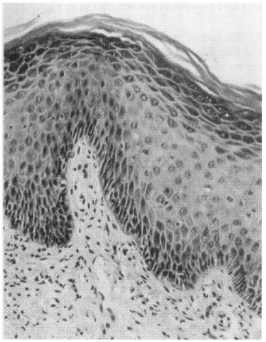

Fig 36.2 Histology of normal vulval skin (× 160).

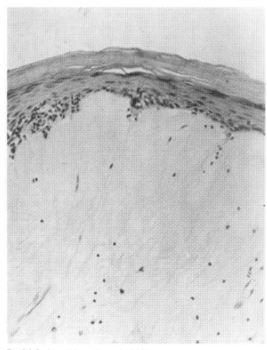

Fig 36.3 Atrophic patterns (× 160).

Mixed dystrophy

The presence of atrophic and hypertrophic areas is associated with this condition.

Dysplasia (vulval intraepithelial dysplasia)

In dysplasia, the appearance of the vulval skin is non-specific. Diagnosis depends on histological assessment. The basal cells of the epithelium are disorderly, showing atypical activity and pleomorphism. The Malpighian layer is thickened with lengthening of the rete pegs, which have abnormal shapes and often show denticulate processes. The subepithelial layer is usually hyalinized and elastic fibres are absent *(Fig. 36.5)*. The degrees of dysplasia may be further divided into categories including vulval intraepithelial neoplasia (VIN). Fewer than 10 per cent of dysplasias progress to vulval carcinoma.

AETIOLOGY

Studies of women who have pruritus vulvae show that this disease has varied aetiology.

General skin diseases

The conditions listed in *Table 36.1* are the usual skin diseases which may manifest as pruritus vulvae. Fungal infections may also cause vulval itch, although the itch is generally intercrural.

General diseases

The most common general disease causing pruritus vulvae is diabetes mellitus. In diabetes, as well as being itchy, the vulva is swollen and dark-red in colour.

Allergic dermatitis

Sensitivity to soap (usually perfumed), some detergents used to wash pantihose, and other contact allergens may cause vulval itch.

Vaginal infections

The most common causes of vulval itch, particularly in younger women, are vaginal infections, particularly

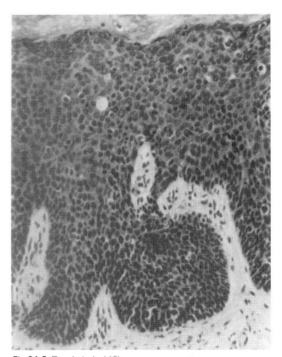

Fig 36.5 Dysplasia (× 160).

The Itchy Vulva: Aetiology	
	Percentage of cases
1. General skin diseases (psoriasis, leucoderma, lichen planus, intertrigo, scabies)	5
2. General diseases (diabetes,? deficiency diseases)	5
3. Allergic dermatitis	5
4. Vaginal discharges Trichomoniasis Candidosis	50
5. Psychosomatic conditions	35

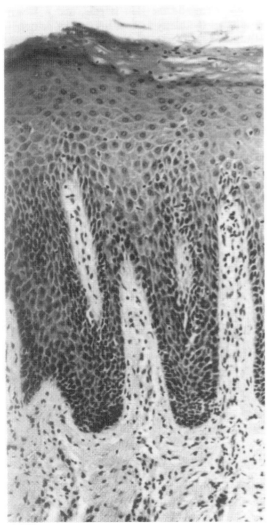

Fig 36.4 Hypertrophic patterns (× 160).

Table 36.1 The itchy vulvae: aetiology.

candidosis and trichomoniasis. As candidal infection of the vulval skin is common, vulval skin scrapings should be taken in cases where general diseases and allergic causes have been eliminated. It may also be helpful to inspect the vulval skin through a magnifying glass or a colposcope.

Psychosomatic causes

Pruritus vulvae is of organic aetiology in more than two-thirds of women with the disease. It is thought that psychosomatic causes account for the remainder of cases.

THE INVESTIGATION OF PRURITUS VULVAE

Steps to be taken include:
- The history will identify if the main area of itch is vulval, anal or intercrural. If it is one of the last two, the cause is probably threadworms, tinea or intertrigo. The woman should be asked about any allergic conditions including contact dermatitis and drug sensitivity. The duration of the pruritus should be determined. If it is longer than 12 months, multiple skin biopsies *(Fig. 36.6)* using a dermatome should be considered, irrespective of the age of the woman or the appearance of the vulva.
- General skin condition should be assessed by examining the patient in a good light, and inspecting all body surfaces including the interdigital folds of the feet and hands.
- General medical causes should be considered, particularly glycosuria. The urine should also be checked for protein. In elderly women a 2-hour postprandial or fasting blood sugar test should be ordered.
- The vagina should be inspected and swabs taken, on more than one occasion, to exclude candidosis and trichomoniasis. A skin scraping for vulval candida infection should be taken if the pruritus has persisted for more than 6 months.

TREATMENT

Any aetiological factor detected should be treated. As a general measure, soap should not be used on the vulval skin and vaginal douches should be avoided.

For all cases except severe dysplasia and carcinoma in situ, medical treatment is preferred. The reason is that if excision of the vulval skin (simple vulvectomy) is made, pruritus recurs in >50 per cent of cases. The patient must be made aware that to obtain a cure, medical treatment must be continued over a long period. During this time attempts should be made to discover any psychological upsets which may have precipitated the pruritus. Owing to the itch-scratch-itch-scratch cycle, a hydrocortisone ointment should be prescribed and applied sparingly. When this is not effective some women benefit if a 2% testosterone propionate ointment is applied. If the itch is severe a sedative should be prescribed to help the woman sleep at night. Elderly women may obtain relief if hormone replacement treatment (see

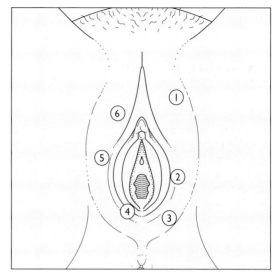

Fig 36.6 Sites from which a biopsy should be made.

page 307) is tried. The patient requires a good deal of support and reassurance over the period of treatment but should be made aware that in time the itch ceases in about 90 per cent of patients.

If the biopsies show severe dysplasia (vulval intraepithelial dysplasia) or carcinoma in situ, vulvectomy is the correct treatment (see Chapter 39).

VULVAL ATROPHY IN YOUNGER WOMEN

Vulval atrophy may occur in a few younger women. It can cause considerable distress not only because it is uncomfortable but because it prevents sexual intercourse, or makes it painful. The woman should be investigated for the presence of impaired glucose tolerance, and allergic conditions sought. Treatment is not very effective. The woman should be advised not to wear pantihose, as these garments prevent ventilation and increase vulval moisture.

Most medications are ineffective, but some success has been obtained using a 2% testosterone propionate ointment or a 2% dihydrotestosterone cream.

CHRONIC VULVAL PAIN

A few women have chronic discomfort or pain in the vulvovestibular area, which can be emotionally distressing. Pain also occurs if sexual intercourse is attempted. The area is tender, and pain or discomfort can be elicited if one or more of the biopsy spots *(see Fig. 36.6)* are touched with a cotton wool swab stick. The vulva usually looks normal. If a skin biopsy is taken it shows nonspecific chronic inflammation. The diagnosis is by exclusion. The aetiology is not known and there is no specific treatment. Psychotherapy may be tried.

37

ENDOMETRIOSIS

Endometriosis denotes the presence of functioning endometrial tissue in an abnormal location, in other words outside the uterine cavity. The development may occur between the muscle fibres of the myometrium (adenomyosis or uterine endometrio- sis), or in various locations in the pelvic cavity. The locations and the approximate chance of the lesion affecting the organ or structure is shown in *Fig. 37.1.*

The incidence of endometriosis is difficult to determine, as in many instances it is only discovered at laparoscopy when the patient presents with infer- tility or obscure abdominal pain. A probable estimate is that between 1 and 7 per cent of women in their reproductive years have endometriosis. Endometriosis is found more commonly among women who are infertile or who delay childbearing until after the age of 30 years.

AETIOLOGY

How the endometrium reaches the ectopic locations is not entirely understood. Adenomyosis is probably caused by direct infiltration of, or lymphatic spread to the myometrium by viable endometrial tissue. Extrauterine endometriosis probably results from the retrograde passage along the Fallopian tubes of endometrial tissue during menstruation. It is now believed that in most women retrograde menstrua- tion occurs, but the development of other than tem- porary endometrial nodules (blisters) only occurs in some women. The retrograde menstruation explains the finding that most endometrial lesions occur on the ovaries or in the cul-de-sac (Pouch of Douglas). Lymphatic or haematogenous spread may be the reason for the rare deposits of endometriosis in distant sites, for example, the umbilicus.

Once viable endometriotic tissue has reached and adhered to the ectopic location, it still has to be explained why it survives and grows in that location, instead of being eliminated by macrophages. A current theory is that there may be a defect in cell mediated immunity which permits the endometrial tissue to survive. In order to grow in these ectopic sites, the endometrial tissue has to respond to

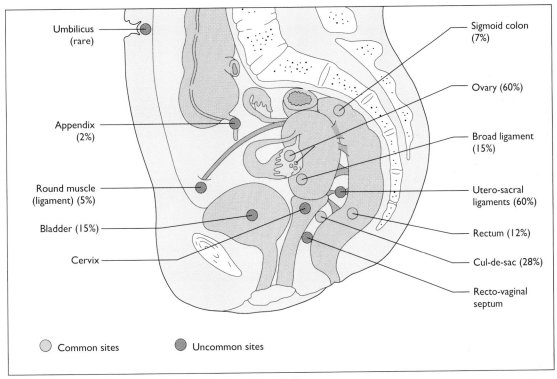

Fig 37.1 Common and uncommon sites of extrauterine endometriosis.

cyclical oestrogen, and to a lesser extent, progesterone. If a constant oestrogen milieu occurs, as in
pregnancy, the lesions tend to be attacked by
macrophages and become fibrotic.

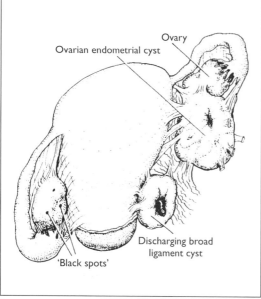

Fig 37.2 Extrauterine endometriosis.

PATHOLOGY

Whatever the location, the ectopic endometrium, surrounded by stroma, implants and forms a miniature
cyst, which responds to the cyclic secretion of oestrogen and progesterone, just as the uterine
endometrium does. During menstruation bleeding in
the cyst occurs. The blood, endometrial tissue and
tissue fluid are trapped in the cyst. Over the next
cycle, the tissue fluid and the blood plasma are
absorbed, leaving dark, thickened blood. The cycle
recurs each month and slowly the cyst enlarges containing increased amount of tarry, chocolate- coloured
inspissated blood. The maximal size of the cyst
depends on its location. Small cysts may remain small
or be attacked by macrophages and become small
fibrotic lesions. Ovarian cysts (endometriomata) tend
to be larger than other cysts, but do not usually
become larger than a medium-sized orange. As the
cyst grows, internal pressure may destroy the active
endometrial lining, making the cyst nonfunctional.

Rupture or leakage of material from even small
cysts is not uncommon. The released inspissated
blood is very irritating with the result that multiple
adhesions surround the cysts. The ectopic endometrium and stromal cells also tend to infiltrate
adjacent tissues, leading to more pelvic adhesions and
fixation *(Fig. 37.2)*. If an ovarian cyst is found which
looks like an endometrioma but there are no adhesions, the diagnosis is unlikely to be endometriosis.

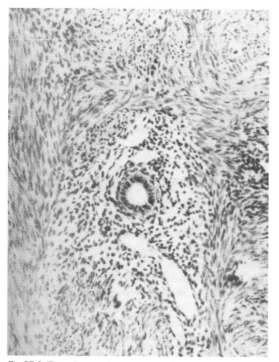

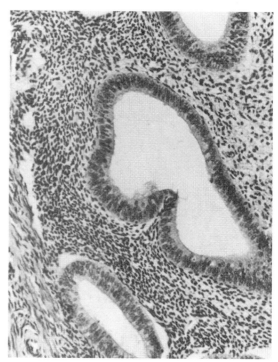

Fig 37.3 The microscopic appearance of adenomyosis. (A) The endometriotic nodule is lying deep in the
myometrium, and both glands and stroma are present (x 160). (B) Another specimen at higher
magnification (x 256) clearly showing the glands and the stroma, which is quite dense.

ADENOMYOSIS (UTERINE ENDOMETRIOSIS)

The cells which infiltrate the muscle derive mainly from the basal layer of the endometrium. As this layer is relatively insensitive to hormonal stimulation, the endometriotic nodules tend to be small, containing little blood, but they provoke a marked stromal reaction. The lesion also appears to stimulate myometrial proliferation, causing the tumour to enlarge slowly *(Fig. 37.3)*. Clinically, adenomyosis may be indistinguishable from a myoma, and both may coexist. As the growth of the clinical adenomyoma takes time, clinical adenomyosis tends to occur later in the reproductive years, often in parous women after a long period of secondary infertility.

EXTRAUTERINE ENDOMETRIOSIS

As mentioned, the ovary is most often involved and ovarian endometriosis may present as small superficial implants (red or black spots) or a larger endometrial cyst. Lesions on the surface of the broad ligament occur either directly from implanting endometrial tissue or as a secondary spread from the ovarian deposit. In these locations the endometrial deposits cause puckering of the peritoneum and adhesions to the posterior surface of the uterus, often fixing it in retroversion. Lesions in the cul-de-sac are of interest as they may not be palpable or visualized by a laparoscope unless the laparoscopy is made during menstruation.

CLINICAL FEATURES

The clinical features of endometriosis are often non-specific. In at least one-quarter of the number of women who have endometriosis the disease is symptomless, and in a further quarter it is found in association with other pelvic conditions. The symptoms also differ depending on whether the lesion is adenomyosis or extrauterine endometriosis.

ADENOMYOSIS

One-third of patients are asymptomatic, the enlarged uterus, which is thought to be a myoma, being detected at routine pelvic examination. In the remaining women, the main symptoms are:
- Progressively increasing pain, often associated with menstruation. In this case the pain increases throughout menstruation, reaching its peak towards the latter stages;
- Menstrual irregularities: premenstrual staining and spotting, increased flow or more frequent periods.

EXTRAUTERINE ENDOMETRIOSIS

The symptoms are often bizarre because of the varying locations of the disease, and do not correlate with the extent of the lesions in many cases. The symptoms include pain, menstrual irregularities, dyspareunia and infertility.

Pain

Typically lower abdominal crampy pain starts premenstrually, reaches its peak in the last few days of menstruation and then slowly subsides. This symptom is often referred to as 'acquired dysmenorrhoea '. If the endometrial cysts are large and adhesions are present, or if lesions involve the peritoneum over the bowel, the woman may complain of constant lower abdominal or pelvic pain which varies in intensity.

Menstrual disturbances

In 60 per cent of affected women menstrual irregularities occur. The woman may complain of 'premenstrual staining' or spotting, heavy menstrual periods (menorrhagia), or more frequent periods which may be heavy.

Dyspareunia

If the endometriotic lesions involve the culdesac, particularly if the uterus is retroverted and fixed by adhesions, the woman may complain of dyspareunia on deep penile penetration, whilst if the peritoneum over the bowel is involved, she may have pain on defaecation.

Infertility

Although endometriosis is associated with infertility, whether it is a cause of infertility is disputed, unless the lesions are severe and distort the anatomy. Usually endometriosis is not suspected until a laparoscopy made during the course of infertility investigations reveals the disease. Mild endometriosis associated with infertility is treated with hormones by some specialists and not by others. In 1992, a group of European experts concluded that there were no reliable data to support treating mild endometriosis with drugs.

CLINICAL EXAMINATION

Abdominal and pelvic examination may show no abnormality if the lesions are small. Larger cysts cause fixed, tender nodular swellings and may be easily palpable.

DIAGNOSIS

It is often difficult clinically to distinguish endometriosis from pelvic inflammatory disease or an ovarian cyst. Because of this it is prudent to examine the pelvis through a laparoscope if endometriosis is suspected. At laparoscopy, the extent of the disease should be determined, which influences treatment *(see Table 37.1)*.

THE MANAGEMENT OF ENDOMETRIOSIS

ADENOMYOSIS

Unless the disease is associated with extrauterine

The Management of Endometriosis		
Stage Characteristics	**Diagnosis**	**Treatment**
I. Minimal and II Mild Small surface nodules with no scarring or peritubal adhesions.	Only by laparoscope in investigation of infertility.	At most, electrocautery or CO_2 laser to lesions. Do not give hormones.
III. Moderate Small scattered surface lesions with scarring; ovarian endometriomata, <2.5cm, few periovarian or peritubal adhesions; nodules in the cul-de-sac or uterosacral ligaments.	Often symptoms but confirmation by laparoscopy needed.	Electrocautery or CO_2 laser to lesions Hormones. Conservative surgery if hormones fail to relieve symptoms.
IV. Severe Ovarian endometriomata >2.5cm; marked adhesions of ovary and/or tubes, cul-de-sac obliteration.	Symptoms and signs. Laparotomy confirms.	Conservative surgery. Hormones. Hysterectomy and salpingo-oophorectomy.
V. Very Severe Stage III plus involvement of bowel, bladder, ureter etc.	Laparotomy. Barium enema. IVP.	Surgery Hormones, if surgery incomplete.

Table 37.1 The management of endometriosis.

endometriosis, it is often misdiagnosed as a myoma. If the woman has no symptoms and the adenomyoma is not large, no treatment is needed. If there are symptoms, hysterectomy is the preferred treatment as the tumour does not respond well to hormone treatment.

EXTRAUTERINE ENDOMETRIOSIS

The management of extrauterine endometriosis depends on the extent of the disease as determined by laparoscopy *(Table 37.1)*, on the symptoms, and on the desire of the woman to retain her fecundity. *Figure 37.4* is an algorithm showing management of this disease, details of which will now be discussed.

HORMONAL TREATMENT

Currently three regimens of hormonal treatment are advocated. The treatments suppress or reduce oestrogen synthesis and release. In consequence menstruation ceases. This inhibits further growth of the lesions, permits the body defenses to absorb the contents of the lesions and leads to their fibrosis.
The hormonal treatments are:
* Danazol.
* Gonadotrophin-releasing hormone agonists (GnRHa).
* Gestrinone.

Danazol

Danazol, an isoxazol derivative of 17-α-ethinyl testosterone, reduces the number of gonadotrophin releasing hormone receptors in the pituitary gland and causes a reduction in the level of sex hormone binding globulin (SHBG). The fall in SHBG causes an increase in free testosterone (T) and a fall in unbound oestradiol. Danazol may also act directly on the ovary to reduce steroid synthesis.

Danazol is given in a dose of 200mg 2 – 4 times a day for 3 – 12 months, depending on the extent of the lesions and on the response. The symptoms are usually relieved in 2 – 6 weeks in three-quarters of women treated. The effect of danazol on the endometriotic lesions is discussed later. Adverse effects are:
* Amenorrhoea in 60 per cent of women and oligomenorrhoea in the remainder.
* Increase in weight, often >3kg.
* Oily skin or acne in 20 per cent of women.
* Deepening voice in 10 per cent of women.

GnRH agonists

GnRH agonists render the pituitary gonadotrophs insensitive to stimulation by endogenous GnRH, with resulting suppression of ovarian steroid secretion. The drug is given in a dose of 200μg intranasally twice daily for 3–6 months or as a long acting injection monthly. The effect on the endometriosis is similar to that of danazol. Adverse effects are:
* Nearly all women experience hot flushes which may be severe.
* Seventy per cent of women develop amenorrhoea.
* Three per cent of women experience bone loss of 2 – 4 per cent over a 6-month period: this is reversible. However, fewer patients are reported to complain of side effects compared with danazol.

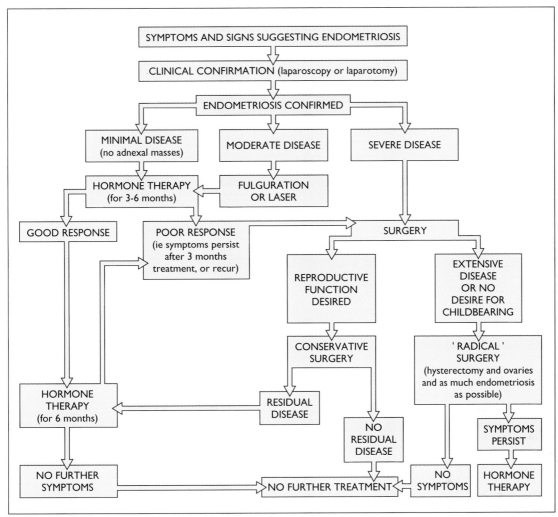

Fig 37.4 The management of endometriosis.

Gestrinone

This is a 'new generation progestogen'. It is prescribed in a dose of 1.2mg twice weekly and, in early studies, seems as effective as danazol. Weight gain occurs in 50 per cent of women.

OUTCOME

The effect of each of these hormonal treatments is similar in terms of relief of pain and reduction in the severity of the endometriosis judged by a second look laparoscopy made after treatment has ceased and the woman has had at least one menstrual period. The results are: in 30 per cent of the women complete regression of the disease will have occurred; in 60 per cent partial regression will have occurred; and in 10 per cent the extent of the disease is unchanged, although the symptoms have been relieved or cured. The findings suggest that further courses of treatment may be needed. It also appears that once hormonal treatment ceases, endometriosis

recurs in about 50 per cent of women over a 5-year period.

It could be argued that surgery gives better results. This is only true if an oophorectomy is performed in addition to other surgery. If the ovaries are conserved endometriosis may recur.

SURGERY

Small lesions detected with laparoscopy can be treated by electrocautery or laser under laparoscopic vision. Larger lesions, particularly those involving the ovaries, require more extensive surgery. The procedure depends on the patient's age, her desire for children and the difficulty of the operation. There is evidence that in extensive endometriosis, a 3-month course of hormone treatment may make the surgery easier. If the woman desires a pregnancy (provided no other bars to conception are present) the aim should be to conserve as much ovarian tissue as possible, by dissecting out or marsupializing the endometrial cysts. In women who have no desire for a further pregnancy, total hysterectomy and oophorectomy may be appropriate treatment, provided that the woman is informed about the procedure and has had the opportunity to think about it and discuss it with the surgeon.

The knowledge that she has endometriosis can cause considerable distress to a woman. In part, this is because of the poor correlation between the size and number of the lesions and the symptomatology and, in part, it is due to the publicity that endometriosis receives in the popular press.

The woman's attending doctor should explain what endometriosis is and what it is not. The differentiation between endometriosis and the premenstrual syndrome needs to be discussed because some of the symptoms are similar. The relationship between endometriosis and infertility also needs to be discussed and treatment stategies outlined. The woman should be made aware of the choices of hormonal treatment and surgery, and of their relative merits. The fact that endometriosis may recur following either treatment needs to be brought to the attention of the woman. However, the doctor should offer qualified optimism about the outcome, and should stress the importance of adequate follow up.

38

BENIGN TUMOURS, CYSTS AND MALFORMATIONS OF THE GENITAL TRACT

Benign tumours or cysts may form in any part of the genital tract. Benign tumours occur most often in the uterus (myomata) and most benign cysts occur in the ovaries. Malformations tend to involve the uterus and the vagina.

MALFORMATIONS OF THE GENITAL TRACT

The Mullerian ducts develop in a female fetus from the paramesonephric ducts, growing caudally on each side. By the 35th day after fertilization, the lower part of the ducts change direction and grow towards the midline where they meet and fuse with each other and then grow caudally once again. By the 65th day they have completed the fusion and their medial walls have gradually disappeared to form a single hollow tube *(Fig. 38.1)*. The most caudal portion which will become the vagina becomes solid and fuses with an ingrowth of entodermal cells from the cloaca. By the 20th gestational week, the solid growth has recanalized and the external genitalia have formed *(Fig. 38.2)*.

Malformations of the genital tract occur when the process described does not occur. The error may be one of failure of the recanalization process or may be a failure of the two Mullerian ducts to fuse.

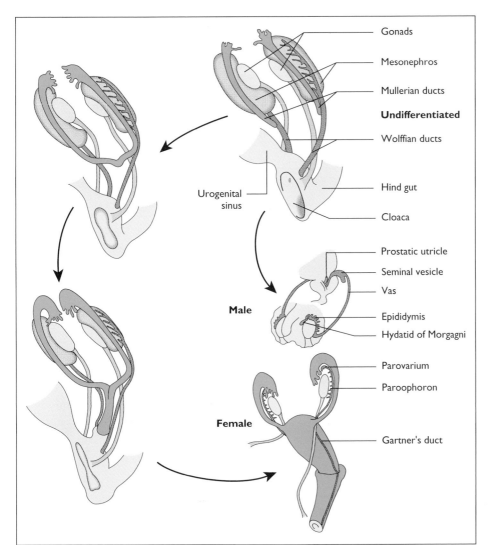

Fig 38.1 The development of the genital organs, from the Mullerian duct in the female and the Wolffian duct in the male.

Gonads
Mesonephros
Mullerian ducts
Undifferentiated
Wolffian ducts
Hind gut
Urogenital sinus
Cloaca
Prostatic utricle
Seminal vesicle
Vas
Epididymis
Hydatid of Morgagni
Male
Parovarium
Paroophoron
Female
Gartner's duct

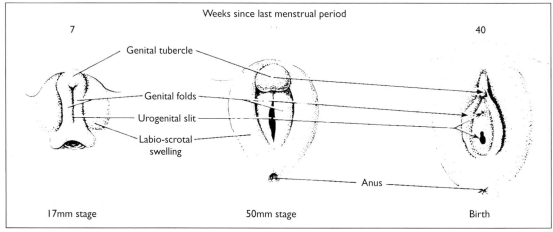

Fig 38.2 Differentiation of the female external genitalia, shown diagrammatically (not to scale).

FAILURE OF RECANALIZATION

The most common defect is an imperforate hymen, which should be detectable during the examination of the neonate. If it is not detected until after puberty, menstrual discharge may collect in the vagina and in long-term cases may distend the uterus and tubes *(Fig. 38.3)*. Treatment is to make a cruciate incision in the hymen and permit the inspissated fluid to escape slowly. Less common defects produce complete or partial vaginal atresia.

FAILURE OF THE DUCTS TO FORM OR TO FUSE

One or other duct may fail to form, only one Fallopian tube and a distorted unicornute uterus being found. If both ducts fail to form the woman will be amenorrhoeic.

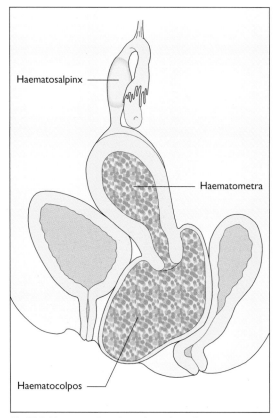

Fig 38.3 Haematocolpos due to imperforate hymen.

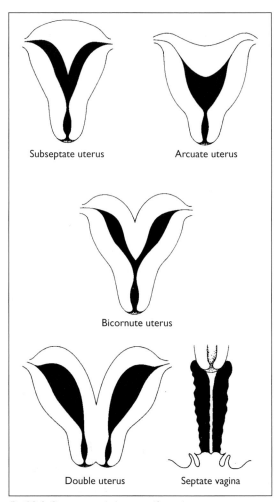

Fig 38.4 Common genital tract malformations.

Failure of the two Mullerian ducts to fuse leads to one of several malformations *(Fig. 38.4)*. Most of these malformations do not reduce the woman's fertility, but should pregnancy occur, late abortion, premature labour or intrauterine fetal death are four times as likely to occur. A subseptate uterus may lead to recurrent abortion, and can be treated by excising the septum by surgery or laser. If the woman has a bicornute uterus and becomes pregnant, the fetus may present as a transverse lie in late pregnancy.

VULVAL TUMOURS

Since the tissues of the vulva are covered by skin, tumours arising in the vulval tissues are similar to those occurring in any part of the integument. A few women develop vulval varicosities which may cause discomfort and are more marked in pregnancy.

VAGINAL TUMOURS

Vaginal cysts are uncommon but occasionally one develops in the lateral wall of the upper vagina. It is a cyst of a remnant of the degenerate Wolffian duct and is referred to as a *Gartner's duct cyst*. A cystic swelling may occur in the anterior wall of the vagina, directly beneath the urethra. This is a *urethral diverticulum*. If it becomes infected the woman complains of dysuria and frequency of urination. Occasionally a *myoma* may develop beneath the vaginal epithelium.

CERVICAL TUMOURS

The most common cervical tumour is a cervical polyp, which occurs as the result of localized hyperplasia of the epithelium and stroma covering a ridge between two clefts in the cervical canal. The columnar epithelium covering the polyp may undergo squamous metaplasia, or ulcerate. Many cervical polyps are symptomless. The main symptom is intermittent bleeding. The diagnosis is made on inspection of the cervix. The polyp can be removed by twisting the pedicle. The tissue should be sent for histopathology. Other tumours which may be detected occasionally are genital papillomata and myomata or fibromyomata.

UTERINE TUMOURS

ENDOMETRIAL POLYPS

Endometrial polyps may occur in association with endometrial hyperplasia and may be a cause of abnormal uterine bleeding. They are detected by curettage provided a ring forceps is also introduced into the uterus *(Fig. 38.5)*; or by hysteroscopy.

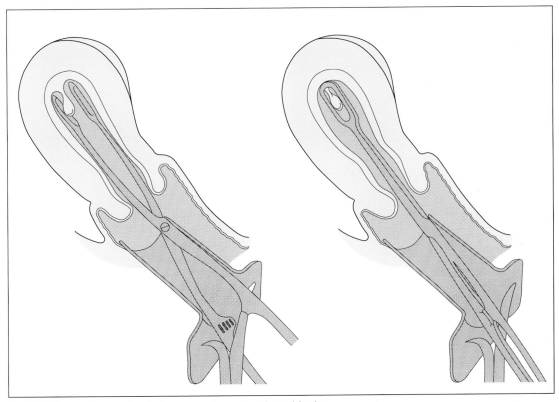

Fig 38.5 The use of sponge forceps to secure and remove endometrial polyps.

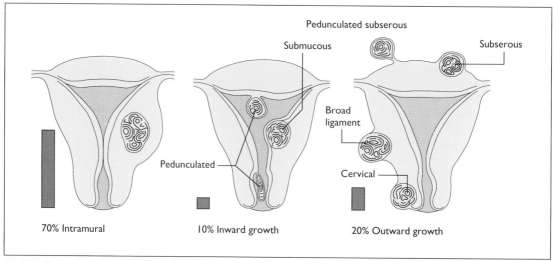

Peducunculated subserous

Submucous

Subserous

Broad ligament

Pedunculated

Cervical

70% Intramural

10% Inward growth

20% Outward growth

Fig 38.6 The development of myomata shown diagrammatically.

UTERINE MYOMATA (FIBROMYOMATA, FIBROIDS)

These are the most common tumours of the genital tract. A myoma is composed of smooth muscle bundles interspersed with strands of connective tissue, surrounded by a thin capsule. The tumour may arise in any part of the Mullerian duct, but occurs most often in the myometrium, where several tumours may develop simultaneously. The tumour can vary from the size of a pea to a football.

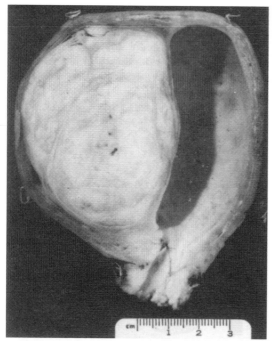

Fig 38.7 The gross appearance of a myoma is shown in the specimen, which also has a pyometra and a carcinoma of the cervix.

Myomata occur in about 5 per cent of women during the reproductive years. The tumours grow slowly and may only be detectable clinically in the fourth decade of life, when the incidence increases to about 20 per cent. They are more common in nulliparous women or women who have only had one child.

Their aetiology is unclear. They may arise from normal muscle cells, from immature muscle rests in the myometrium or from embryonal cells in the walls of uterine blood vessels. Whatever their origin, the tumours begin as tiny multiple seedlings which are scattered through the myometrium. The seedlings grow very slowly but progressively (over years rather than months), under the influence of circulating oestrogens, and unless detected and treated, as most are today, may form a tumour weighing 10kg or more. At first the tumour is intramural, but as it grows it may develop in several directions. This is shown in *Fig. 38.6*. After the menopause, as oestrogen is no longer secreted in any quantity, myomata tend to atrophy.

Pathology

If the tumour is cut, it pouts above the surrounding myometrium as its capsule contracts. Whitish-grey in colour, it is composed of whorled intertwining bundles of muscles, in a matrix of connective tissue *(Fig. 38.7)*. At its periphery the muscle fibres are arranged in concentric layers, and the normal muscle fibres surrounding the tumour are similarly oriented. Between the tumour and the normal myometrium, a thin layer of areolar tissue forms a pseudocapsule, through which the blood vessels enter the myoma.

On microscopy, groups of spindle-shaped muscle cells with elongated nuclei are separated into bundles by connective tissue *(Fig. 38.8)*. As the entire blood supply of the myoma is derived from the few vessels entering from the pseudocapsule, the growth of the tumour means that it often outstrips its blood supply. This leads to degeneration, particularly in the central portion of the myoma. Initially *hyaline degeneration* occurs, which may become *cystic,* or *calcification* may occur over time – 'the womb stones' of nineteenth century gynaecologists. In pregnancy a rare complication (*red degeneration*) may occur. This follows extravasation of blood though the tumour, giving it a raw beef appearance. In fewer than 0.1 per cent of tumours, sarcomatous change occurs.

Symptomatology

The symptoms depend on the size and the position of the myoma. Most small myomata and some larger ones are symptomless and are only detected during a routine examination. If the myoma is subendometrial, it may be associated with menorrhagia. If the heavy bleeding persists the woman may become anaemic. As the uterus contracts, it may cause crampy pains. Subendometrial myomata which become pedunculated may cause a persistent bloody discharge from the uterus.

Irrespective of their position in the uterus, large myomata may cause pressure symptoms in the pelvis, dysuria and frequency, and constipation or backache if the enlarged uterus presses on the rectum. A cervical myoma may cause pelvic pain and make sexual intercourse impossible *(Fig. 38.9).*

Diagnosis

Abdominal and vaginal examination may show a 'knobbly' uterus, or a smooth enlargement of the uterus. On moving the cervix the whole firm mass moves. In some cases the diagnosis is obvious, in others the smooth enlargement may be due to a pregnancy or to an ovarian mass. A pelvic ultrasound examination will establish the diagnosis.

Management

Four choices exist:
- To continue to observe the myoma.
- To perform a myomectomy.
- To perform a hysterectomy.
- To offer the woman gonadotrophin releasing hormone analogue (GnRHa).

Observation. Symptomless myomata less than the size of a 14-week pregnancy may be observed, with a few exceptions. The latter are:
- If the myoma distorts the uterine cavity and is considered a factor in the couple's infertility.
- If the myoma is situated in the lower part of the uterus or the cervix which would complicate childbirth.
- If the myoma grows rapidly which might suggest sarcomatous change.

If the myoma is associated with menstrual disturbances, the woman has the choice to have a hysteroscopy or a careful diagnostic curettage, to exclude intrauterine pathology, or to have surgical treatment.

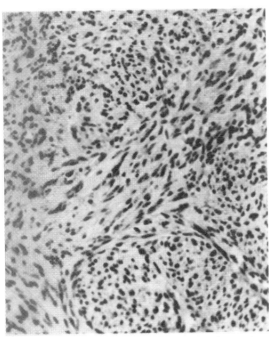

Fig 38.8 The microscopic appearance of a myoma. The bundles of spindle-shaped muscle cells run in several directions and tend to form a whorl-like pattern (× 160).

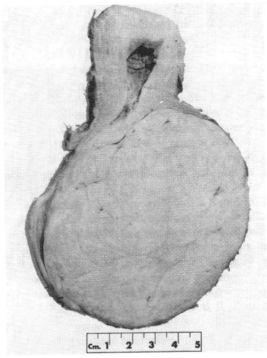

Fig 38.9 A large cervical myoma.

Myomectomy. If the woman is desirous of preserving her reproductive function, myomectomy may be chosen. The operation removes all detected myomata and reconstitutes the uterus. The woman must accept that if problems arise during myomectomy the surgeon may have to proceed to hysterectomy. Following myomectomy, 40 per cent of women who have the opportunity to conceive will do so. Against this is the fact that in 5 per cent of women, the myomata recur and a similar number of women continue to have menorrhagia which necessitates the use of hormones (see page 215), hysteroscopic resection or hysterectomy.

Hysterectomy. Total hysterectomy is the treatment of choice in older women, women who have no wish for a further pregnancy and women who have menorrhagia or marked pressure symptoms. A patient should not be rushed into making a decision to have a hysterectomy. She should be given time to think and to ask questions about hysterectomy. The gynaecologist should also make sure that misconceptions about the operation are addressed. This was discussed on page 221.

GnRH analogue. Given by injection at intervals, the drug will suppress oestrogen secretion and consequently the myomata will atrophy. Unless the drug is continued the myomata grow again. GnRH analogue has a small place in the treatment of selected cases of symptomatic myomata prior to myomectomy, or if the woman is nearing the menopause. However, this drug produces a hypo-oestrogenic state, bone loss may increase and predispose the woman to osteoporosis.

MYOHYPERPLASIA

Occasionally vaginal examination shows an enlarged uterus which does not contain myomata as determined by ultrasound. The condition is termed myohyperplasia *(Fig. 38.10)* and it is thought that it may be caused by psychosomatic factors, but no clearly identified problem has been detected. The uterus rarely exceeds the size of a 10-week pregnancy and the endometrium may be hypertrophic or normal. Myohyperplasia is often symptomless, but may be associated with menorrhagia. Treatment for menorrhagia is discussed on page 213.

MYOMAS AND PREGNANCY

The incidence of myomas complicating pregnancy is 1 in 200, but the majority of myomata are small and cause no problems. The complications which may occur depend on the number, the size and the position of the myomata in the uterus.

The effect of pregnancy on the myomata

The increased vascularity of the uterus together with the increased circulating levels of oestrogen often lead to an increase in size and a softening of a myoma. If the growth of the myoma increases too fast, it may outstrip its blood supply, causing degenerative changes in the tumour. The most serious outcome is necrobiosis (red degeneration). The patient may complain of pain and low grade fever usually in the second quarter of pregnancy. Palpation reveals that the myoma is very tender. Treatment is to give analgesics. The pain resolves within a few days and the pregnancy continues.

The effect of the myoma on the pregnancy

This depends on the size and position of the tumour. If it distorts the uterine cavity the risk of spontaneous abortion is doubled and there is an increased chance that labour will start prematurely. Large tumours in the myometrium may also distort the uterine cavity causing malposition or malpresentation of the fetus. Tumours in the lower part of the uterus may obstruct the birth canal, preventing vaginal delivery. Large tumours may cause pressure symptoms on the bladder or the rectum.

Diagnosis

If the patient presents early in pregnancy, the myoma may be felt on vaginal examination. A single fundal myoma may cause diagnostic difficulty but this can be resolved by an ultrasound examination.

Management

In most cases no treatment is needed during pregnancy. Myomectomy is inadvisable as the operation is attended by marked bleeding, and haemostasis can be difficult. In late pregnancy the position of the myoma in relation to the fetal presenting part and the pelvic cavity will permit a decision to be made

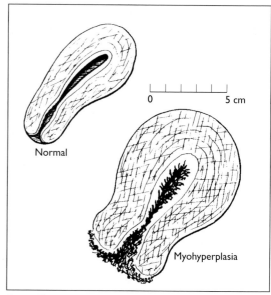

0   5 cm

Normal

Myohyperplasia

Fig 38.10 Myohyperplasia.

about the method of delivery. The patient and her partner should be involved in the discussion and the reason for the final decision explained.

As the tumour usually is the upper segment of the uterus, vaginal delivery is possible for most patients. A few women with low-lying myomata which obstruct the birth canal require caesarean section. Myomectomy should not be performed during the same operation because of the dangers of haemostasis and infection.

FALLOPIAN TUBE TUMOURS

Benign tumours and cysts of the Fallopian tubes and the broad ligament are rare. Occasionally cysts are found in remnants of the Wolffian duct at surgery (hydatid of Morgagni). Parovarian cysts are often large and may be thought to be ovarian until exposed at surgery.

BENIGN OVARIAN CYSTS AND TUMOURS

The ovary consists of:
- Coelomic epithelium.
- Oocytes, derived from primitive germ cells.
- Mesenchymal elements which forms the medulla.

These tissues are particularly dynamic, being affected by hormonal stimuli from puberty to the menopause. This may be the reason why so many benign cysts and tumours may arise in the ovary.

CLASSIFICATION OF BENIGN OVARIAN CYSTS AND TUMOURS

There is no entirely satisfactory classification of ovarian cysts and tumours. This is because of the complexity of ovarian new growths and because the distinction between some of them can only be made after histological examination. In *Table 38.1*, a classification is presented and the proportions of benign cysts and tumours encountered is shown.

Functional cysts

A follicle cyst is an enlargement of an unruptured Graafian follicle which has continued to secrete fluid. The cyst is usually unilateral and <5cm in diameter. The cells may secrete oestrogen or be relatively quiescent. Because of this the symptoms vary. The woman's menstrual cycle may be lengthened and menorrhagia may occur, or it may be of normal length or shorter.

Multiple follicle cysts may occur following the use of clomiphene or gonadotrophins for inducing ovulation.

Corpus luteum cysts occur when, instead of degenerating when implantation of the embryo fails to occur, the corpus luteum survives and grows. *Theca lutein cysts* occur in gestational trophoblastic disease (see page 138)

If the clinical findings are insufficient to reach a diagnosis a transvaginal ultrasound examination will help to diagnose an ovarian cyst. However, small cystic enlargements should not be reported as ovarian cysts without qualification. For example just before ovulation, follicles may measure 20mm (+ or - 10mm). A simple cyst measuring <30mm on ultrasound scanning is better described as a follicle, to avoid unnecessary investigations and perhaps surgery.

Treatment. The cyst should be observed for 2 or 3 months during which time it will probably disappear. Should it still persist and is unilocular, showing no solid areas on ultrasound, it may be aspirated under ultrasonic or laparoscopic guidance. If needle aspiration shows bloodstained fluid a laparotomy is needed. Multilocular persistent cysts require surgical removal.

Benign ovarian neoplasms

Mucinous cystadenoma and serous cystadenoma account for 40 per cent of benign ovarian cysts and tumours. Both derive from the multipotential coelomic epithelium. This epithelium forms the Mullerian duct and can imitate tubal, uterine or cervical epithelium.

A Classification of Benign Ovarian Cysts and Tumours			
Tumour (benign)	**Cell origin**	**Type**	**Proportional incidence per cent**
Functional cysts (follicle, corpus luteum)	Normal follicle	Cystic	24
Serous cystadenoma	Coelomic epithelium	Cystic	20
Mucinous cystadenoma	Coelomic epithelium	Cystic	20
Teratoma (dermoid cyst)	Oogonia	Cystic	15
Endometriomata	Ectopic endometrium	Cystic	10
Fibroma (inc. Brenner's tumour)	Mesenchyme	Solid	5

Table 38.1 A classification of benign ovarian cysts and tumours.

Mucinous cystadenoma

The cysts occur most frequently between the ages of 35 and 55. They can grow to a considerable size, and are multilocular *(Fig. 38.11)*. They are usually unilateral and rarely become malignant. The cyst is lined with tall columnar cells, each of which has a basal nucleus and cytoplasmic mucin *(Fig. 38.12)*. Mucin is constantly secreted into the cyst so that its wall becomes tense. Often a portion of the wall bulges outwards and a depression may form at the neck of the bulge, which may become occluded, forming a daughter cyst *(Fig. 38.13)*. Occasionally the cyst may rupture releasing mucinous cells, which may become attached to the peritoneum and omentum leading to an intraperitoneal accumulation of mucin (*pseudomyxoma peritonei*)

Serous cystadenoma

These cysts are also more frequently detected in women aged 35–55. They are lined with cuboidal epithelium, resembling that of the oviduct *(Fig. 38.14)*. The cells secrete thin watery fluid, but the quantity secreted is not great. In consequence the tension inside the cyst is low and the epithelial cells proliferate to form intracystic papillomata *(Fig. 38.15)*. In some cases the cells penetrate the cyst wall to form external papillary projections. Serous cystadenoma are uni- or parvilocular and are bilateral in 30 per cent of cases. They only grow to a moderate size. Malignant changes occur in one-third of cases, usually when the woman is in her 50s.

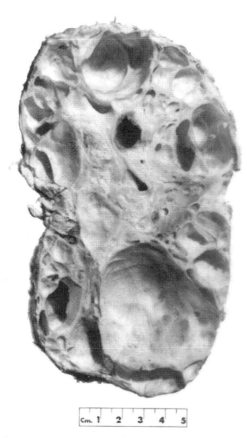

Fig 38.11 Mucinous cystadenoma.

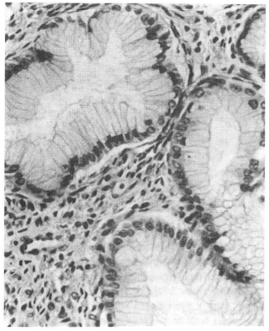

Fig 38.12 The microscopic appearance of mucinous cystadenoma – note the cells lining the tumour resemble those of the endocervix (x 256).

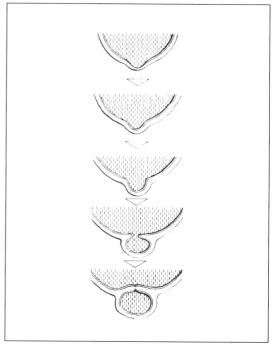

Fig 38.13 Diagram to show how daughter cysts form in the wall of a mucinous cystadenoma.

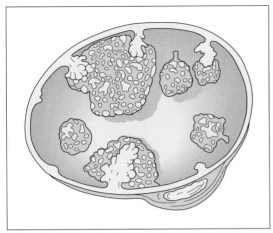

Fig 38.14 Gross appearance of a serous cystadenoma.

Endometriomata
These ovarian tumours (chocolate cysts) are usually associated with other evidence of endometriosis. They rarely become malignant. Endometriosis is discussed on pp 259.

Benign teratoma (dermoid cyst)
Deriving from germ cells, benign teratomata are relatively common. The cyst contains epithelial, mesodermal and endothelial elements. Thus the dermoid may contain hair, teeth and pultaceous material from sebaceous glands. The tumour is bilateral in 10 per cent of cases. It may occur at any age, but most are detected when the woman is aged between 20 and 40 years. The nature of the tumour is confirmed by ultrasound examination or radiology.

Connective tissue neoplasms
Fibromata constitute 5 per cent of benign ovarian neoplasms. The tumour may consist entirely of connective tissue or may be found in association with serous cystadenoma, or with the rare Brenner tumour. Fibroma are usually small, and are bilateral in 10 per cent of cases. Rarely, the fibroma is associated with hydrothorax and ascites (Meigs syndrome).

THE DIAGNOSIS OF OVARIAN TUMOURS
Benign ovarian cysts and tumours grow silently and are often undetected for some years. They do not cause pain, but if large may cause discomfort. They rarely affect menstrual function. Periodic abdominal and vaginal examinations will detect benign tumours. A painless cystic or solid mass in the cul-de-sac, or in the position of an ovary, or distending the abdomen, which is cystic to firm on palpation suggests an ovarian tumour. The diagnosis can be confirmed by an abdominal or transvaginal ultrasound scan, which differentiates the tumour from pregnancy, obesity, pseudocyesis, a full bladder or cystic degeneration of a myoma *(Fig. 38.16)*.

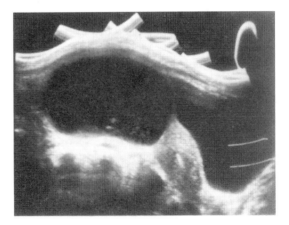

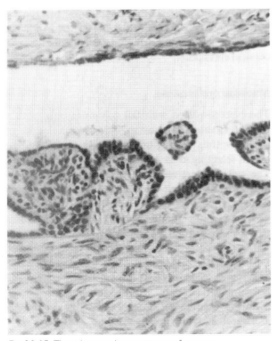

Fig 38.15 The microscopic appearance of a serous cystadenoma. Note that the cells lining the tumour resemble those of the endosalpinx (× 256).

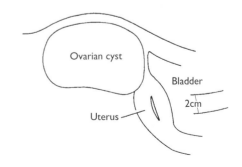

Fig 38.16 Ovarian cyst (ultrasound-sagittal scan). Line drawing showing the identification of relevant points.

MANAGEMENT OF BENIGN OVARIAN TUMOURS

The treatment of mucinous cystadenoma is surgical, the extent of the operation depending on the age of the patient. In younger women ovarian cystectomy is possible, the ovary being reconstructed after the tumour has been shelled out. A similar approach can be used in cases of serous cystadenoma, but in women over the age of 40, bilateral salpingo-oophorectomy and total hysterectomy is preferred, because of the possibility of malignant change. Endometriomata and benign teratomata can often be shelled out of the normal ovarian tissue and the ovary reconstructed, as can fibromata.

OVARIAN TUMOURS AND PREGNANCY

One pregnancy in 1500 is complicated by a clinically detectable ovarian tumour, measuring >50mm in diameter. If an ultrasound examination of the pelvis is made routinely, an ovarian tumour is detected in 1 in 200 pregnancies. Most of them are cysts, usually an enlarged corpus luteum which resolves spontaneously.

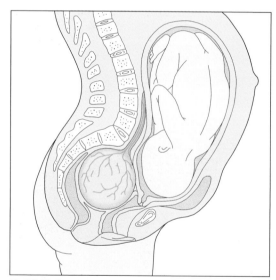

Fig 38.17 Ovarian cyst obstructing labour.

Neoplastic tumours are less common in pregnancy. Most are serous cystadenomas, a few are mucinous cystadenomas and these two account for 65 per cent of all neoplasias complicating pregnancy. Teratomas account for 25 per cent. The remaining 10 per cent is made up of a wide variety of ovarian tumours.

The effect of the pregnancy on the tumour

The size of the tumour does not change during the pregnancy, but the growing uterus may displace it so that it becomes more obvious. Rarely, torsion of the ovary containing the tumour may occur. Even more rarely the tumour may rupture.

The effect of the tumour on the pregnancy

The only problem is that the tumour may become incarcerated in the cul de sac and obstruct the birth canal *(Fig. 38.17)*.

Diagnosis

In early pregnancy a vaginal examination may reveal two masses, the pregnant uterus and the ovarian tumour. If any doubt exists, a pelvic ultrasound examination will clarify the diagnosis.

Treatment

Treatment depends on the size and consistency of the tumour and its appearance on ultrasound examination. Ovarian tumours less than 80mm in diameter and echo-free, can be observed, repeat scans being made to see if the tumour increases in size. If treatment is decided upon, the cyst may be aspirated or an ovarian cystectomy performed. A multilocular cyst or a tumour >80mm in size which is thick walled or semi-solid, requires surgical removal, after the 12th gestational week. A tumour detected after the 30th gestational week may be difficult to remove surgically and premature labour may follow. The decision to operate can only be made after careful consideration and involvement of the patient and her partner. If the tumour obstructs the birth canal and cannot be moved digitally, the patient should receive caesarean section and an ovarian cystectomy performed.

39

MALIGNANCIES OF THE FEMALE GENITAL TRACT

Only four cancers can be either prevented or diagnosed at a stage when treatment is curative in most cases. Skin cancer can be prevented by avoiding excessive exposure to the sun; lung cancer can largely be prevented by avoiding smoking tobacco. The other two cancers – cancer of the uterine cervix and breast cancer – can be detected, in most cases, at a stage when treatment is curative.

In this chapter cancers of the genital tract will be discussed, the most common being mentioned first. Rare cancers such as vaginal cancer and cancer of the Fallopian tubes will not be discussed.

CERVICAL PRECANCER AND CANCER

The cervical epithelium undergoes changes through the menstrual cycle and is readily accessible for examination. The epithelium covering the ectocervix is stratified and identical with that of the vagina (Fig. 39.1). It is separated from the underlying stroma by an apparent basement membrane. Superior to this is a layer of basal cells from which the other cell layers differentiate. Above the basal layer are five or six layers of parabasal cells. Above them are intermediate and superficial cell layers. The intermediate cell layer consists of large cells, each with reticulated nuclei and vacuoles of glycogen in the cytoplasm. The superficial cell layer varies in thickness, depending on the oestradiol: progesterone ratio present. The superficial cells are flattened and have small nuclei, the cytoplasm containing glycogen (Fig. 39.2). A small amount of keratin is produced in some of the cells, which become 'cornified'. During the reproductive years, the superficial cells are constantly shed or exfoliated into the vagina, and differentiation of cells from the basal layer also proceeds constantly.

The characteristics of the superficial cells can be studied by taking a smear from the cervix and staining it with Papanicolaou's stain. In some women the nuclei become abnormally shaped or dyskaryotic which may indicate a 'precancerous' change; this can be detected by cervical smears.

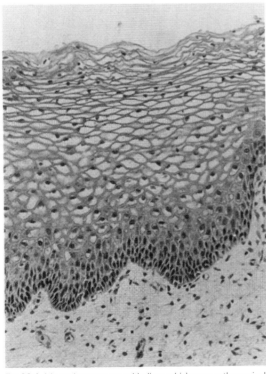

Fig 39.1 Normal squamous epithelium which covers the vaginal portion of the cervix (× 160).

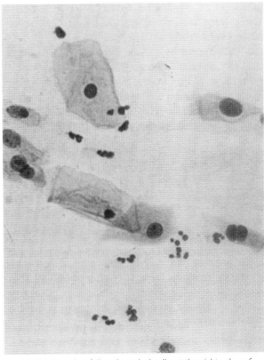

Fig 39.2 Normal exfoliated cervical cells; at the right edge of the illustration two ciliated endocervical cells can be seen (× 400).

THE EPIDEMIOLOGY OF CERVICAL CANCER

Cervical cancer occurs almost exclusively among women who are or have been sexually active, but the cause of cervical cancer is not known. There is increasing evidence that infection by certain strains of the human papillomavirus (HPV) is a factor. The genital tract (including the vulva) of between 10 and 30 per cent of sexually active women has been infected with HPV by the age of 30, and in most the infection is symptomless (see page 246). The initial infection may be vulval or vaginal, from which the virus spreads to the uterine cervix; the cervix may, however, be infected directly.

The genesis of HPV infection is complex as the presence of cervical cell infection by the virus does not mean that it is always transmitted by sexual intercourse; nor that it necessarily leads to cervical cancer. If cervical cancer does develop it may manifest itself soon or many years after the HPV infection.

This suggests that if cervical carcinoma develops it must be due to the added effect of a co-agent. One theory is that the HPV sensitizes the cells and acting with another agent (such as tobacco smoking) may reduce the effectiveness the woman's immune system to deal with the virus, permitting the development of the abnormal cells. Other theories exist, which indicate that the real relevance of HPV infection in the genesis of cervical carcinoma is unclear. On the one hand, over 80 per cent of women who have cervical carcinoma have evidence of HPV (particularly strains 16 and 18) as demonstrated by cytology. On the other hand, in 5 to 20 per cent of women who have clinically and cytologically normal cervical cells, HPV infection of the cells can be demonstrated by DNA hybridization.

CERVICAL EXFOLIATIVE CYTOLOGY

As dyskaryotic cells found on a cervical (pap) smear suggest that the woman may develop cervical cancer, it is recommended that all sexually active women should have pap smears made regularly. The first smear should be made soon after the woman starts sexual intercourse and should be repeated after one year, as abnormal cells may be missed in a single smear. If no abnormality is found on either smear, regular smears at 2-year intervals should be made, at least until the woman reaches the age of 65.

In women aged 40 and over, the doctor or nurse taking the smear should also examine the woman's breasts, teach her breast self-examination and measure her blood pressure.

The technique of taking a cervical smear

A tray is provided on which a Cusco vaginal speculum, some slides, a spray-on fixative plastic, a modified Ayre spatula and an endocervical brush are placed. Before performing a vaginal examination, the warmed speculum is inserted to expose the cervix. The cytobrush is inserted into the cervical canal and

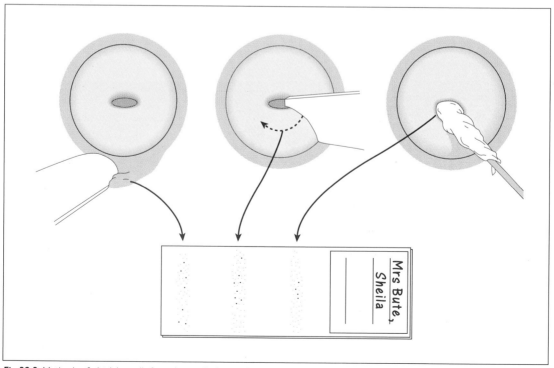

Fig 39.3 Methods of obtaining cells from the cervix for cytological examination, (1) using a special wooden spatula, and (2) using a cotton-tipped swab stick.

rotated. The sample is smeared onto the slide. The ectocervix is sampled with the Ayre spatulum by rotating it through 360° twice and the sample is smeared on to a slide *(Fig. 39.3)*.

The smears are sent to a reliable, quality assured cytological laboratory for examination.

Cytologists have agreed that nuclear abnormalities should form the basis of a cytological diagnosis. They have agreed to report smears as follows:

- *Unsatisfactory*. In these slides a diagnosis cannot be made because there are too few cells, there are no endocervical cells or the slide has been processed incorrectly. The smear should be repeated 4 weeks later.
- *Inflammatory or inconclusive*. In these slides the nuclei are distorted by the effects of vaginal infections, such as trichomoniasis and gardnerella. The referring doctor is asked to treat the infection appropriately and then to repeat the smear.
- *Normal*. Repeat the smear in 1–3 years.
- *Mild dyskaryosis*. The slide may show HPV infection with no dyskaryosis; HPV infection and dyskaryosis; or dyskaryosis without HPV infection.
- *Moderate dyskaryosis*.
- *Severe dyskaryosis*. (Fig. 39.4).

To confuse matters further some cytologists now use an American classification (the Bethesda Classification). Smears showing abnormal cells are placed in two categories: low grade and high grade squamous intraepithelial lesions (SIL). Low grade SIL includes HPV infection and mild dyskaryosis. High grade SIL includes moderate and severe dyskaryosis. Recently, concern has been expressed that the simplified classification may lead to overtreatment.

TELLING THE PATIENT

The result of the smear should be reported to the woman by phone and/or by letter. This applies to all smears not just 'abnormal' ones. If an abnormal smear is reported the need to counsel and explain is imperative.

To many women the finding of a dyskaryotic smear suggests the presence of cancer. If HPV is found many women question their own and their partner's previous sexual behaviour. Either finding can lead to guilt, misery and anxiety. Doctors should be aware of this and should talk with the woman explaining the meaning of the result of the smear and that HPV is not always sexually transmitted. The woman should also be told, in clear non-jargon language, what procedures may be needed. In one reported study the term 'precancer' was perceived as threatening, and the authors suggested that a better term would be 'early warning cells'.

MANAGEMENT OF ABNORMAL CERVICAL SMEARS

HPV infection with no evidence of dyskaryosis

Take smears at 6-monthly intervals until the smear is negative for HPV, then annually for two years. If there is no evidence of HPV at this time revert to smears every two years. If dyskaryosis appears in any smear, treat as recommended below.

Mild dyskaryosis with or without HPV

The treatment for this condition is controversial: no concensus having been reached. The reason is that there is no agreement what proportion of cases of mild dyskaryosis progress to, or on biopsy are in a more severe form. One group of gynaecologists believe that the risk is high and that, in many cases, an immediate biopsy will show moderate or severe dysplasia. They recommend that patients are referred for immediate colposcopy and cervical biopsy.

The other group believe that no immediate action need be taken for six months when a second smear is made (some delaying for a third smear at 12 months). They believe that only if either or both of these smears show dyskaryosis, colposcopy and biopsy need be performed.

Increasingly the concept of immediate treatment is gaining ground, in spite of the strain it will place on colposcopy services.

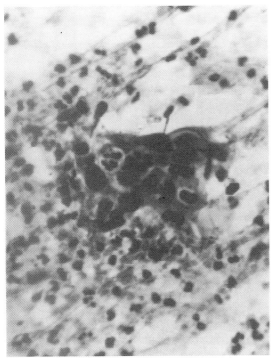

Fig 39.4 Exfoliated cervical cells showing 'severe dyskaryosis' (× 400).

Moderate and severe dyskaryosis

These degrees of dyskaryosis require referral for colposcopy and cervical biopsy.

COLPOSCOPY

Dyskaryosis is a cytological diagnosis and observer error is not uncommon. For this reason a colposcope often is used to verify abnormal findings. A colposcope is a system of lenses which magnifies the cervix 5 – 20 times and enables a trained observer to translate changes in colour tone, opacity, surface

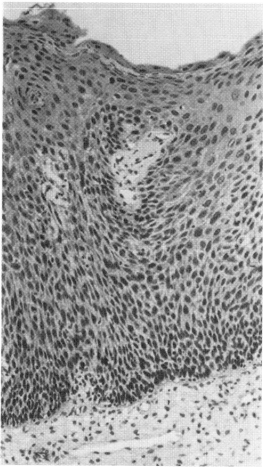

Fig 39.5 Dysplasia (moderate) CIN 2 (× 160).

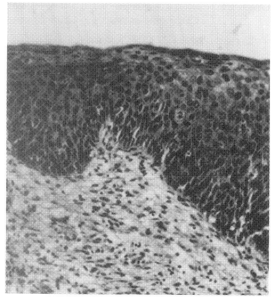

Fig 39.6 Dysplasia (severe) CIN 3 (× 160).

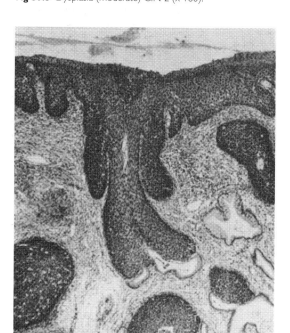

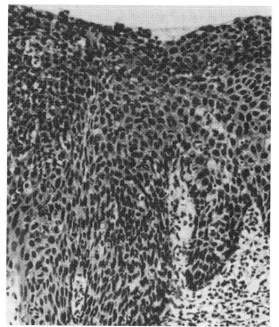

Fig 39.7 Cervical biopsy from the patient whose cervical smear is shown in **Fig 39.4**. Carcinoma-in-situ was found. (A) (× 40) There appears to be invasion of the tissues but in reality the cells have only crept into endocervical crypts. (B) (× 160) The lack of stratification and pleomorphism of the cells is seen.

configuration, vascular pattern and intercapillary distance into a diagnosis.

Abnormal epithelium is white in colour after application of aqueous acetic acid solution (acido-white epithelium); white keratotic patches may be seen; and the blood vessels may appear as punctate dots or as a mosaic arrangement. Bizarre branching vessels usually denote invasive cancer. A trained observer can differentiate between the minor and major cervical precancer lesions and carcinoma with a reasonable degree of accuracy. The predicted diagnosis is confirmed by punch biopsies which are examined histologically.

HISTOLOGY

Mild dysplasia is characterized by nuclear abnormalities in the basal third of the epithelium; the upper layers are not affected. In *moderate dysplasia* some dyskaryotic nuclei are found in the upper layers of the epithelium and abnormal nuclei are more common *(Fig. 39.5)*. In *severe dysplasia* the abnormal nuclei occupy all the epithelial layers, and there is a high nuclear-cytoplasmic ratio *(Fig. 39.6)*. Severe dysplasia may be difficult to differentiate from carcinoma in situ. In *carcinoma in situ* there is no differentiation as the surface layers are reached; the nuclei vary in size and stain deeply, the cells are crowded and the cytoplasm is scanty *(Fig. 39.7)*.

CERVICAL INTRAEPITHELIAL NEOPLASIA (CIN)

In some cases there is uncertainty about the exact histological diagnosis and whether the identified lesion will regress, persist or progress. This has led to

CIN Classification		
Grade 1	Mild dysplasia	{ Dysplasia of low degree
Grade 2	Moderate dysplasia	
Grade 3	Severe dysplasia/ Carcinoma-in-situ	{ Dysplasia of high degree

Table 39.1 CIN Classification.

a classification which includes all grades of dysplasia, the CIN classification *(Table 39.1)*.

THE NATURAL HISTORY OF CIN

The current belief about the natural history of CIN is shown in *Fig. 39.8*.

THE MANAGEMENT OF CIN

The management of CIN depends on the age of the woman, her desire to reproduce and on the location and extent of the lesion.

Current recommendations for treatment are:

CIN grade 1

There is a lack of agreement about the management if colposcopically controlled biopsy shows mild dysplasia (CIN 1). Increasingly gynaecologists are recommending that the lesion be obliterated using one of the methods outlined in the managemnt of CIN 2 and 3.

CIN grades 2 and 3

These major grade lesions require either local destructive treatment or excision of the suspect area. Local destructive treatment includes laser, cryosurgery, and electrocoagulation diathermy. Each

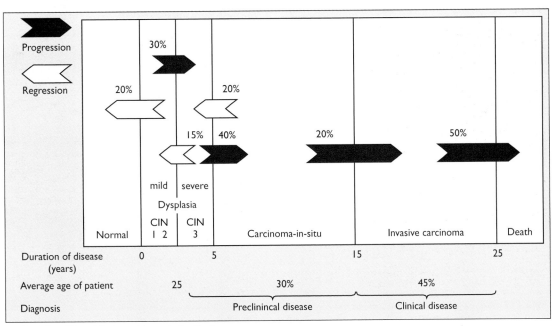

Fig 39.8 The 'life cycle' of unstable cervical epithelium.

of these choices has its ardent advocates. Selection of patients is important. The whole lesion must be visible and invasive cancer must have been excluded. All treatments can be given under local anaesthesia (2ml lignocaine 2% in normal saline) or general anaesthesia depending on the patient's and the gynaecologist's preference. Laser protagonists claim that the accuracy of the method and the absence of cervical scarring makes it the preferred method, although they admit the equipment is expensive and requires regular maintenance.

Proponents of other modalities claim that their results are as good as those following laser therapy (over 90 per cent of women have normal smears and normal colposcopic findings after 5 years of follow-up), and that the techniques are simpler, quicker and cheaper.

Each of these treatments may be followed by bloodstained or other discharge for one to three weeks. About 5 per cent of women have vaginal bleeding. Some women complain of pain or severe discomfort. Sexual intercourse and the use of tampons should be avoided for 4 weeks to allow complete healing. The treatments do not affect the woman's fertility or alter the course of a subsequent pregnancy.

Some CIN 2 and 3 lesions require more extensive excisional treatment so that the tissue can be examined histologically to exclude invasive cancer, particularly if the suspect areas extend up the cervical canal and their upper limit cannot be identified by colposcopic inspection. The whole transformation zone and some of the cervical canal area is excised using cutting laser or a low-voltage diathermy loop (large loop excision of the transformation zone), with ball cautery of the exposed area if needed, to achieve haemostasis after excision of the tissue. An alternative is for the gynaecologist to use knife conization. Knife conization, usually with suturing

to repair the cervix, is associated with a 10 per cent chance of postoperative haemorrhage. If the woman becomes pregnant there is an increased risk of miscarriage in the second quarter of pregnancy and she may give birth to a preterm baby, as a result of an incompetent cervix. The risk increases with the size of the cone excised.

Depending on age, the presence of other gynaecological conditions (for example, myoma or menorrhagia), and personal preferences, some women with CIN 3 may choose hysterectomy.

As mentioned, follow-up is essential. The woman should be reviewed 6 and 12 months after treatment when a cervical smear is taken and a colposcopic examination is made. If the cytology is negative and the colposcopy normal, annual smears are made from then on. Following hysterectomy for CIN, 6-monthly smears should be made for the first year and thereafter every 2 years as abnormal cells may be found in the upper vagina signifying vaginal CIN.

THE PHYSIOLOGICAL EFFECTS OF CIN ON WOMEN

Many women diagnosed as having CIN become depressed and upset, particularly if a health professional implies that the woman has been sexually promiscuous.

The woman may be concerned that her partner has been or is continuing to be unfaithful. Her attitude to sexual intercourse may change and she may want to avoid sex.

The anxieties and uncertainty should be resolved as far as possible by giving the woman a full explanation of CIN and letting her have the opportunity to ask questions. She may also need continued psychological support.

CERVICAL CARCINOMA

Carcinoma of the uterine cervix is the second most common gynaecological cancer (after breast cancer). The annual risk for women over the age of 35, is 16 per 100 000. The peak incidence is between the ages of 45 and 55, with a recent trend towards a younger

Staging of Carcinoma of the Uterine Cervix	
Stage 0	Carcinoma in situ
Stage I	The carcinoma is confined to the cervix Ia. Preclinical carcinoma on diagnosis by microscopy Ib. Invasion >5mm
Stage II	The carcinoma extends beyond the cervix but has not extended to reach the pelvic wall or the lower vagina IIa. No obvious parametrial involvement IIb. The cancer involves the parametrium
Stage III	The cancer has spread to reach the pelvic wall or the lower third of the vagina
Stage IV	The cancer has spread beyond the true pelvis or has invaded the bladder

Table 39.2 Staging of carcinoma of the uterine cervix (Modified from the FIGO classification, which should be consulted).

Squamous Carcinoma of the Cervix – Lymph Node Involvement and Survival Rates

Stage	Lymph node involvement	5-year survival
0	0	100
I(a)	<1	100
I(b)	15	85
II(a)	25	75
II(b)	35	55
III	55	35
IV	>65	<15

Table 39.3 Squamous carcinoma of the cervix – lymph node involvement and survival rates.

age. Cervical cancer usually grows outwards becoming a fungating mass; occasionally it grows inwards enlarging the cervix. More than 85 per cent of cervical cancers are squamous cell carcinomas, the remainder being adenocarcinomas which arise from the cells lining the cervical canal or its clefts. With time the cancer spreads either by direct extension upwards to involve the uterine cavity, or downwards to involve the vagina or via the lymphatic drainage to the external iliac lymph nodes (47 per cent of cases); the obturator lymph node (20 per cent of cases); the hypogastric nodes (7 per cent of cases) or the paracervical nodes (2 per cent of cases). The spread of the cancer detected on clinical examination and CAT scan, enables an oncologist to stage the cancer and to recommend treatment on the staging *(Table 39.2)*. The higher the stage on the initial examination, the greater is the chance of lymph node involvement and the poorer the prognosis *(Table 39.3)*. In early stage disease (Stage IB and IIA, see later) lymph node metastases are present in 25–30 per cent of cases.

DIAGNOSIS

In its earliest stage, an abnormal smear is the only way to detect cervical cancer as symptoms tend to occur only with established invasive disease. Irregular bleeding per vaginam, particularly after sexual intercourse, or a pink vaginal discharge, particularly after urination, demand investigation by a vaginal examination using a speculum and a cervical smear. Diagnosis is confirmed by a cervical wedge biopsy or if gross evidence of cervical cancer is evident by biopsy and endocervical curettage.

TREATMENT

The best results of treating of cervical cancer are obtained in oncological units staffed by pelvic surgeons and radiological oncologists. Microinvasive (Stage Ia) cancer is treated by simple total hysterectomy. Stage Ib cancer may be treated either by radical hysterectomy or by radiotherapy. Radical hysterectomy includes removal of the parametrium and pelvic lymphadenectomy, whilst radiotherapy includes a combination of external beam and intra cavity radiation. Both give similar 5-year survival rates. The choice should be made after a senior doctor has talked with the woman, during which the benefits and drawbacks of each method are discussed. More advanced cervical carcinoma is treated by radiotherapy, although in some centres chemotherapy is being tried.

As follow-up after treatment is usually in the hands of the woman's GP, there must be good and regular communication between the staff of the oncological unit and the woman's doctor.

ENDOMETRIAL CARCINOMA

Endometrial carcinoma is a disease of women in their middle years, the peak incidence occurring in the 55–65 age group. Women whose menopause is delayed beyond the age of 55, who are relatively infertile, and overweight or hypertensive are more likely than other women to develop endometrial cancer. This profile suggests that unopposed oestrogen may play a role in the development of the cancer.

The tumour may originate in any part of the endometrium, and grows slowly, tending to spread over a part of the endometrium before invading the myometrium. If the growth starts in the lower part of the uterus, the fungating mass may block the cervix and fluid or pus may collect in the uterus (pyometra). Various histological patterns of adenocarcinoma are found on the histological examination of an endometrial biopsy or a curettage. The more undifferentiated the endometrial cells, the worse is the prognosis. The cancer is staged using the International Federation of Obstetrics and Gynaecology (FIGO) classification *(Table 39.4)*.

CLINICAL FEATURES

The usual symptoms of an endometrial carcinoma are a bloody discharge per vaginam, or irregular bleeding, which is slight in amount and recurrent. Some women have a watery vaginal discharge, but this is uncommon. Examination usually shows a normally sized uterus, unless there are associated myomata or a pyometra. Any peri- or postmenopausal woman who has symptoms of irregular bleeding per vaginam or a bloody vaginal discharge must be examined and endometrial tissue sampled. With the development of the hysteroscope, the uterine cavity can be inspected and a biopsy taken under vision. However, curettage should be performed in most cases, either using a biopsy curette

Surgical-Pathological Staging of Endometrial Carcinoma (FIGO, 1989)	
Stage	
Ia	Tumour limited to endometrium
Ib	Invasion to <1/2 myometrium
Ic	Invasion to >1/2 myometrium
IIa	Endocervical glandular involvement only
IIb	Cervical stromal invasion
IIIa	Tumour invades serosa and/or adnexae and/or positive peritoneal cytology
IIIb	Vaginal metastases
IIIc	Metastases to pelvic and/or para-aortic lymph nodes
IVa	Tumour invades bladder and/or bowel mucosa
IVb	Distant metastases including intra-abdominal and/or inguinal lymph node

Table 39.4 Surgical-pathological staging of endometrial carcinoma (FIGO, 1989).

(this can be done with the woman as an outpatient) or a formal curettage under general anaesthesia. Two biopsy curettes are currently used (Gynnescan and Pipelle). They are introduced through the cervix and rotated in the uterine cavity. The procedures are said to be relatively painless but 60 per cent of women experience discomfort or pain.

SCREENING FOR ENDOMETRIAL CANCER

Some authorities in the USA perform an endometrial biopsy on all postmenopausal women before prescribing hormone replacement treatment. As endometrial cancer in the age group 50–59 is about 1 in 1000 it is questionable if this invasive procedure is cost effective.

Studies are in progress to find out if transvaginal ultrasound using a technique which measures the thickness of the endometrium will help detect endometrial carcinoma rather than having to resort to the invasive methods mentioned. It is currently thought that if the endometrium is less than 5mm thick, carcinoma is not present, whilst an endometrium thicker than 5mm needs to be investigated further.

TREATMENT

Over 75 per cent of cases are diagnosed when the cancer is at an early stage. Total hysterectomy and bilateral oophorectomy is the treatment of choice in these cases. As lymphatic spread is late, pelvic lymphadenectomy can be avoided, although the fact that 10 per cent of Stage 1 cases have lymph node involvement has led some authorities to advocate pelvic lymphadenectomy for surgical staging and as a guide to prognosis. The excised uterus is examined histologically and if the myometrium has been invaded to more than half its thickness, either whole pelvis irradiation (50Gy over 5 weeks) or hormone treatment is given. Some gynaecological surgeons arrange for intravaginal irradiation 3 – 4 weeks after the hysterectomy, giving 40Gy. The objective is to prevent recurrence in the vaginal vault. Problems with this approach are that the vaginal vault may become stenosed making intercourse uncomfortable and bladder or rectal symptoms may occur from radiation damage.

If the patient is unfit for surgery or if the cancer is advanced, hormone treatment may be used as an alternative or an adjuvant. Most medical oncologists give a progestogen, such as medroxyprogesterone acetate 200–400mg orally daily, on a continuous basis. This treatment may cause negative mood change, which is a progestogenic side effect, and may occasionally contribute to thrombophlebitis and thromboembolism.

PROGNOSIS

The prognosis depends on the stage of the disease, the histological grade of the tumour and the age and health of the woman *(Table 39.5).*

CARCINOMA OF THE VULVA

Vulval carcinoma accounts for 3 per cent of genital tract cancers and affects elderly women. The growth usually starts as a lump or an ulcer on one labium majus (50 per cent of cases) or on a labium minus (25 per cent of cases). In some cases multiple areas are affected. In recent years, a number of younger women have been presenting with malignant change in a vulval condyloma.

The affected person may have complained of vulval itching for months or years or may have had few symptoms and has only noticed the lump or the ulcer recently.

CLINICAL

The lesion presents as a hard nodule or an ulcer with a sloughing base and raised edges which may be small or large depending on the duration of the disease *(Fig. 39.9).* If the cancer is large, lymph node involvement will have occurred in more than 50 per cent of cases.

Treatment is either simple vulvectomy with postoperative irradiation of the inguinal lymph nodes, or radical vulvectomy with inguinal, femoral and pelvic

The Recommended Treatment and 5-Year Survival Rate of Endometrial Cancer Related to the Stage of the Disease		
Stage	Recommended treatment	5-year survival rate
I, G1, 2	Hysterectomy	80 per cent
I, G3	Hysterectomy, post-operative radiation	60 per cent
II	As for carcinoma of the uterine cervix	50 per cent
III	Hormone therapy + megavoltage irradiation of the entire pelvis	30 per cent
IV	Hormone therapy 5-year	10 per cent

Table 39.5 The recommended treatment and 5-year survival rate of endometrial cancer related to the stage of the disease.

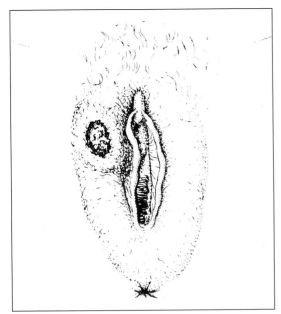

Fig 39.9 Drawing of a vulval carcinoma in the anterior part of the vulva.

lymphadenectomy. Wound necrosis is a troublesome complication after radical vulvectomy and persistent leg oedema occurs in 20 per cent of women.

CANCER OF THE OVARY

Malignant ovarian tumours are rarely diagnosed early and, in consequence, carry a high mortality. About 6 per cent of ovarian tumours are found to be malignant at surgery, the proportion increasing as a woman grows older.

The tumour may arise in several ways as is shown in *Table 39.6*.

Primary ovarian carcinoma accounts for about 20 per cent of all gynaecological cancers. In more than 70 per cent of cases the growth has spread beyond the ovaries when first detected. By this time the prospect of 5-year survival of the affected women is less than 25 per cent.

CLINICAL

The woman, who is usually aged 50 or more, may notice that her abdomen is becoming larger (from the mass or from ascites), or she may complain of pressure symptoms on her bladder or rectum. Adbominal discomfort and gastrointestinal symptoms may be present. She may have lost weight and have no appetite. In most cases the symptoms are few and the tumour is detected during a routine examination. Germ cell malignancies can affect women under the age of 30. The most common germ cell cancer is disgerminoma.

MANAGEMENT

Ovarian malignancies should be treated in oncological units, not by a general gynaecologist or a surgeon. The initial management is surgical, as much malignant tissue being removed, including the omentum, as is surgically possible without causing severe damage. The exception to surgery is the disgerminoma for which radiotherapy appears to be more effective. Following surgery, chemotherapy is initiated. There is no consensus as to the most effective chemotherapy. The current trend is to give a combination of several chemotherapeutic agents (including cisplatin). The response is measured by a reduction in tumour size. Some pelvic surgeons make a 'second look' laparotomy after 6 courses of treatment to assess the response and possibly to 'debulk' persisting or recurrent disease.

Combination chemotherapy is toxic: 60 – 80 per cent of patients have severe nausea and vomiting during treatment; severe hair loss occurs in 50 – 60

A Classification of Malignant Ovarian Tumours		
Tumour	**Type**	**Proportional incidence per cent of all ovarian tumours**
Secondary change in serous cyst-adenoma, occasionally in a mucinous cystadenoma (includes endometrioid carcinoma)	Cystic or semi-solid	5

Rare tumours:
  Feminizing: granulosa-theca cell
  Virilizing: androblastoma
  Neuter: disgerminoma
  Teratoma (embryoma)
	Solid	0.5

Secondary carcinoma:
  Krukenberg, from stomach
  Adenocarcinoma, from uterus
	Solid	0.5

Table 39.6 A classification of malignant ovarian tumours.

per cent; peripheral neuropathy in 5 – 30 per cent and renal toxicity in 15 – 60 per cent.cecause of the high death rate following a diagnosed ovarian cancer, studies are being made to determine if a cancer can be detected at an early stage in a post-menopausal woman. Currently transvaginal ultra-sound, the measurement of CA 125 antigen and Doppler colour flow mapping (to detect the early angiogenesis which occurs in a malignant tumour) are being investigated. Preliminary results are disappointing.

TELLING THE PATIENT WHO HAS GYNAECOLOGICAL CANCER

The fear of cancer is widespread in the population, many people believing that it is a death sentence. If cancer is diagnosed the woman and her family may be devastated. The doctor should understand the patient's fears, and anticipate her possible reaction to the news (anger, distress with crying, silence etc.).

Before talking with the woman and, if she wishes, her husband or partner or a near relative, the doctor should have the case records, including test results, available. The discussion should take place in a quiet, private room. The doctor should identify him or herself. The information (including providing an honest appraisal of the prognosis) should be given in nonjargon language, and time should be allowed for the information to sink in. The patient's understanding of her condition should be checked in a supportive, empathetic manner, and time given for her to react. If the reaction is anger, the doctor should respond by being sympathetic. If she responds by showing shock, or distress or crying, the doctor should let her recover and not try to stop her releasing her emotions. Time should be given for her or her near relative to ask ques-

tions. Most importantly the patient should be offered the opportunity to have a further talk with the doctor as she may be so upset by the news that she is unable to ask questions which concern her.

THE PSYCHOSEXUAL IMPLICATIONS OF GYNAECOLOGICAL CANCER

During and following treatment for gynaecological cancer many women become depressed, which may adversely affect their relationship with their husband or partner. Surgery of the genital tract, especially if it involves the vagina or vulva threatens the woman's identity. Her vagina may be shortened, her vulva mutilated, she may no longer lubricate when sexually stimulated and she may perceive her sexual activity as inappropriate. Her husband may be concerned that sexual intercourse may damage her or lead to him developing cancer. He may find difficulty in accepting his 'mutilated' wife as a sexual partner. Women who have cervical cancer may be concerned that the disease is a result of past sexual behaviour. These feelings are commonly associated with reduced or absent sexual desire.

Strategies to reduce these psychosexual concerns include preoperative explanation of the effects of the surgery or radiotherapy, sexual counselling, and the use of oestrogen vaginal creams, tablets or ovoids when the surgery involves the vagina, or the ovaries are extirpated or irradiated. Sexual explanation and counselling should include information about ways other than sexual intercourse to obtain sexual pleasure, such as cuddling and kissing, oral sex, and masturbation by the other partner. The counselling session should include both partners and be conducted in a non-threatening environment with ample time for discussion.

40

UTEROVAGINAL DISPLACEMENTS, DAMAGE AND PROLAPSE

UTERINE DISPLACEMENTS

The uterus is an organ which normally pivots about an axis formed by the cardinal ligaments at the level of the internal cervical os. In 90 per cent of women, the uterus is anteflexed and anteverted, lying on the urinary bladder and moving backwards as the bladder fills. In 10 per cent of women the uterus is retroflexed and may be retroverted *(Fig. 40.1)*. This is a developmental occurrence. The uterus is mobile and can be moved by inserting a finger in the posterior vaginal fornix. In spite of anecdotal statements, a mobile retroverted uterus is not a cause of infertility, abortion or backache.

Acquired uterine retroversion may occur, but is less common. It is associated with endometriosis of the uterosacral ligaments or the cul de sac; with adhesions resulting from pelvic inflammatory disease; or caused by a tumour in front of the uterus pushing it backwards.

SYMPTOMS

Developmental retroversion is symptomless; only when the retroverted uterus is 'fixed' may symptoms occur. These include the symptoms associated with the underlying cause. In addition the woman may complain of dyspareunia on deep penetration, pelvic pain and low backache. A few women who have chronic pelvic pain and are told by their doctor that their uterus is retroverted, will obtain some relief if the uterus is manipulated to become anteverted. They often remain pain-free when the uterus becomes retroverted again, as it usually does.

DIAGNOSIS

A clinical finding that the uterus is retroverted and is accompanied by symptoms, should alert the medical practitioner to determine if the retroversion can be corrected by manipulation. *(see Fig. 40.2)*. If it can, it is not the cause of the symptoms. If it cannot be manipulated it *may* be the cause of the symptoms.

TREATMENT

In most cases the woman needs reassurance that the retroverted uterus is not the cause of any symptoms she may have and does not require treatment. If the uterus is 'fixed' and the woman has symptoms of deep dyspareunia or chronic pelvic pain, operation may be suggested, but the patient should be told that although it may correct the position of the uterus, the symptoms may not be relieved permanently. Of the many operations possible the one chosen is to shorten and plicate the round ligaments; at the same time any pelvic pathology is treated.

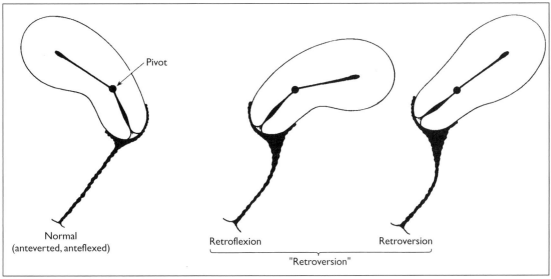

Fig 40.1 Retroversion and retroflexion of the uterus.

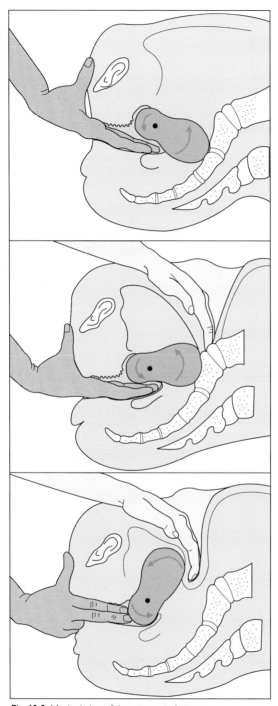

Fig 40.2 Manipulation of the retroverted uterus.

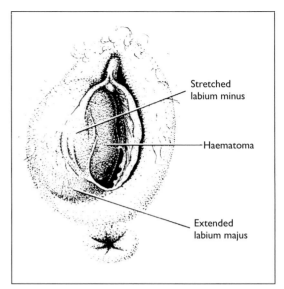

Fig 40.3 A large vulval haematoma.

Stretched
labium minus

Haematoma

Extended
labium majus

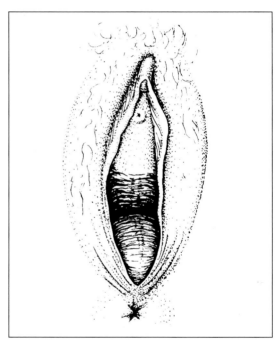

Fig 40.4 Marked perineal deficiency.

UTEROVAGINAL DAMAGE AND INJURIES

Injury may occur to the vulvovaginal area if a girl or woman falls astride some object or is kicked. The vagina may be damaged or a haematoma may form in the vulva *(Fig. 40.3)*. Injury may also occur if a young girl or a postmenopausal woman is sexually assaulted.

During the first sexual intercourse, the hymen is stretched and torn and a small amount of bleeding results; very occasionally more severe bleeding occurs if a larger blood vessel is damaged.

Injury resulting from childbirth is discussed on pages 65 and 79. Occasionally a vaginal tear is not sutured immediately, and the woman attends a medical practitioner some time later. On inspection the vaginal entrance is seen to gape and the perineal muscles are separated *(Fig. 40.4)*. The woman may complain that water enters her vagina when she bathes, or that vaginal flatus occurs.

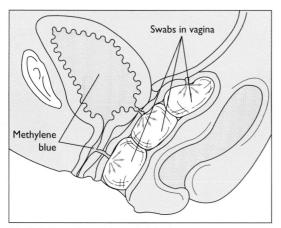

Fig 40.5 Detecting a vesicovaginal fistula.

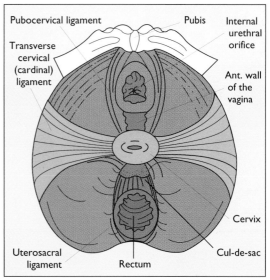

Fig 40.6 The transverse cervical 'ligament'.

Vaginal burns may occur following a very hot vaginal douche, or the deliberate insertion of a caustic agent, such as rock salt, to procure an abortion or, in a few cultures, to tighten the vagina after childbirth to make sexual intercourse more satisfying to the man.

Cervical damage may occur during rough cervical dilatation. The laceration is usually small but may extend from one or other lateral angle of the external cervical os. This may cause marked bleeding. Cervical damage may also occur during childbirth and is discussed on page 65.

GENITAL TRACT FISTULAE

Genital tract fistulae may follow childbirth, but in developed countries usually occur during surgery or following radiotherapy. Fistulae are very uncommon in the developed countries. They may occur between the vagina and uterus and any adjacent organ. The most frequently encountered fistulae are between the vagina and the bladder (vesicovaginal fistula) or between the vagina and rectum (rectovaginal fistula).

Obstetrical and surgical fistulae occur immediately after the procedure or 5–14 days after the operation, when the traumatized ischaemic tissue sloughs. The woman complains of continuous leakage of urine in cases of a vesicovaginal fistula, or faeces in the case of a rectovaginal fistula. If the fistula is large it can be seen on vaginal inspection with a Sims speculum, the woman lying in the left lateral position. Small fistulae may require tests to pinpoint the damaged area. One such test is shown in *Fig. 40.5*. Closure of small vesicovaginal fistulae may occur if the bladder is drained continuously for 14 days, but rectovaginal fistulae and larger fistulae require surgery.

UTEROVAGINAL PROLAPSE

Uterovaginal prolapse is defined as a descent of the uterus and/or vagina. A vaginal prolapse may occur independently of any uterine descent, but a prolapsed uterus always carries some part of the upper vagina with it.

To understand how uterovaginal prolapse occurs requires some knowledge about the supports of the uterus. The uterus is supported in the midpelvis by three structures. These are:
- The vagina, the walls of which lie in apposition and are muscular.
- The transcervical (cardinal) ligaments, which stretch from each pelvic wall and attach to the uterus at the level of the supravaginal cervix. They are not ligaments in the true sense as they are composed of a felted mass of collagenous connective tissue through which blood vessels pass to supply the uterus and bladder *(Fig. 40.6)*. The cardinal ligaments act as the middle support of the uterus and their function can be explained in terms of chicken wire. If the strain is not too great the ligaments have considerable tensile strength, but if the strain is increased or the ligaments are damaged, they stretch *(see Fig. 40.7)* Posteriorly, on each side, condensations of the tissue form the uterosacral ligament.
- The upper supports of the uterus are the relatively weak round ligaments, which operate mostly by maintaining the uterus in an anteverted position so that the increase in intra-abdominal pressure on straining forces the uterus onto the bladder rather than directly down towards the vulva.

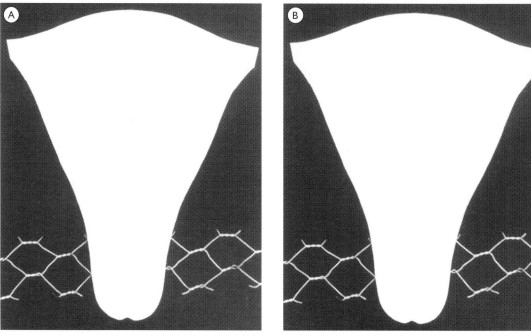

Fig 40.7 The 'chicken wire' analogy. In (A) the areolar tissue is not stretched; in (B), because of the uterine descent, condensation of the tissue occurs, with the appearance of a ligament.

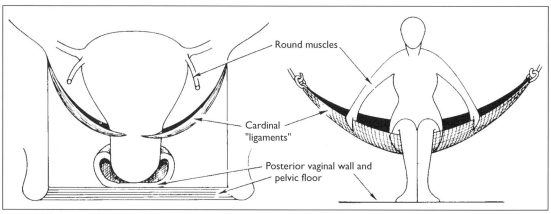

Fig 40.8 Mechanism of prolapse – if the 'holding apparatus', or the 'supporting apparatus' is stretched, some descent of the uterus, or of the vagina, will occur, particularly if the intra-abdominal pressure is increased.

Acting in conjunction, these supports prevent uterine prolapse *(Fig. 40.8)*. However, this state of affairs may be altered if the supports are stretched during childbirth. This may occur if the woman tries to expel the fetus before the cervix is fully dilated, strains for a long time in the second stage of labour, or if undue force is used to expel the placenta. In these circumstances the cardinal ligament may be stretched, making a uterine prolapse more likely. This may only become apparent after the menopause when, deprived of oestrogen, the collagen tissue of the ligaments diminishes and the vaginal muscle becomes weaker, permitting the prolapse to occur.

A further way in which prolapse occurs in a very few nulliparous women, is through the supporting tissues failing to develop properly.

DEGREES OF UTERINE PROLAPSE
For descriptive purposes utero-vaginal prolapse in divided into three degrees of increasing severity *(Fig. 40.9)*. In each of the three degrees the cervix elongates and may become congested or oedematous.

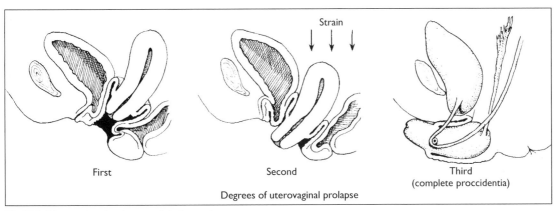

Fig 40.9 Diagram showing degrees of uterine prolapse.

First

Second

Strain

Third
(complete proccidentia)

Degrees of uterovaginal prolapse

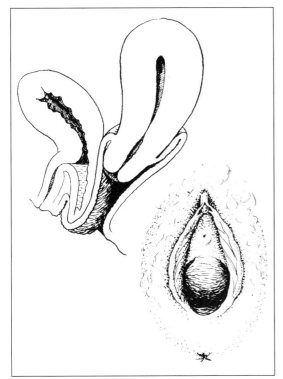

Fig 40.10 Cystocele.

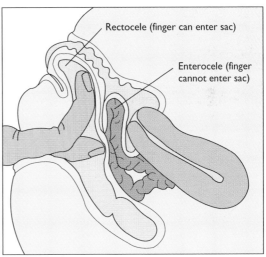

Rectocele (finger can enter sac)

Enterocele (finger cannot enter sac)

Fig 40.11 Enterocele and rectocele.

PROLAPSE OF THE ANTERIOR VAGINAL WALL (CYSTOCELE)

This occurs during childbirth when the fibres of the levator ani muscle which support the vagina are stretched. The weakened anterior vaginal wall bulges into the vagina, bringing the adjacent bladder with it *(Fig. 40.10)*.

PROLAPSE OF THE POSTERIOR VAGINAL WALL (RECTOCELE)

In this case the supporting tissues of the distal posterior wall, including the perineal muscles, are stretched or damaged during the delivery of the baby. With diminished support, the posterior vaginal wall, together with the anterior rectal wall, bulges into the vagina *(Fig. 40.11)*.

If the supports of the proximal vaginal wall are weakened (for example after hysterectomy) it may bulge into the vagina, often containing bowel. This is termed an enterocele.

When the cervix protrudes from the vagina as in the 3rd degree of prolapse, the cervical epithelium becomes dry and its superficial layers are keratinized.

Uterovaginal prolapse is more common in the later reproductive years and after the menopause. In most cases it is due to damage to the supporting tissues and pudendal nerve damage occurring during childbirth, but not apparent until the tissues atrophy in middle age. An additional cause may be chronic constipation leading to straining to evacuate stools.

With better obstetric care the frequency of uterovaginal prolapse is diminishing and severe cases are not often seen.

SYMPTOMS AND DIAGNOSIS

Many women have no symptoms but are concerned that 'something is bulging in my vagina'. Some women feel dragging pains in the lower pelvis, and have difficulty or discomfort when they try to micturate or defaecate. Other women are mildly incontinent.

The type and degree of uterovaginal prolapse can be diagnosed by looking at the woman's vulvovaginal area when she coughs or strains. A vaginal examination using a Sims speculum will confirm the prolapse. A rectal examination may be needed to differentiate a rectocele from an enterocele.

TREATMENT

Treatment depends on the age of the woman, her desire to have further children and the degree of the prolapse. Younger women with mild degrees of symptomless prolapse can delay treatment until the prolapse worsens or the menopause is reached. It is preferable not to treat a prolapse surgically if the woman wishes to have a further child, as the delivery must then be by caesarean section to avoid damage to the repair. If the woman has a cystocele, a midstream urine sample should be taken to exclude bacteriuria. If the urine is sterile, surgery is not required unless the woman desires it. She should be checked periodically.

If the prolapse is marked and is causing symptoms, surgery can be recommended. There are two choices, which should be discussed with the woman. The first is vaginal hysterectomy and vaginal repair. The second is the Manchester operation, which involves shortening the cervix and the cardinal ligaments and plicating them in front of the shortened cervix (to keep the uterus anteverted) and then performing a vaginal repair. If urinary incontinence is present it should be treated.

Elderly women should be given oestrogen for 4–6 weeks before operation to improve the quality of the vaginal tissues. Old frail women, or women who refuse an operation, may choose to have a polythene ring pessary introduced into the vagina. The size chosen should prevent descent of the vaginal walls or the uterus and be comfortable. The woman should have the ring pessary removed at intervals for cleaning and then replaced.

The treatment of a cystocele or a rectocele is to repair the vagina by excising a triangular piece of the anterior or posterior vaginal wall, depending on whether a cystocele or a rectocele is present, pushing the bladder or rectum proximally and suturing the supporting muscles beneath it and then rejoining the cut edges of the vagina.

41

THE URINARY TRACT AND ITS RELATIONSHIP TO GYNAECOLOGY

The close connection of the bladder to the vagina and the short urethra give rise to more problems in a woman's urinary tract than a man's. The anatomy of the urinary tract is described on page 3. The function of the urinary tract is to permit waste products of metabolism to be removed from the body in the urinary flow. For this reason the mechanics of micturition will be discussed first.

THE MECHANICS OF VOLUNTARY MICTURITION

The bladder fills as urine trickles down the ureters. To accommodate the urine, the bladder distends, and can accommodate 300–400ml of urine without any increase in the resting intravesical pressure, which remains below 10cm of water. In the resting state the vesico-urethral junction is flat and there is an angle of about 90° between the bladder and the urethra (the urethro-vesical angle) *(Fig 41.1A)*.

Continence is maintained because of the inherent tone of the urethra and by the muscles which envelop the urethro-vesical junction and the proximal urethra, which keep the intraurethral pressure 7–10cm higher than the pressure within the bladder.

When more than 350ml of urine distends the bladder cholinergic muscarinic stretch receptors in the bladder wall are stimulated. This causes the detrusor muscle to contract and the intravesical pressure rises. Paradoxically, the extension of the detrusor muscle which surrounds the proximal urethra in a spiral fashion relaxes so that the intraurethral pressure falls below the intravesical pressure. By the age of 5 most children have learned to inhibit the detrusor contractions and to keep the urethra closed, so that micturition can be delayed until an appropriate time. In some women this higher centre control cannot be maintained and micturition occurs inappropriately. A second line of defence against involuntary micturition is provided by the muscles forming the external urethral sphincter and the fibres of the pubococcygeal muscle which surround and support the distal urethra.

When the person is ready to pass urine, the detrusor muscle is permitted to contract strongly, which raises the intravesical pressure above the intraurethral pressure. The detrusor contractions also cause funnelling of the bladder base and obliterate the urethrovesical angle *(Fig. 41.1B)*. (The funnelling mechanism is currently in dispute).

At the same time, the person contracts the abdominal muscles which raises the intravesical pressure further. These changes and the relaxation of the proximal urethral muscle permit urine to pass into the urethra. The person now relaxes the muscles surrounding the distal urethra, and urine is voided until the bladder is empty. When this occurs the detrusor ceases to be stimulated and relaxes, and the urethro-vesical angle is restored. The proximal urethra contracts from its distal end to the urethro-vesical junction, 'milking' back a few drops of urine into the bladder. Finally the external sphincter closes.

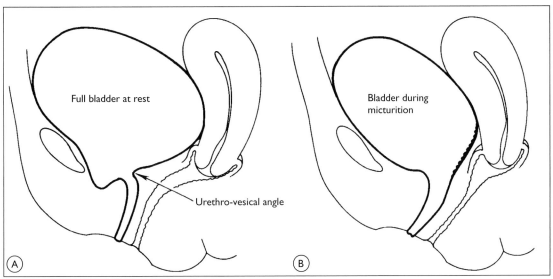

Fig 41.1 Tracing from radiographs of the bladder and urethra. (A) At rest; (B) During micturition.

URINARY INCONTINENCE (INVOLUNTARY MICTURITION)

As women grow older the incidence of urinary incontinence increases, often causing social isolation or psychological problems. In the age group 35–50, 5 per cent of women are incontinent at least once each week. By the age of 60, 15–20 per cent of women complain of urinary incontinence, and by the age of 80 one woman in four is incontinent.

In women two main and two subsidiary forms of urinary incontinence occur. The two main forms are:
- *Urge incontinence.*
- *Urethral sphincter incontinence* (genuine stress incontinence).

The two subsidiary forms are:
- *Reflex incontinence.*
- *Overflow incontinence.*

Of the subsidiary forms, *reflex incontinence* is an involuntary loss of urine due to abnormal reflex activity in the spinal cord in the absence of a desire to pass urine. *Overflow incontinence* (urinary retention with overflow) occurs in:
- Motor neurone disease.
- Urethral obstruction, which is rare in women.
- Cases of chronic bladder distension.

The proportion of women complaining of the two main forms of incontinence is not known. The best estimates are shown in *Table 41.1*.

URGE INCONTINENCE (THE UNSTABLE BLADDER)

In this condition the detrusor muscle contracts involuntarily. There are two categories of urge incontinence. In the first, *sensory incontinence*, the woman passes urine, not because of involuntary detrusor activity but because it hurts if she does not empty her bladder. The woman has to micturate frequently, often several times at night as well as during the day, and may have dysuria. In some cases there is obvious urinary tract infection. In others no evidence of this is found.

In the second category, *motor urgency (detrusor instability)*, the urge to micturate before the bladder is full occurs at variable intervals and variable amounts of urine are voided. This may be accompanied by urinary frequency and incontinence if the woman is unable to reach a toilet. At night she may wet the bed. Pain on micturition is not a feature.

The two forms may be differentiated by urodynamic studies to evaluate detrusor activity during bladder filling, although it is doubtful if this is worth doing as both forms are treated in the same way.

Urge incontinence is a psychosomatic, not a psychological problem, as women with the condition are no more likely to demonstrate psychiatric morbidity than other incontinent women.

URETHRAL SPHINCTER INCONTINENCE

In urethral sphincter incontinence, involuntary loss of urine occurs when the intravesical pressure exceeds the intraurethral pressure in the absence of detrusor activity. Two defects are thought to be present. The first is that the proximal urethra has been displaced downwards through the urogenital diaphragm. When the abdominal pressure rises, as when a woman sneezes, coughs or jolts, the pressure it is not transmitted to the urethra, with the result that the intravesicular pressure rises while the intraurethral pressure does not. The second mechanism is that either because of defective development of the urethral supporting muscles, or damage to the bladder neck supports during childbirth, when the bladder is at rest its base is funnelled, not flat. This impairs the normal closure mechanism at the urethro-vesical junction.

The combined effect of these mechanisms is to increase the intravesical pressure above the intraurethral pressure in the absence of a voluntary pressure increase. This results in a leak of urine into the urethra when only a small increase in intra-abdominal pressure occurs.

Clinical findings

The mechanisms explain the clinical findings which are that the woman complains that a small amount of urine leaks if she laughs, coughs or jumps. The leak can be confirmed if her doctor asks her to cough when she has a full bladder.

DIAGNOSTIC MEASURES TO DETERMINE THE CAUSE OF THE INCONTINENCE

A woman presenting with a complaint of urinary incontinence requires careful examination. The social inconvenience caused by the incontinence should be evaluated. The woman should be asked if she is taking any medications, as some drugs, for example, tricyclics, prazosin and lithium may cause symptoms

The Types of Urinary Incontinence and Their Proportions		
Type of incontinence	Proportion related to the woman's age	
	<70 years old	>70 or more
Urethral sphincter	50%	26%
Urge incontinence	20%	33%
Mixed	30%	41%

Table 41.1 The types of urinary incontinence and their proportions.

of urinary incontinence. General medical conditions, such as parkinsonism, multiple sclerosis and diabetic neuropathy must be looked for and excluded, as should local bladder causes, such as bladder stone or pressure on the bladder from a myoma. The physical examination should include assessment of the perineal reflexes of segments S1–S4, and the anal sphincter tone should be tested. A specimen of midstream urine should be obtained and sent to a laboratory to exclude the possibility of bladder infections.

To try to identify the main (or the only cause) of the incontinence tests should be arranged.

The pad test

The woman is asked to place a weighed pad (with a waterproof backing) over her vulva. She drinks 500ml of sodium-free liquid over a 15-minute period. For the next 30 minutes she performs a range of activities such a climbing a flight of stairs, walking, standing up from sitting and washing her hands under running water. The pad is then removed and weighed again, any weight difference being urinary loss. A more sophisticated pad test, which demands considerable patient compliance is to test for 48 hours, the woman keeping the pads and bringing them to the doctor for weighing.

Urinary diary

If urge incontinence is suspected, the woman is asked to record her daily fluid intake and output each time she drinks or passes urine.

Urodynamic studies

If the diagnosis is still uncertain the woman should be asked to attend a urodynamic clinic so that objective evaluation of the problem may be made, by uroflowmetry and cystometry. Some elderly women are reluctant to undergo urodynamic testing because of embarrassment. They and all postmenopausal women who are not taking hormone replacement treatment, may obtain considerable improvement in their urinary incontinence if they are prescribed a vaginal oestrogen (a cream or an ovoid) for a few months. In about 35 per cent of them, the incontinence is relieved, obviating the need for urodynamic testing.

TREATMENT
Urge incontinence

Several strategies are recommended but the success rate is variable. Bladder drill may help. The woman tries to increase the time between passing urine, no matter how difficult she finds it. The objective is to retrain her bladder to contain more urine before detrusor activity is stimulated. Bladder drill takes time and application. Considerable support and help, preferably from a trained person is needed.

Drugs may help. As detrusor activity is under cholinergic control, anticholinergic drugs are chosen. The currently preferred drug is oxybutynin (2.5–5.0mg three times a day). A number of women cannot take oxybutynin because of the anticholinergic effects of dry mouth, dry skin, blurred vision or constipation. These women may find relief if they take dicyclomine 30mg four times a day.

Urethral sphincter incontinence

Unless the incontinence is severe, the choice of medical or surgical treatment should be offered to the patient. Obese women should try to reduce their weight as this has been found to relieve incontinence in some women. Pelvic floor exercises have been found to help *(Table 41.2)*. The exercises must be continued for several months. An alternative, which many women may find more convenient, is the use of vaginal cones. Weighted vaginal cones (in sets of 5 weighing from 20 to 90g) are purchased. The woman inserts the lightest cone into her vagina. It is kept in by contraction of the levator ani muscle. She progresses from the lightest cone to the heaviest. In addition, postmenopausal women should use a vaginal cream (containing oestriol or oestradiol) or oestrogen pessaries daily for 6 weeks.

Pelvic Floor Exercises

These exercises help a person strengthen the muscles which act as a sling to keep the bladder, the genital organs and the rectum in their correct position.

You should try to do the exercises at least once an hour when you are awake, for the rest of your life.

At first you may find the exercises a little tiring but persevere and you will find them easy to do. The pelvic floor exercises only take about two minutes of each hour and relieve your urinary problems.

The exercises are easy to learn. No one can detect that you are doing them so they may be done in company, when you are watching TV, washing the dishes, cleaning the house, at work, etc.

The exercises have three components:

1. When sitting down, contract the pelvic floor muscles, as if you were trying to lift your genital organs from the seat. Hold the contraction as you count slowly (5 seconds). Then relax. Repeat the exercise 10 times.
2. Stand up and contract the pelvic floor muscles as if you were trying to stop the flow of urine midstream, or if you were tightening your vagina. Hold the contraction for 5 seconds. Then relax. Repeat the exercise 10 times.
3. Finally do a fast version of the exercises, contracting and relaxing every second 10 times.

You can check your progress if you wish and can make sure that you are contracting the right muscles by inserting your finger into your vagina and feeling the strength of the contraction.

If you do the exercises as described, after a week or two you will be pleased with the improvement of the grip.

Table 41.2 Pelvic floor exercises.

These measures effectively relieve urinary sphincter incontinence in up to 50 per cent of affected women. If they fail or the woman chooses surgery, several surgical approaches are possible. Most gynaecologists prefer an operation which elevates the bladder neck so that it lies within the abdominal pressure zone *(Fig. 41.2)* and provides support under the urethro-vesical junction. One example is shown in *Fig. 41.3*. The operations have similar success rates of over 90 per cent in the immediate postoperative years, but long-term studies show that 6 years after the operation only 75 per cent of women are continent. In addition, utero-vaginal prolapse is increased among some treated women. Whether this is due to the operation or to a general weakness of the utero-vaginal supports, which also caused the incontinence, is not known.

If surgery fails to elevate the bladder neck, glutaraldehyde crosslinked bovine collagen (GAX-collagen), may be injected into the tissues on each side of the bladder neck. This relieves the incontinence in some women but is still experimental.

URINARY TRACT INFECTION

The short urethra and its intimate relationship with the vagina increases the chance that a woman will develop urinary tract infection. When the woman becomes sexually active, penile thrusting may move bacteria which have colonized the lower urethra upwards to infect the bladder. This may lead to symptomatic infection or to symptomless bacteriuria (>100 000 organisms per ml of urine), which affects 3–8 per cent of sexually active women. Provided that the woman empties her bladder regularly, the condition is without consequence, but should urinary stasis occur, as in pregnancy, the bacteria may grow in the urine causing clinical acute infection. Initially the infection is confined to the bladder causing *cystitis*, but the infection may spread, either along the ureter or via the lymphatics to infect the kidney, causing *pyelonephritis*.

CLINICAL ASPECTS

The symptoms of lower urinary tract infection (UTI) are frequency of micturition and dysuria; whilst if the kidneys are involved, the woman will be febrile and may have rigors and loin pain.

INVESTIGATIONS

The woman should be asked if she has had previous attacks of UTI and whether she has an irritating vaginal discharge, which if present should be investigated. Her recent sexual activity should be explored and a urethral discharge looked for. A mid-stream specimen of urine is obtained and sent for examination and culture.

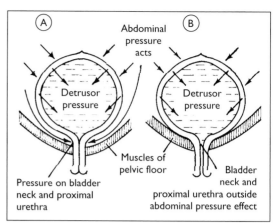

Fig 41.2 The effect of the position of the bladder neck on stress incontinence. In (A) the urethrovesical junction is normally situated. An increase in abdominal pressure acts *equally* on the detrusor pressure and on the bladder neck pressure, so that the pressure gradient is maintained and a positive 'closure' pressure is present. In (B) the urethrovesical junction is *outside* the effects of abdominal pressure as the junction is below the pelvic floor. An increase in abdominal pressure is transmitted only to the detrusor pressure, which exceeds momentarily the intra-urethral pressure. The positive closure pressure is lost and the patient passes a small amount of urine.

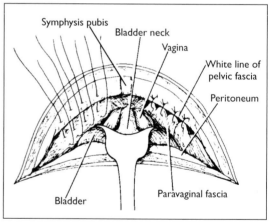

Fig 41.3 Modified colposuspension (retropubic approach). Sutures are placed between the paravaginal fascia and the ileopectineal ligaments. These sutures elevate the bladder neck. The sutures on the right have been tied; those on the left are ready to be tied. During exertion the intra-abdominal pressure rises and compresses the urethra against the symphysis pubis, thus controlling the incontinence.

TREATMENT

Antibiotics are prescribed. The antibiotic chosen depends on local conditions. Norfloxacin 800mg in a single dose, or Augmentin are currently recommended. If the patient has pyelonephritis aggressive treatment is needed. Cephalexin 1g parenterally, followed by 500mg six-hourly is favoured.

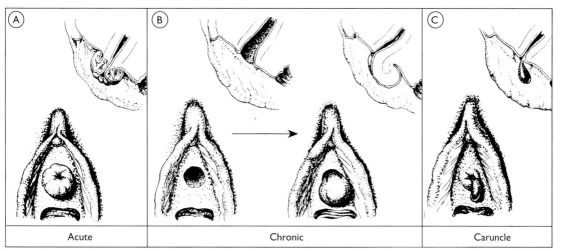

A	B	C
Acute	Chronic	Caruncle

Fig 41.4 Urethral prolapse and urethral caruncle.

THE URETHRAL SYNDROME

In this syndrome the woman complains of dysuria, frequency and pain, which usually start 12–36 hours after sexual intercourse. The symptoms last for 1–4 days and recur when sexual intercourse is resumed, although not every time. If the symptoms are severe and recur frequently they can cause a considerable disruption to the relationship and often sexual frustration.

Investigation includes taking a careful history. Vaginal swabs should be taken as some women with the syndrome are found to have vaginitis. A midstream specimen of urine is also taken. This either fails to show any bacterial growth, or a concentration of bacteria $<10^2$/ml.

TREATMENT

Many women are cured if they drink 500ml of water before intercourse, and empty the bladder completely 20–30 minutes after having sex. If this simple measure fails to cure the condition, cinoxacin 250mg taken after each act of sexual intercourse may be tried or the woman may be prescribed trimethoprim 100mg or nitrofurantin 50mg, each taken daily. (Nitrofurantin should not be taken for more than 6 months because of the possible development of fibrotic alveolitis). In the past the condition was believed to be caused by trigonitis, which was treated by cauterizing the trigone. However, this treatment has been outmoded.

URETHRAL PROBLEMS

URETHRAL PROLAPSE

In the *acute form* the entire circumference of the urethra suddenly everts and becomes engorged as the venous return is impeded *(Fig. 41.4A)*. The woman, who usually is elderly, complains of pain, dysuria and frequency. The immediate treatment is to reduce the prolapse and insert a catheter. Surgery may be offered later.

In the *chronic form* atrophy of the urethral tissues may permit the external urinary meatus to gape, and allow the posterior urethral wall to prolapse *(Fig. 41.4B)*. It appears as a small red swelling and is painless. If it becomes infected it becomes larger and painful. Treatment is to apply an antiseptic ointment and an oestrogen cream. If the symptoms persist, surgery should be suggested.

URETHRAL CARUNCLE

This is a pedunculated polyp, arising from the posterior margin of the urinary meatus *(Fig. 41.4C)*. It is vascular, dull red in colour and tender. The patient complains of pain, frequency and dysuria. Treatment is to excise the caruncle and cauterize its bed.

42

THE BREAST

The adult breast is of varying size and is divided into 15 to 25 lobes separated from each other by fibrous septa which radiate from the nipple. Each lobe has its own duct system which terminates in a dilated area beneath the nipple and then opens on to the surface of the nipple as a punctate orifice. Each lobe is divided into lobules, each of which contains 10 to 100 acini surrounded by fatty tissue, lymphatics and blood vessels.

During the menstrual cycle the female breast undergoes cyclical changes induced by oestradiol and progesterone. Oestradiol induces growth of the acini and combined with progesterone in the luteal phase of the menstrual cycle, causes duct development, increased vascular congestion and fluid transudation into the breast tissues. The result is that in the late luteal phase the breasts are fuller, heavier and may be painful.

DISORDERS OF SIZE AND SHAPE

Current fashion decrees that to be beautiful a woman's breasts should be large (but not too large), full and well supported. Many women have small breasts and some have breasts which are large and pendulous. A woman who has breasts which she perceives as too small or too large may seek medical aid. In most cases the woman is secreting normal quantities of oestrogen, so oestrogen ointments or creams will not increase breast size nor will any hormone decrease breast size.

SMALL BREASTS

The size of the breasts may appear larger if the woman has a good posture and contracts her pectoral muscles. Increase in breast size may be obtained by inserting a shaped 'form' behind the breast tissue and in front of the pectoral muscle, via an incision at the lower margin of the breast. Until 1992 the form was filled with silicone, but with recent concern that silicone may leak and cause damage, this has now been prohibited. A saline-filled implant may be chosen, but this too may cause problems. Augmentation mammaplasty should only be undertaken by an experienced cosmetic surgeon.

LARGE BREASTS

Large pendulous breasts not only appear unattractive (or so some women believe) but may cause shoulder pain. Treatment is to wear a supporting bra or to undergo a reduction mammaplasty.

BREAST DISEASES

In some women the normal cyclical enlargement of the breasts is exaggerated so that the duct systems increase in size and the breasts become tender and nodular. The change may affect one segment of each breast, usually the upper, outer segment, but may involve all segments.

The condition is termed benign breast disease, which has replaced the previous diagnostic terms of mazoplasia, fibroadenosis and chronic mastitis. Benign breast disease may be localized or diffuse. Its aetiology is not known.

LOCALIZED BREAST DISEASE

This variety is usually found among women aged 25 – 45 and in premenopausal women when single large cysts are found. The woman has few if any symptoms, but the discovery of the breast lump causes fear of cancer. The breast should be examined carefully, an ultrasound image made and a mammogram arranged. Once cancer has been excluded, treatment is reassurance.

DIFFUSE BREAST DISEASE

This form is found most often in women aged 30 – 50. The symptoms vary from mild discomfort to severe tenderness and pain. They are worse in the luteal phase of the menstrual cycle, but may persist throughout. Palpation of the breasts reveals coarse nodular areas as if bundles of string were in the breast.

There appears to be a considerable psychological element in the cause of breast tenderness and pain. Many of the women have or have had 'chronic pelvic pain' and PMS. For this reason it is often helpful to explore the woman's lifestyle and to talk about relationship problems. As in the management of PMS, it often helps if the woman keeps a daily diary of her symptoms, their severity and duration, before any treatment is offered. This is because treatment is not very effective, although some women find relief by wearing a well-fitting bra day and night. Some authorities claim that a low-fat diet reduces the problem, but there is no clear evidence that this is true.

By the time that the woman seeks medical help she will probably have tried reducing her caffeine intake and dieting and have purchased over-the-counter medications, such as vitamin B1 and evening primrose oil, or have been prescribed diuretics. Double-blind studies using these medications have shown them to have no benefit over placebo, which emphasises the psychosomatic nature of the complaint.

If the mammary dysplasia causes severe breast tenderness and pain and the above treatments have been used, the woman may choose to try a hormonal approach.

One such approach is to prescribe one of two antioestrogenic, antiprogestogenic, androgenic drugs, danazol and gestrinone, both of which reduce FSH secretion with consequent falls in oestrogen and progesterone. The drugs relieve the pain either completely or partially in 40 – 50 per cent of users. Danazol is given in a dose of 200 mg twice daily from day 12 –26 of the menstrual cycle, or continuously for 6 months in a dose of 200mg daily. Gestrinone is given in a dose of 2.5mg twice weekly for 3 months or longer. Unfortunately both drugs have androgenic side effects, as discussed on page 262.

A second hormonal treatment is to prescribe dydrogesterone 10mg daily from day 12 – 26 of the menstrual cycle on the presumption that the cause of the disease is progesterone deficiency. A third is to prescribe the prolactin antagonist, bromocriptine 2.5 – 5.0mg daily throughout the menstrual cycle. About 8 per cent of women treated stop using bromocriptine because of side effects, usually nausea.

No method of treatment seems superior to any other, and if one fails to relieve the symptoms another may be suggested. Studies have shown that breast pain or discomfort is not relieved by any of the available treatments in one-third of patients.

Patients should be given a full, clear explanation of the possibility that treatment will not be successful and the opportunity to talk with their doctor.

A recent study has found that a woman who has benign breast disease has a slightly increased risk of developing breast cancer in the premenopause. It would be wise to encourage such women to have mammograms regularly from the age of 40.

DUCT ECSTASIA

The pain is localized to an area below the areola or an inner quadrant of the breast. The pain may occur at any time during the menstrual cycle and is increased in cold weather. Flame-shaped shadows may show on mammography. Treatment is to exercise the affected wedge-shaped area.

FIBROADENOMA OF THE BREAST

Benign encapsulated tumours may arise in the breasts of women aged less than 30. Fibroadenoma are symptomless and are detected by accident or by breast self-examination. The lump is smooth and is very mobile. It has been called a 'breast mouse'. Treatment is to exercise the fibroadenoma.

THE TIETZE SYNDROME

Some women complain of breast pain which is, in reality, due to an enlarged costochondrial junction of one of the ribs. The pain is localized, chronic and not related to the premenstruum. There is no effective treatment.

BREAST CANCER

Breast cancer is the second most common cancer in women, and affects one woman in 14, usually after the age of 50. Early detection is the only way to control the disease as, by the time the cancer can be palpated easily, spread is likely to have occurred.

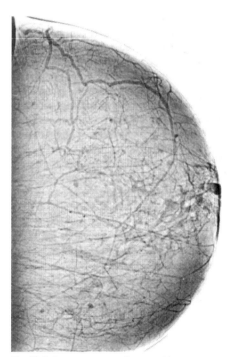

Fig 42.1 A mammogram of a normal breast.

For this reason programmes to persuade women to learn and practise breast self-examination have been developed in many countries. In addition, health authorities recommend that women over the age of 35 have an annual breast examination by a doctor. This should be supplemented by mammography between the ages of 40 and 45, then annually from the age of 50 *(Fig. 42.1 and 42.2)*. About 95 per cent of women who have mammographic and clinical screening will have no evidence of breast cancer; 5 per cent will require further investigation, and 1 per cent will need a breast biopsy to establish or exclude breast cancer.

The aetiology of breast cancer has not been elucidated. A genetic factor exists as breast cancer tends to be found in families. Childbearing before the age of 30 seems to be protective.

TREATMENT

Early breast cancer is best treated by breast conserving surgery and radiation therapy to the axilla. The effectiveness of adjuvant treatment using chemotherapy or tamoxifen is being studied. A recent meta-analysis of over 75,000 women with early breast cancer has shown that women who received additional treatment following surgery had a higher 5- and 10-year survival rate. For women under the age of 50, adjuvant chemotherapy for 6 months or ovarian ablation or tamoxifen for 2 years had approximately equal efficacy in prolonging survival. The treatments increased the 10-year survival rate by 10 per cent. For women over 50, tamoxifen or chemotherapy increased the survival at 10 years by 12 per cent. Tamoxifen had fewer adverse effects.

More advanced breast carcinoma is treated by modified radical mastectomy or radiotherapy. Survival is increased if the woman is given adjuvant treatment with chemotherapy or tamoxifen if she is aged 50 or more.

These treatments eliminate oestrogen secretion with the result that the patient is likely to suffer severe menopausal symptoms (hot flushes, dry vagina, bone loss) which may interfere with her social and sexual life. For this reason each patient should be given sufficient information to enable her to make an informed choice.

Following breast-conserving surgery or a modified radical mastectomy the majority of women have no psychiatric or sexual problems, provided full explanation of the extent of and problems associated with surgery has been given by the surgeon. Breast conservation is marginally better in preserving body image and perhaps sexual enjoyment. About 25 per cent of women have significant depression or anxiety.

An increasing number of women of premenopausal age are receiving chemotherapy or anti-oestrogen treatment after surgery, so menopausal symptoms are causing more problems because of hot flushes and failure of vaginal lubrication. In addition, some women find difficulty in accepting the alopecia, weight changes and pallor following chemotherapy. The anti-oestrogen, tamoxifen, appears to cause fewer menopausal symptoms, possibly because it has mild oestrogenic effects on the vagina.

Most women following treatment for breast cancer are helped if they (and their partners) can talk with an experienced clinician about the problems they may develop. Questions will relate to how each partner sees the woman's body; how to find comfortable ways to have sex and to use a water based lubricant to avoid vaginal dryness; and what sexual enjoyment other than sexual intercourse can be experienced by the couple.

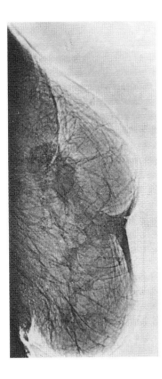

Fig 42.2 A mammogram of a breast containing an advanced carcinoma. Note the retracted nipple and skin thickening.

43

GYNAECOLOGICAL PROBLEMS IN CHILDHOOD AND ADOLESCENCE

INTERSEX

The first question a mother asks after her baby has been born is 'Is it a boy or a girl?'. The answer is given after looking at the infant's genitals. In 2 in 10 000 neonates, the genital sex is ambiguous. The child is judged as being intersex.

Most neonates with ambiguous genitals are genetically female and have congenital adrenal hyperplasia. A few have an adrenal tumour or drug induced virilism. In rare cases the neonate is a hermaphrodite, having a testis and an ovary, the external genitals being ambiguous.

CONGENITAL ADRENAL HYPERPLASIA

This condition affects 1 in 10 000 neonates and is due to a group of enzyme defects which prevent the synthesis of cortisone from progesterone. The lack of circulating cortisone permits the hypothalamus–pituitary to release quantities of corticotrophins which stimulate the adrenal gland to secrete androgens, with resulting virilization of the external genitals *(Fig. 43.1)*.

The most common enzyme defect is C-21-hydroxylase deficiency (found in >90 per cent of cases). In three-quarters of cases ambiguous external genitals are the only sign of the condition, but in a quarter of cases aldosterone production is lost and the patient has a salt-losing syndrome.

Any child with ambiguous genitals should be investigated for CAH, by determining the chromosomal sex from a buccal smear and by measuring the 17-hydroxyprogesterone level, a level of >7mmol/L confirming the diagnosis. Treatment is urgent or death may supervene from salt loss. The infant is treated with cortisone or one of its derivatives. Careful follow-up is essential but surgical correction of the external genitals should be delayed for 3–4 years.

OTHER CAUSES OF INTERSEX

Other varieties of intersexuality are not diagnosed until after puberty, when menstruation fails to start. They include *gonadal dysgenesis* (Turner's syndrome); *testicular feminization* (androgen insensitivity syndrome) and *Klinefelter's syndrome* (seminiferous tubular dysgenesis).

GONADAL DYSGENESIS

Two varieties of this condition exist. They are pure gonadal dysgenesis and Turner's syndrome.

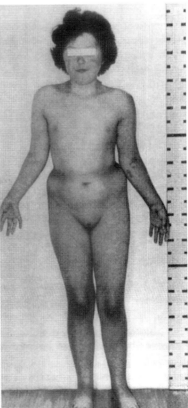

Fig 43.2 Gonadal dysgenesis (Turner's syndrome). The patient is of short stature, has a 'webbed' neck and cubitus valgus, and is sexually infantile. Pelvic examination showed a vagina, a rudimentary uterus, but palpable gonads. (By kind permission of the Author and the Publishers of 'Triangle', The Sandoz Journal of Medical Science, 1967, 8, 37.).

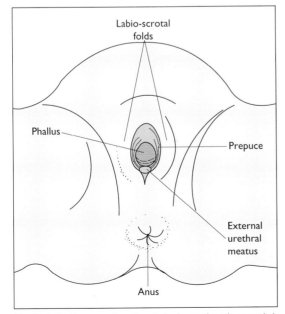

Fig 43.1 Ambiguous external genitalia due to the adrenogenital syndrome.

Pure Gonadal dysgenesis

In this condition genital hypoplasia is detected in a girl who has normal breast development. A chromosome analysis shows a mosaic 46, XO/XX

Turner's Syndrome

The adolescent girl is short in stature having failed to experience a marked prepubertal growth spurt. She may have a webbed neck or other deformities *(Fig. 43.2)*. She seeks medical help when she fails to menstruate. Investigations show that she has raised FSH and LH levels and a chromosome analysis reveals a karyotype of 46, XO. Treatment is undertaken by a paediatrician who will prescribe hormone replacement treatment (see p 307) to help the development of her breasts and genital tract and to prevent osteoporosis in later life. As the ovaries contain no follicles, the girl is sterile. She is helped by counselling. She needs to be reassured of the benefits of hormone replacement, and helped to accept her short stature and sterility. The counsellor should stress that neither of these should reduce her sexuality and sexual enjoyment.

TESTICULAR FEMINIZATION

Physically the person is female with female external characteristics, including good breast development *(Fig. 43.3)*, and has been reared as a girl. She and her parents are concerned when she fails to menstruate. Examination shows that she has a short vagina which ends blindly. A karyotype is 46, XY, as she is genetically male. The gonads are in the abdominal cavity or in a hernial sac. They synthesize testosterone but the body tissues lack alpha reductase enzyme to covert it to dihydroxytestosterone and receptor cells in genital tract tissues and skin may be missing. As the testes may become malignant they should be removed and hormonal replacement treatment given.

KLINEFELTER'S SYNDROME

The person is a tall phenotypically male whose puberty is delayed and who has a small penis and testes. The chromosome count is 47,XXY or 46,XY/XXY. The person may have a low libido. The young man needs sympathetic support, counselling and encouragement to become more assertive. Testosterone implants may improve his libido, but his small penis may prevent him from forming a full sexual relationship.

THE 'GENITAL CRISIS'

In a few female infants, because of tissue sensitivity, maternal oestrogen thickens the vaginal and uterine epithelium. After birth the oestrogen is withdrawn and the child has a small withdrawal bleed per vaginam, the so-called genital crisis. Similarly a few female infants may secrete a small amount of watery milk. The parents require reassurance.

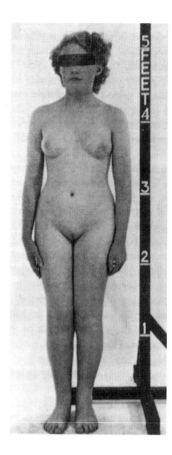

Fig 43.3 Testicular feminization. Although apparently a female, the vagina ends in a blind pouch and the gonad is, in fact, a testis. (Reprinted from the *Brit. Med. J.,* 1955, I, 1174, by permission of the Author (Dr C.N. Armstrong) and Editor).

FUSION OF THE LABIA MINORA

The labia may be seen to be adherent at the neonatal examination or this may occur when the girl is a toddler. The treatment is to separate the labia with the fingers and for the mother to apply an oestrogen cream to the separated labia for 2–3 weeks to encourage epithelization.

VULVOVAGINITIS IN PREPUBERTAL CHILDREN

Vulvovaginitis may occur at any age. The child is brought by the mother complaining of an inflamed tender vulva and perhaps a vaginal discharge. The causes are listed in *Table 43.1*. The vulval area should be inspected and an anal swab taken for pin and thread worms. A swab should be taken from the vagina. If an intravaginal foreign body is suspected and cannot easily be detected the child should be referred to a gynaecologist who deals with children, for examination with a vaginoscope.

Treatment is:

- To treat an identified specific cause appropriately.
- To encourage vulval general cleanliness (and the avoidance of soap), followed by careful vulval drying and the wearing of cotton panties day and night.

Vulvovaginitis: Causes	
	Percentage
I Non-specific	60
2 Specific	
(a) Bacterial: E. coli 12	
N. gonorrhoeae 2 } 20	
Other 6	
(b) Fungal (Candida)	10
(c) Protozoal (trichomonad)	5
(d) Foreign body	5
(e) Helminthic/viral	1

Table 43.1   Vulvovaginitis: causes.

- If the condition persists for >2 weeks in spite of these treatments oestrogen cream may be applied to the vulva with vaginal introitus twice daily for 5 days.

PRECOCIOUS PUBERTY

Precocious puberty indicates that sexual maturation has occurred before the age of 9. Most cases are constitutional in origin but ovarian or adrenal hormone-secreting tumours must be excluded. The investigations include:

- Full history and physical examination.
- Bone age studies.
- Ultrasound, CAT scan or MRI to exclude an ovarian or an adrenal tumour, and a brain scan.

Management is psychological and endocrinological. The girl (and her parents) need considerable psychological support as the girl perceives herself as different from her peers and may be teased. If the girl's bone age is advanced, she will be taller initially but as the epiphyses fuse earlier will be shorter than her peers. Several hormone treatments are being tested to treat precocious puberty. The most promising is a GnRH analogue given daily by nasal sniffs or as a depot preparation each month, to reverse the physical changes.

THE PHYSICAL CHANGES OF PUBERTY AND EARLY ADOLESCENCE

The endocrinological changes which occur before and after puberty were detailed in Chapter 3. These changes manifest in physical changes (Table 43.2). If they do not parallel fairly closely the changes in their peers, some girls become anxious and seek reassurance. Other girls develop an eating disorder.

By the age of 17 over 99 per cent of adolescents will have reached menarche. Delay after this age may be constitutional or have a recent cause (Table 43.3). Investigations include:
- A full careful history.
- A full physical examination including a pelvic examination.

The history and examination may indicate special examinations, for example, imaging of the skull, and/or the pelvic organs; nuclear sex chromatin; laparoscopy. Treatment is discussed in Chapter 30.

Time of Appearance of Sexual Characteristics in Australian Girls	
Age	**Characteristics**
9–10	Growth of bony pelvis begins Fat deposition initiates beginnings of female contour Budding of the nipples
10–11	Budding of the breasts Appearance of pubic hair (androgens are responsible for pubic and axillary hair)
11–13	Growth of internal and external genitalia Glycogen content of the vagina increases; the height of the epithelium increases with change in cell type, and the pH is lowered. Occasionally a vaginal discharge is noted.
12–14	Pigmentation of the nipples Growth and rounding of the breasts
13–15	Axillary hair appears Menarche occurs (mean 13 years, range 9 to 16) Pubic hair increases in amount Acne present in 60 per cent of adolescents
16–18	Cessation of skeletal growth

Table 43.2   Time of appearance of sexual characteristics in Australian girls.

Primary Amenorrhoea	
	Percentage of cases
Gonadal dysgenesis (inc. Turner's syndrome)	45
Congenital absence of uterus or vagina	15
Low body weight (inc. anorexia nervosa)	10
Congenital adrenal virilism	5
Testicular feminization	5
Other (inc. hypothyroidism 4 per cent; systemic disease, 4 per cent)	15
No cause (i.e. constitutional delayed menarche)	5

Table 43.3   Primary amenorrhoea.

MENSTRUAL DISTURBANCES IN ADOLESCENCE

Menstrual disturbances have been discussed in Chapter 30. As mentioned, in the first 2 years after the menarche, some young women experience oligomenorrhoea, whilst in others menstruation occurs at longer or shorter intervals. Unless the disorder persists, treatment is to reassure the young woman that it will settle.

Later in the teenaged years, dysfunctional uterine bleeding affects a small number of young women. Many of the invasive investigations listed for older women are inappropriate for teenagers. For example, diagnostic curettage is invasive and usually not necessary. Treatment using hormones is the main modality, as endometrial ablation and hysterectomy are inappropriate. Hormonal treatment or treatment with NSAIDs for 3 – 6 months usually controls the menstrual disturbance, after which the reciprocity of the hypothalamic-pituitary-ovarian axis re-establishes itself, but in 5 per cent of affected adolescents, the dysfunctional uterine bleedings recur.

Dysmenorrhoea affects many adolescent women and is considered on pp 220.

44

A WOMAN'S MIDDLE YEARS: MENOPAUSE

A woman's middle years extend from the age of 40 to 65. The most important landmark during this time is the menopause. Menopause means the cessation of menstruation, but the term is commonly used to include the perimenopausal years and the 10 or more years following the cessation of menstruation. The period is more correctly called the climacteric.

From the mean age of 40 (±5) years a woman's ovaries become less receptive to the effects of FSH and LH, either because the number of receptor binding sites on each follicle are decreasing or because increasing numbers of follicles are disappearing, or because of both. The effect is that oestrogen secretion declines and fluctuates, anovulation becoming more frequent. The fluctuations are a major factor in causing the menstrual disturbances which occur in some women in the years preceding the menopause (Chapter 30). In addition, the negative feedback to the hypothalamus and pituitary gland is less effective, with the result that FSH levels begin to rise.

As the years pass fewer follicles are left in the ovaries and the levels of oestrogen begin to fall more rapidly. When this occurs FSH levels continue to rise as do LH levels, reaching a peak in the immediate postmenopause. The high circulating levels of gonadotrophins persist from this time on.

The remaining ovarian follicles become increasingly resistant to the higher FSH levels and oestrogen secretion is reduced still further until oligomenorrhoea, and later, amenorrhoea results. If the amenorrhoea persists for 6 months, with or without menopausal symptoms, the menopause has been reached. If the clinician is doubtful if the menopause has occurred it can be confirmed by measuring serum FSH on several occasions. A level of >40IU/L indicates menopause. The measurement of oestrogen levels is not helpful, as the levels of oestrone, oestradiol and oestriol fluctuate even after the menopause, particularly in the first 12 months. A change in the ratio of oestradiol : oestrone occurs, oestrone becoming the dominant circulating oestrogen. After the menopause any circulating oestrogen detected is synthesized in the peripheral fat by aromatization of androstenedione, derived mainly from the adrenal cortex, with some from the ovarian stroma.

Oestrone ↑

CHANGES IN THE GENITAL TRACT AFTER THE MENOPAUSE

The decline in circulating oestrogen to low levels after the menopause leads to atrophy of the organs of the genital tract and the breasts *(Fig. 44.1)*. The *ovaries,* the *Fallopian tubes* and the *uterus* become progressively atrophic. In the uterus the muscle fibres are converted into fibrous tissue and any myomata present atrophy. The *vaginal epithelium*

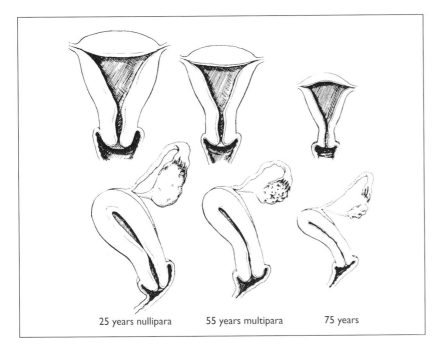

Fig 44.1 To show the reduction in the size of the uterus in old age.

25 years nullipara   55 years multipara   75 years

becomes thinner and less rugose and intermediate cells replace superficial cells. The vaginal secretions diminish as does the vaginal acidity, and pathogenic organisms grow more easily. The *urethral mucosa* may become atrophic. In some women urinary symptoms of frequency, dysuria and incontinence result (see Chapter 41). The *pelvic floor muscles* lose their tone as their blood supply is reduced; relaxation of the muscles increases and uterovaginal prolapse may become evident (Chapter 40). The *external genitals* slowly become atrophic, and in old age the labia majora may lose their fat, revealing the labia minora.

THE SYMPTOMS OF THE CLIMACTERIC

The symptoms experienced by menopausal women result from the low levels of oestrogen. The two true menopausal symptoms are hot flushes and vaginal symptoms of 'burning', dryness and dyspareunia. Other symptoms are listed but most are not exclusively the result of oestrogen deprivation.

HOT FLUSHES

During a hot flush (hot flash in the USA) the woman experiences a feeling of heat centered on her face, which spreads to her neck and chest and may become generalized. This flushing is associated with peripheral vasodilatation and a temporary rise in body temperature of 3°C. The cause of the hot flush is unknown.

Each hot flush lasts for 1 - 3 minutes and is often accompanied by sweating. Hot flushes may occur many times during the day and night. If they occur at night when the woman is in bed, sweating tends to be profuse and sleep is disturbed; the next day she may feel fatigued.

Hot flushes may begin in the months before the menopause, but are worse after it, reaching a peak incidence 1–2 years after the menopause. Approximately one-third of climacteric women experience no or mild symptoms; one third have moderate symptoms but usually do not seek medical advice and one-third have severe disabling symptoms. The hot flushes may persist for a number of years after the menopause.

VAGINAL SYMPTOMS

The vaginal symptoms owing to oestrogen deprivation tend to occur later in the climacteric, if they occur at all. Vaginal dryness and 'burning' are usually reported, but some women experience marked dyspareunia which may affect their relationship with their partner considerably. Women who have regular sexual intercourse are less likely to develop dyspareunia.

OTHER SYMPTOMS.

Of many other symptoms listed as 'due' to the menopause, few are. Some menopausal women lose interest in sex, but this may be as much a function of their poor relationship as due to a hormonal deficiency. Contrary to popular belief, depression is no more common in the menopausal years than at other times. As a woman grows older her skin becomes less elastic, particularly it is photodamaged. Lack of oestrogen in the postmenopausal years makes the wrinkling and dryness more apparent; however, this may respond, to some degree, to hormonal treatment.

LONG-TERM EFFECTS OF OESTROGEN DEFICIENCY

As well as symptoms occurring at or soon after the menopause, long term effects of oestrogen deficiency occur which reduce life expectancy and the quality of life. These are an increased risk of ischaemic heart disease and osteoporosis.

Ischaemic heart disease. At all ages of life, women have a lower mortality from cardiovascular disease than men. In the postmenopausal years the gap closes. These observations suggest that oestrogen offers a woman some degree of protection against developing heart disease.

Osteoporosis. As women and men grow older, there is an increased tendency for their bones to become osteopenic and spinal fractures occur, leading to symptoms of backache and a reduction in height. Other women sustain fractures of the wrist or hip from falls that would previously have been trivial. These women have osteoporosis. Postmenopausal women, deprived of oestrogen, develop osteoporosis earlier in life than men, who are protected at least until the age of 75 by circulating testosterone.

THE PSYCHOLOGICAL SYMPTOMS OF THE CLIMACTERIC

The perception of the menopause as threatening is culture-based. In some societies women welcome the menopause as they are no longer able to bear children and have greater freedom. In many Western culture, where the stress is on youth, the menopause is often perceived negatively. Relationships with a partner and children may have deteriorated, the woman may be anxious about the future,or she may feel that she is becoming less attractive.

SEXUALITY AFTER THE MENOPAUSE

Sexual desire and drive are unchanged in 60 per cent of postmenopausal women, at least up to the age of 65-70. Sexual desire and drive are increased in 20 per cent and reduced in 20 per cent of postmenopausal women. The most important influence on a postmenopausal woman's sexuality is the pattern established in the reproductive years: if it was good then it will continue to be good! As men grow older, however, their sexual desire and response changes. The man may desire sex less often, it takes longer to stimulate him and his erection is less firm and prolonged. Doctors who are consulted about a sexual problem by a postmenopausal woman may have to explain the changes. As women live longer than men, more elderly women have no partner and may seek 'permission' from a doctor if they use self stimulatory methods to obtain sexual pleasure.

THE MANAGEMENT OF THE CLIMACTERIC

The management of menopausal women includes:
- Providing an explanation of the changes which are occurring.
- Giving advice about nutrition and diet and answering concerns about weight.
- Discussing the benefits of hormone (oestrogen) replacement treatment.

Hormone replacement treatment / therapy – HRT

Before prescribing HRT the doctor should make a general medical check, if this has not been made in the previous year. The physical examination should include: an estimation of the body mass index; a breast examination, including a mammogram; a measurement of the blood pressure; and a vaginal examination, including a pap smear.

There are compelling data which show that if a menopausal woman takes small daily doses of an oestrogen she will:
- Be relieved of the flushes and vaginal symptoms;
- Experience a feeling of well being;
- Reduce the risk of having a heart attack by 30 – 50 per cent, provided she takes the other measures recommended: stopping smoking; eating a prudent diet; and taking regular enjoyable exercise, such as walking;
- Prevent bone loss and consequently delay the onset of osteoporosis.

There are several choices of oestrogen replacement treatment. The woman may choose, for example, to take a daily oestrogen tablet, or apply an oestrogen transdermal patch every 3rd day. The dose of oestrogen is adjusted so that the symptoms are relieved. A few women, particularly those who have had a hysterectomy, choose to have an oestradiol implant every 6 months.

If the woman has not had a hysterectomy, unopposed oestrogen treatment increases the risk that she will develop an endometrial carcinoma (from 1 per 1000 women per year to 3 – 4 per 1000 per year). Women who have retained their uterus should be prescribed a progestogen for the first 12 days of each month. During the time the woman takes the progestogen she may experience symptoms similar to

those of the premenstrual syndrome, and at the end of the course usually she will have a withdrawal bleed, which lasts 3-4 days. The effects of progestogen and the withdrawal bleeds deter many women from taking HRT, in spite of the clear benefits of the treatment. Two strategies are available to overcome the problem. The first is for the woman to be prescribed a combination of oestrogen and progestogen to be taken each day; the second is for the woman to take tibolone (Livial) daily. In each case irregular bleeding may be expected for the first 4 – 6 months of treatment but after that amenorrhoea is usual.

The doctor should try to persuade the woman to continue with HRT for 10 years as a protection against osteoporosis; and probably longer to protect her from having a heart attack.

If the woman's main problem is atrophic vaginitis, oestrogen pessaries or cream may be preferred, at least until the symptoms are relieved.

Should irregular bleeding occur during HRT the woman should have an endometrial biopsy or curettage performed (or have a Doppler transvaginal ultrasound examination made to determine endometrial thickness, although this is experimental at present).

POSTMENOPAUSAL BLEEDING

Irregular bleeding per vaginam may also occur in women not taking HRT. The causes are listed in *Table 44.1*. As 15 per cent of women who have postmenopausal bleeding will be found to have a malignancy, investigations include inspection of the vagina, a pap smear and an endometrial curettage or biopsy, even if the clinical diagnosis appears to be atrophic vaginitis or a cervical polyp. Treatment depends on the cause.

Causes of Postmenopausal Bleeding (800 Reported Cases)	
	Percentage
No demonstrable lesion	25
Oestrogen therapy	20
Atrophic vaginitis	15
Endometrial carcinoma	15
Endometrial polyp or hyperplasia	15
Cervical carcinoma	4
Benign cervical lesions (polyp)	4
Ovarian tumour (mostly malignant)	1
Bleeding from urinary tract	1

Table 44.1 Causes of postmenopausal bleeding (800 reported cases).

OSTEOPOROSIS

With an aging population osteoporosis is becoming a major public health problem. Estimates show that between 20 and 30 per cent of women living in the developed countries will have an osteoporotic fracture if they live into their 70s. The cost in diminished quality of life and the cost to the community to treat the fractures is large and increasing.

Once osteoporosis is established, treatment is not particularly effective. The strategy must be to prevent or delay its onset.

The chance that a woman will develop osteoporosis depends on genetic inheritance, her peak bone mineral density (which is reached between the age of 15 and 25), and the rate at which she loses bone. Until the age of 40 bone loss is balanced by bone formation; after the age of 40, about 0.5 per cent of the bone mass is lost annually. Following the menopause, bone loss varies from 1 to 7 per cent a year depending on the individual, averaging 3 per cent a year. This amount of bone loss continues for 10 years and then reduces to between 0.5 and 1.0 per cent per year.

PREVENTION OF OSTEOPOROSIS.

Adolescent and young women should be persuaded to take at least 1g of calcium each day, (preferably in food) so that they may achieve their peak bone mass.

A young woman who is amenorrhoeic for >6 months (for example, a woman with anorexia nervosa or who is a compulsive exerciser) should be prescribed oestrogen, the Pill being a good choice.

A woman on reaching the menopause should be advised to have HRT, as oestrogen effectively prevents bone loss. (An alternative under investigation is nasal calcitonin.) A woman who chooses not to have HRT should undergo a bone densitometry made and, depending on the result, should be advised whether she needs treatment or can continue without.

ESTABLISHED OSTEOPOROSIS

Once clinical osteoporosis has been diagnosed, either by bone densitometry or following a fracture, treatment is more difficult. Drugs used to treat established osteoporosis act either by preventing bone resorption or by stimulating bone formation. Drugs preventing bone resorption such as those used in HRT, calcitonin, calcitriol and bisphosphonate etidronate (Didronel) intermittently with calcium, are being investigated. The anabolic steroid nandrolone decanoate, (Deca-Durabolin) which stimulates bone formation and prevents resorption to some extent is also under study. Until the benefits and adverse effects of these drugs have been evaluated, prevention holds the most promise for reducing the adverese health effects of osteoporosis.

45

THE ANATOMY OF THE FEMALE GENITAL TRACT

By the time the student studies gynaecology, he or she has been well grounded in the disciplines of anatomy and physiology, and only a brief review of the anatomy of the female genital tract will be made here.

THE VULVA *(FIG 45.1)*

The *labia majora* are two large folds containing sebaceous and sweat glands embedded in adipose and connective tissue and covered by skin. They form the lateral boundaries of the vulval cleft, and are the homologues of the scrotum. Anteriorly they unite in an adipose pad over the symphysis pubis, to form the mons veneris. In the adult female the mons is covered with hair, which terminates cephalically in a horizontal upper border. Hair also grows on the outer, but not the inner, surface of the labia majora. Posteriorly the labia majora unite to form the posterior commissure. In childhood the labia majora contain little adipose tissue, and in age the adipose tissue disappears. At the extremes of life, therefore, the labia majora are relatively small.

The *labia minora* are flat, delicate folds of skin containing connective tissue and some sebaceous glands, but no adipose tissue. On their medial aspect the keratinized epithelium of the skin changes into poorly keratinized squamous epithelium, containing many sebaceous glands. Anteriorly the labia minora split into two parts, one passing over the clitoris to form the prepuce of the organ, the other passing beneath to form the homologue of the frenulum of the male. Posteriorly they fuse to form the fourchette, which is always torn during parturition. In the reproductive years the labia minora are hidden by the labia majora, but in childhood and old age they appear to be more prominent as the labia majora are relatively small. The size of the labia minora varies considerably in different women, but this is of little clinical importance.

The cleft between the labia minora is called the *vestibule*, and contains the *external urethral meatus* and the *hymen*, which lies just inside and surrounds the vaginal orifice. The vestibule is surmounted by the *clitoris*, which is the homologue of the penis, and is composed of erectile tissue. As with the penis, it becomes enlarged and stiffens during sexual excitement. The clitoris is one of the major erotic zones of the female. Only the glans and prepuce of the clitoris are normally visible, but the corpus can be palpated along the lower surface of the symphysis pubis as a cord-like structure.

The *hymen* is a thin, incomplete membrane surrounding the vaginal orifice, and has one or more apertures in it, which allow menstrual blood to escape. The apertures are of various shapes and sizes. The hymen varies considerably in elasticity, but is generally torn during a first coitus. An 'intact' hymen is considered a sign of virginity, but this is not reliable as in some cases coitus fails to cause a tear,

Fig 45.1 The vulva of a virgin.

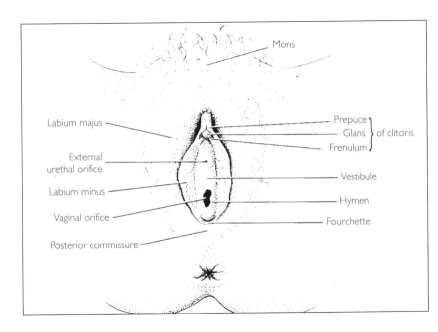

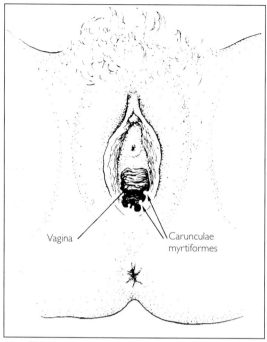

Fig 45.2 The vulva of a parous woman.

a much greater tearing of the hymen, and after parturition only a few tags remain. These are carunculae myrtiformes *(Fig 45.2)*. Just lateral to the hymen, surrounding the vaginal orifice on each side, and deep to the bulbocavernosus muscle (the sphincter vaginae), are two collections of erectile tissue — the *vestibular bulbs*. Embedded in the posterolateral parts of the bulbs, on each side is Bartholin's gland *(Fig 45.3)*, which is the homologue of Cowper's gland in the male. The gland is pea-sized and not palpable unless infected. It is connected to the posterior part of the vestibule, between the hymen and the fourchette, bya duct some 2cm in length. It is lined by columnar cells, which secrete a mucoid substance during sexual excitement.

VASCULAR SUPPLY OF THE VULVA

Arteries
The external genitalia are very vascular, and are supplied by branches of the internal pudendal arteries, which originate from the internal iliac arteries, and by the pudendal arteries, deriving from the femoral arteries.

Veins
The veins of the vulva form large venous plexuses, which become dilated during sexual excitement, and to an even greater degree during pregnancy, when varicosities are not uncommon. Most of the veins accompany the corresponding arteries, but those draining the clitoris join the vaginal and vesical venous plexuses.

and in others the hymen may be torn by digital interference. In attempting to make a decision regarding viriginity, palpation to feel a circular ridge of hymenal tissue is more accurate than inspection. Although the hymen is relatively avascular, tearing at first coitus may be accompanied by a small amount of bleeding, which ceases rapidly. Childbirth causes

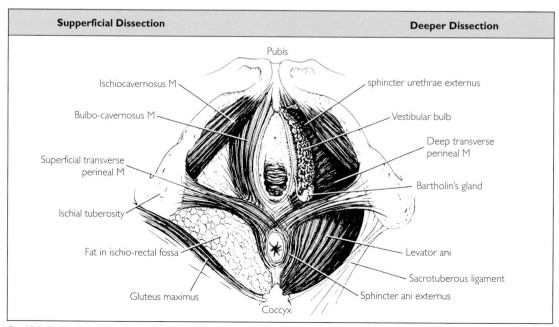

Fig 45.3 Dissection of the perineum to show the superficial muscles, the position of Bartholin's gland and the vesticular bulb.

Lymphatics

Lymphatic vessels form an interconnecting meshwork which extends through the labia minora,

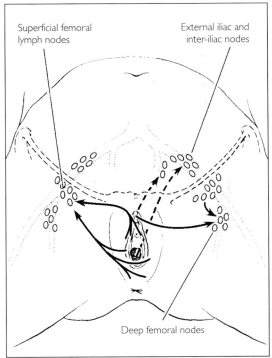

Fig 45.4 Schematic diagram showing the distribution of the lymphatics of the vulva. It shows that an extensive intercommunications exists between the lymphatics of each side.

the prepuce, the fourchette and the vaginal introitus. These vessels join to form 'trunks'. The anterior trunks join with a lymphatic meshwork over the mons (which also drains the glans of the clitoris). The anterior collecting trunks pass to reach the ipsilateral and contralateral superficial femoral nodes. The lymphatics form the labia majora also form trunks and pass to the superficial femoral nodes. There are connections between the superficial and the deep femoral nodes, which then connect with the nodes along the external iliac vessels.

The lymphatics from the clitoral shaft (which interconnect with those of the glans) pass directly to inter-iliac nodes in the pelvis *(Fig. 45.4)*. The lymphatics anastomose with those of the opposite side, and consequently bilateral or contralateral involvement is not uncommon in malignant tumours of the vulva. The vulval lymphatics also anastomose with the lymphatics of the lower third of the vagina, which drain into the external iliac nodes.

THE VAGINA

The vagina is a fibromuscular sheath, extending upwards and backwards from the vestibule, at an angle of about 85° to the horizontal, and parallel with the plane of the pelvic brim when the woman is erect *(Fig. 45.5)*. The walls of the vagina, as well as being muscular, contain a well-developed venous plexus. Normally the walls are in apposition, the vagina being a potential cavity, and having an H-

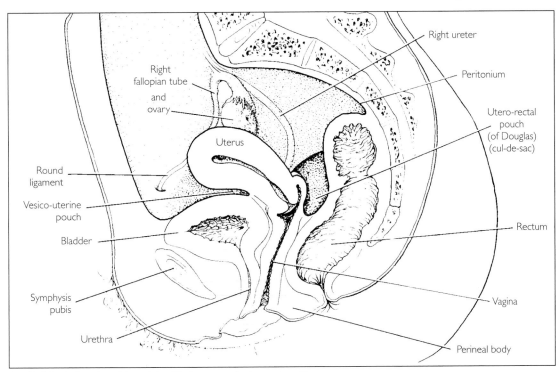

Fig 45.5 Sagittal section of the pelvis, with the woman in the erect position.

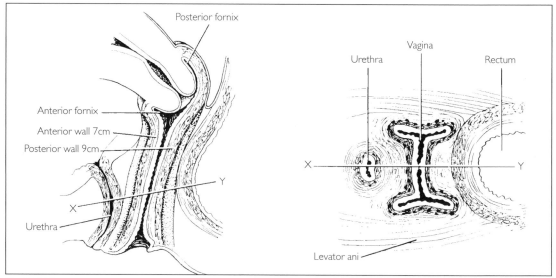

Fig 45.6 The vagina in cross-section. Note the greater length of the posterior wall and the 'H' shape on a cross-section. It can be seen that the vaginal walls are normally in apposition.

shape in cross-section in the middle third *(Fig 45.6)*. In the lower third, the widest diameter of the vagina is the anteroposterior diameter, but above this the widest diameter is the transverse diameter. Knowledge of this is of importance when introducing a vaginal bivalve speculum. Because of the well-developed walls, the lining epithelium tends to be lifted into ridges, or rugae, which run in a circumferential manner from two longitudinal columns running sagittally the length of the anterior and posterior vaginal walls. The formation of rugae in this

manner permits the great distension without damage of which the vagina is capable. The length of the anterior vaginal wall is 7cm, and its upper end is invaginated by the cervix. Because of this, the posterior vaginal wall, which ends blindly, is 2cm longer. The vaginal vault is divided into four areas, which are related to the projecting cervix. These are the shallow *anterior fornix*, the capacious *posterior fornix* and the shallow *lateral fornices*. Although the vagina varies considerably in length and width, its functional size is largely determined by the tone in its muscular wall

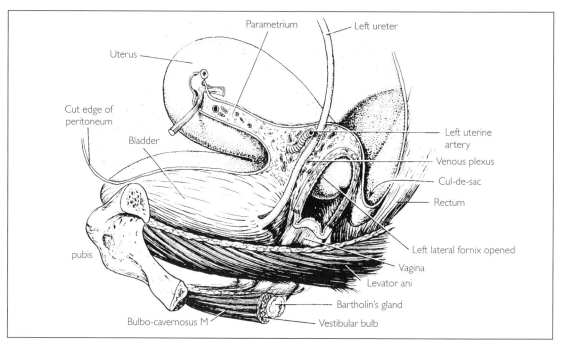

Fig 45.7 The relationship of the parametrium to the vagina and other pelvic organs.

and the contractions of the surrounding muscles. These are under voluntary control. Unless the vagina has been injured or shortened at operation, anatomical variations in size do not cause difficulty or pain (dyspareunia) during coitus; and most cases of dyspareunia are psychosomatic in origin.

The vagina is surrounded by several important structures. The anterior wall is in contact with the urethra, to which it is closely bound, and above this with the base of the bladder. Posteriorly the lower one-third is separated from the rectum by the complex of muscles and fascia which constitutes the perineal body, but above is in direct contact with the rectum. The upper one-quarter, including the posterior fornix, is covered by the peritoneum of the utero-rectal pouch (pouch of Douglas or cul-de-sac). The upper third of the lateral walls are in intimate contact with the pelvic connective tissue, and the fornices abut the parametrium which contains a rich venous plexus. Lying about 1cm above each lateral fornix are the uterine artery and the ureter *(Fig. 45.7)*. In the middle third, the lateral wall blends with the levator ani muscles, which together with the muscular vagina form one of the supports of the

uterus. In the lower third the walls are related to the bulbocavenosus muscle, the bulb of the vestibule and Bartholin's glands.

HISTOLOGY OF THE VAGINA

The vagina is lined with stratified, squamous, non-keratinized epithelium, some 10 to 30 cells deep, which rests upon a basement membrane and is continuous at the upper end with an identical epithelium covering the vaginal portion of the cervix. Should the epithelium be exposed to the dry external atmosphere, keratinization occurs. The cells are all derived by differentiation from the basal cells which lie upon the basement membrane. Three main cell types are described, (1) parabasal cells, (2) intermediate cells, and (3) superficial cells. The superficial cells, and some intermediate cells, contain glycogen. The entire epithelium shows cyclic changes during the menstrual cycle, and in pregnancy, and cellular development and differentiation is controlled by the ratio of circulating oestrogens, progesterone and androgens *(Fig. 45.8)*. The cells do not secrete mucus, but secretions seep between the cells to moisten the vagina, and the superficial cells are con-

	Vaginal				
	Oestrogen	Epithelium	Glycogen	pH	Flora
New born	+	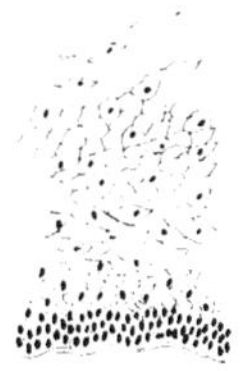		Acid 4–5	Sterile ↓ Doderlein's bacilli Secretion abundant
Month-old child	−	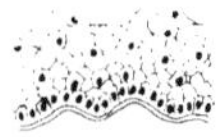	+	Alkaline >7	Sparse, coccal and varied flora. Secretion scant
Puberty	Appears	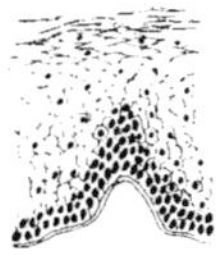	− ➡ +	Alkaline ↓ Acid	Sparse, coccal ↓ Rich bacillary
Mature	+ +	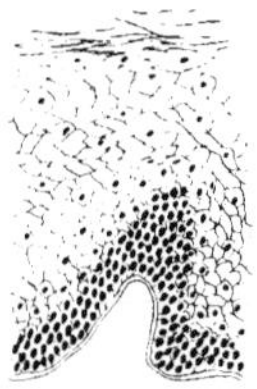	+	Acid 4–5	Doderlein's bacilli Secretion abundant
Post menopause	+ ➡ −	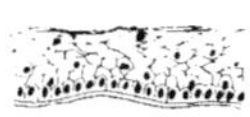	−	Neutral or alkaline 6– >7	Varied Dependant on level of circulating oestrogen Secretion scant

Fig 45.8 Cyclic changes in the vagina related to age.

stantly exfoliated. The exfoliated cells release the contained glycogen, which is acted upon by Döderlein's bacillus, a normal inhabitant of the vagina, to produce lactic acid. This causes the normal acidity of the vagina, and explains the relative resistance of the vagina to infection. The vaginal epithelial cells can also absorb drugs, particularly oestrogens.

The epithelium rests upon a connective tissue layer containing elastic tissue, nerves, lymphatics and blood vessels, and external to this are the thick layers of interdigitating muscle fibres, which cross in a spiral manner, the main direction being oblique rather than circular. Outside the muscle is a well-developed sheath of connective tissue, which is condensed anteriorly to form the so-called pubocervical (or vesicovaginal) fascia, and posteriorly to form the rectovaginal fascia. The condensed connective tissue fuses with, and is part of, the visceral layer of the pelvic fascia.

VASCULAR CONNECTIONS

The arterial blood supply is from the vaginal and uterine arteries, which are branches of the internal iliac artery, and which form a plexus around the organ. A median artery arises from this plexus on the anterior and on the posterior walls. The arteries are called azygous vaginal arteries *(Fig. 45.9)*. The venous drainage, which goes to the internal iliac veins, is from a rich venous plexus situated on the muscular wall of the vagina, which is especially well developed at the lower end of the vagina, and which communicates with the vesical, pudendal and haemorrhoidal venous plexuses.

The lymphatic drainage of the lower third of the vagina is to the inferior gluteal nodes, near the ischial spine. Lymphatics also link with those of the upper vagina. The lymphatic drainage from the upper two-thirds of the vagina passes to the internal iliac, the obturator and the sacral nodes.

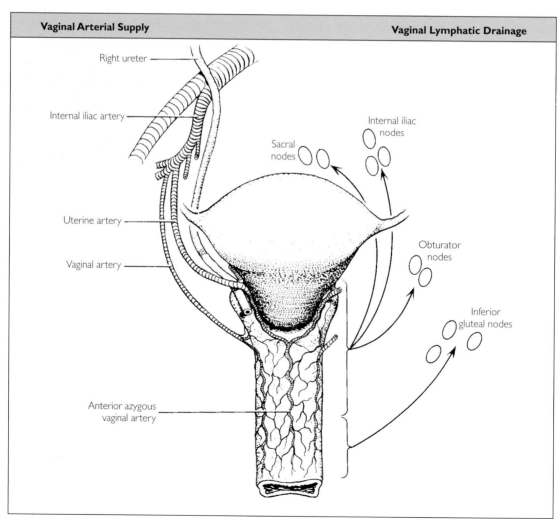

Vaginal Arterial Supply

Vaginal Lymphatic Drainage

Right ureter

Internal iliac artery

Uterine artery

Vaginal artery

Anterior azygous vaginal artery

Internal iliac nodes

Sacral nodes

Obturator nodes

Inferior gluteal nodes

Fig 45.9 The vaginal arterial blood supply and lymphatic drainage shown diagrammatically. Note that the uterus is angled forward at about 90° to the vagina, and appears foreshortened.

THE UTERUS

The uterus is a thick-walled, hollow, muscular organ, shaped like a pear, its apex forming the cervix which projects into the vaginal vault *(Fig. 45.10)*. It is located in the middle of the true pelvis, lying between the bladder and the rectum. It is flattened from before backwards, and its muscular anterior and posterior walls bulge into the cavity so that the walls are in apposition. Viewed from the front, the cavity has a triangular shape. It communicates with the peritoneal cavity via the Fallopian tubes (or oviducts) above, and with the exterior via the vaginal tube below. The uterus varies in size, being largest during the reproductive years and in women who have had children. The 'average' uterus of a nulliparous woman, measures 9cm in length, 6cm in width at its widest part, and 4cm from before backwards, and it weighs 40 to 60g. The wall is 1 to 2cm thick, and hence the length of the cavity measures 7cm. All these dimensions are increased by about 1.5cm in women who have borne children.

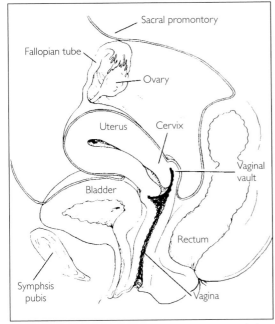

Fig 45.10 The uterus from the side showing the anatomical relations.

STRUCTURE

Externally the uterus is covered with peritoneum on the anterior and posterior aspects, and this forms the serosal layer. Deep to the serosal layer is the muscle layer, the myometrium, which is composed of three interdigitating layers of muscle. The outer, mainly longitudinal, layer and the inner, mainly circular, layer are poorly developed, and the bulk of the myometrium is formed from the middle layer, which is composed of obliquely interdigitating strands of muscle. Deep to the myometrium is the endometrium, which is a soft layer of variable thickness made up of tubular glands, which dip into a stroma of cells held in a fine meshwork of connective tissue. A well-developed vasculature is derived from the myometrial vessels.

The uterus is made up of a *body*, or *corpus*, and *isthmus* and a *cervix (Fig. 45.11)*. The body is further divided into the area which lies above the insertion

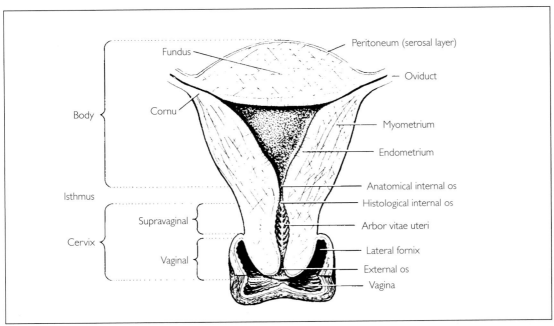

Fig 45.11 Coronal section of the uterus showing the cavity and the cornual areas.

of the oviducts, and is called the *fundus*. The area where the oviducts join the uterus on each side is termed the *cornu*. The body (including the fundus) comprises the greater portion of the organ, and is formed of thick bundles of muscle. The isthmus is a constricted, annular area, 0.5cm wide, which lies between the corpus and the cervix. The proportion of muscle begins to diminish in the isthmus, and connective tissue appears in increasing amounts. The constriction at the upper end of the isthmus is called the *anatomical internal os*, and the line at the lower end of the isthmus where the endometrium changes into columnar cervical epithelium is termed the *histological internal os*. On the surface of the uterus the anatomical internal os is marked by the reflection of the peritoneum which covers the uterus, onto the superior surface of the bladder.

The *cervix* is fusiform or cylindrical in shape, and measures 3cm from above downwards, half projecting into the vagina. The proportion of muscle tissue decreases rapidly in the cervix, and in its mid portion only 10 per cent of its bulk is made of muscle, the rest being connective tissue. The supra-vaginal portion of the cervix is surrounded by pelvic fascia, termed the parametrium, except posteriorly where it is covered with the peritoneum of the uterorectal pouch. The vaginal portion of the cervix is cone-shaped and projects into the vagina *(Fig. 45.7)*. It is covered with stratified squamous epithelium, which joins the columnar epithelium of the cervical canal at or near the external os. The cervical canal is spindle-shaped, and connects the cavity of the uterus to the vaginal cavity *(Fig 45.11)*. The mucous membrane lining the canal is thrown up into anterior and posterior folds, from which circular folds radiate to give

the appearance of a tree-trunk and branches. The folds are given the name *arbor vitae uteri*. The epithelium dips into the underlying stroma in a complicated system of clefts and crypts. The endocervical epithelium consists of columnar cells which secrete mucus, but the quality and quantity of this are under the control of the sex hormones.

RELATIONS

The uterus normally lies bent forward at an angle of 90° to the direction of the vagina, but is freely mobile, rotating about a fulcrum at the level of the supravaginal cervix. Anteriorly the uterus is separated from the bladder by the vesico-uterine pouch, and posteriorly is in contact with coils of bowel and the omentum. The anterior and posterior surfaces are covered with peritoneum, but its narrow lateral surfaces are in direct contact with the broad ligament and, below, with the connective tissue, venous plexuses, arteries, nerves and the ureter, which make up the substance of the parametrium. The peritoneum which covers the anterior and posterior walls, joins at the lateral margins of the uterus to form the two leaves of the *broad ligaments*; and these two sheets of peritoneum remain in close proximity, except where they contain the ascending uterine artery, and where they diverge to accommodate the round ligament (more accurately, the round muscle) and the infundibulopelvic ligament. The broad ligament extends from the lateral uterine border to the pelvic wall. Its upper border is formed by the peritoneum covering the oviduct, and below it merges anteriorly with the peritoneum of the pelvic floor and posteriorly with the peritoneum covering the recto-uterine shelf and the uterosacral ligaments *(Fig. 45.12)*.

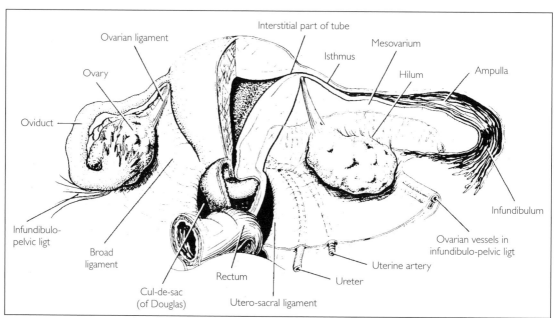

Fig 45.12 The female pelvic organs viewed from behind. On the left the oviduct and ovary are in the position found in vivo; on the right dissection has been made.

UTERINE SUPPORTS

These are discussed more fully in Chapter 40, but in summary are as follows: the uterus is supported from below by the muscular vagina and the fibres of the levator ani muscles vagina and the fibres of the levator ani muscles which interdigitate with the middle third of the muscular vaginal sheath. An additional support of great significance is the collection of connective tissue, muscular-walled blood vessels and areolar tissue, which forms a fan-shaped sheet on each side of the supravaginal cervix, and

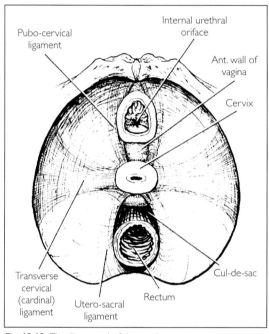

Fig 45.13 The 'ligaments' of the cervix.

stretches from the fascia lining the pelvic wall to join the fibromuscular cervix. This fan-shaped sheet is condensed posteriorly to form the *uterosacral ligaments*, and medially to form the *cardinal ligament*, or the *transverse cervical ligament (Fig. 45.13)*. Anteriorly the fascia sweeps forward down the anterior wall of the vagina beneath the bladder base. This condensation is called the pubocervical fascia. Laterally the broad ligament has a steadying effect on the uterus, whilst the round muscles play some part — although a minor one — in keeping the uterus in an anteverted position.

VASCULAR CONNECTIONS

The uterus is supplied by the uterine arteries which arise from the internal iliac artery. Each vessel runs forwards and inwards in the base of the broad ligament, and crosses the ureter above it and at right angles to it ('water *under* the bridge'), 1cm lateral to the supravaginal cervix. It gives off a descending branch which anastomoses with the ascending branches of of the vaginal artery, and which supplies the lower cervix; and a circular branch to supply the upper cervix. The main trunk changes direction and passes upwards, coiled and tortuous, between the layers of the broad ligament adjacent to the lateral uterine wall, and supplies branches to the myometrium at intervals. It ends by anastomosing with the ovarian artery *(Fig. 45.14)*. Each branch supplying the uterus divides in the outer muscular layer, to send anterior and posterior branches to the myemetrium, and to anastomose with those from the opposite side. These arteries give off branches at right angles, which penetrate and supply the myometrium, and, entering the endometrium, form the basal arteries.

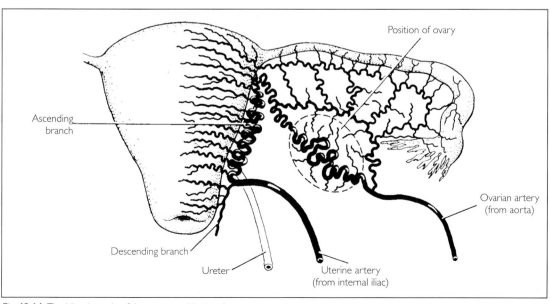

Fig 45.14 The blood supply of the uterus, oviduct and ovary.

The veins of the uterus accompany the uterine artery and form pampiniform plexuses of great complexity, particularly in the parametrium where they communicate with the veins of the bladder. The pampiniform plexus drains into the uterine vein and the ovarian vein, and has communications with the vertebral plexus of veins.

LYMPHATIC DRAINAGE

The lymphatic drainage of the uterus consists of three communicating networks: the deepest network lies in the endometrium, the second lies in the substance of the myometrium and the superficial network is subperitoneal. The networks form collecting trunks, which pass from the corpus between the layers of the broad ligament along with the ovarian lymphatics. They then pass through the infundibulopelvic fold, and ascend on the posterior abdominal wall to join the nodes of the para-aortic group. A few channels pass along the round muscle to the superficial femoral nodes. The lowest two trunks communicate with the collecting trunks from the cervix, which pass through the base of the broad ligament to an inconstant node lateral to the parametrial node, to the nodes along the internal iliac arteries (the internal iliac or hypogastric nodes), and

to the obturator nodes anteriorly. A few channels pass backwards along the uterosacral ligaments to the sacral nodes (Fig. 45.15).

THE OVIDUCT

The oviducts, or Fallopian tubes, are two small muscular tubes, one on each side, which extend for about 10cm from the uterine cornua towards the pelvic wall, forming the upper border of the broad ligaments. The outer half of each oviduct lies in contact with the ovary, curving over its superior surface to end in the abdominal ostium. Since the tube is hollow, a direct connection exists between the peritoneal cavity and the uterus. The mucous membrane lining of the tube is thrown up into folds which almost obliterate the lumen, and which are prolonged through the abdominal ostium to form the fimbriae of the tube. The oviduct can be divided into four parts. The *infundibulum* is the outermost portion of the tube. It includes the trumpet-shaped abdominal ostium, and lies in close proximity to the ovary. The *ampulla* is the longest segment of the oviduct, is normally rather tortuous, and has a relatively thin dilatable wall. The *isthmus* is a straight, narrow, relatively thick-walled segment, and the

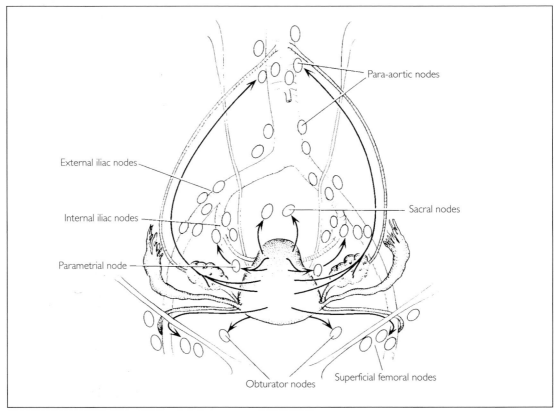

Fig 45.15 The lymphatic drainage of the female genital organs. For clarity, the lymphatic channels have been omitted and are indicated by arrows.

interstitial portion is the short, narrow portion within the uterine wall. The size of the lumen decreases from the infundibular to the interstitial portion, where it is only 1mm in diameter; whilst the complexity of the folds in the mucous membrane increases from the interstitial to the infundibular portions *(Fig. 45.16)*.

The mucous membrane is lined with epithelial cells, about half of which are mucus-secreting and half ciliated. The mucus secreted into the lumen is propelled towards the uterus by the action of the cilia and by peristaltic movements of the musculature of the tube. The mucus is rich in protein, and may provide nourishment for the fertilized ovum during its passage down the oviduct.

THE OVARY

The two ovaries are the homologues of the testes, and are ovoid-shaped organs. Each ovary normally lies in a shallow peritoneal fossa adjacent to the lateral pelvic wall, with its long axis in a vertical plane, but its position is influenced by movements of the uterus and broad ligament *(Fig. 45.17)*. The ovaries have an irregular surface, pinkish-grey in colour, and vary in size in different women, and at different times of the cycle. In the infant the ovary is a delicate, elongated structure, with a smooth, glistening surface. The ovary of a neonate contains little stroma and mainly consists of primordial follicles. As infancy and childhood progress increasing numbers of follicles degenerate, and there is a progressive

increase in stroma, up to puberty. During puberty the ovary enlarges, and in the reproductive period it averages 3.5cm in length, 2cm in breadth, 1cm in thickness, and weighs about 7g. Post-menopausally it undergoes rapid regressive changes, becoming wrinkled, white in colour and less than half the size it was in the reproductive era. Each ovary is attached to the posterior leaf of the broad ligament by a fold of peritoneum called the mesovarium, through which pass the ovarian vessels and nerves *(Fig. 45.12)*. The peritoneum stops where the mesovarium joins the ovary, and this part of the ovary is called the hilum. The remainder of the ovarian cortex is covered by a single layer of low columnar epithelium under which is a layer of connective tissue, called the tunica albuginea. This layer increases in density with increasing age.

VASCULAR CONNECTIONS OF OVARY AND OVIDUCT
The arterial, venous and lymphatic connections of both ovary and oviduct are similar, and the two organs are often referred to as the *adnexae* or uterine appendages.

The *arterial* supply is from the long, slender, ovarian artery, a branch of the abdominal aorta, which arises immediately below the renal artery and crosses the inferior vena cava, the ureter and the psoas muscle on the right side, and the left psoas muscle on the left side. The vessel crosses the external iliac artery at the pelvic brim, runs between the two layers of the infundibulopelvic fold and

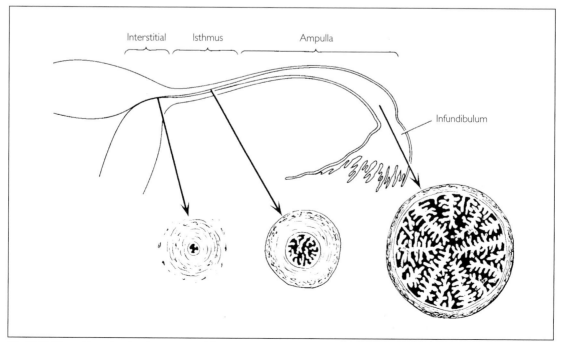

Fig 45.16 The oviduct, showing the structure of the mucosal layer.

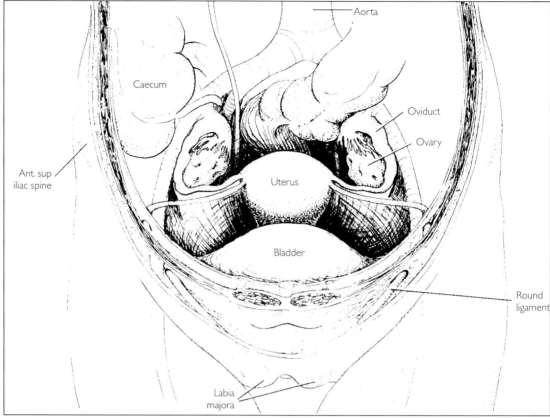

Fig 45.17 The position of the ovary, viewed from in front in the erect patient.

enters the broad ligament. Within the broad ligament it runs 0.5cm below the tube, and gives off branches to the ovary via the mesovarium, and to the oviduct between the layers of the broad ligament. It ends by joining the terminal branch of the uterine artery to form an arterial arcade. The *venous drainage* is into a pampiniform plexus, and then to the ovarian veins. The right ovarian vein joins the inferior vena cava, the left ovarian vein usually enters the left renal vein.

The *lymphatics* of each adnexa drain to the para-aortic nodes, and there is some evidence of communicating trunks to the contralateral ovary via the subperitoneal lymphatic plexus of the fundus of the uterus.

The *nerve supply* of the ovary is very well developed, and arises from a sympathetic plexus which surrounds the ovarian vessels in the infundibulopelvic ligament. Its fibres derive from branches of the aortic and renal plexuses. Sensory nerves follow the arteries and are relayed in the spinal cord at the level of the tenth thoracic segment. This well-developed nerve supply accounts for the extreme sensitivity of the ovary to squeezing.

ANATOMY OF THE URINARY TRACT

The urethral meatus lies in the anterior part of the vestibule, and the urethra runs upward and backward for 4cm to join the bladder base at an angle. It is intimately connected with the anterior vaginal wall, and a series of small crypts open into its posterior surface in the kowest third. These crypts are known as Skene's tubules and lie between the lateral urethral wall and the vagina. They are homologues of the male prostate, and may become the site of chronic infection.

The bladder is a muscular organ with a considerable capacity for distension. The base is relatively flat, lies parallel with the axis of the vagina, and contains the internal urinary meatus and the orifices of the ureters *(Fig. 45.18)*. The triangular area between these three openings constitutes the trigone. The dome, or fundus, of the bladder varies in shape and position depending upon the degree of distension. It is lined by transitional epithelium, and external to this is the muscular layer. The involuntary muscle which forms the bladder can be divided into two parts, that forming the fundus, which is

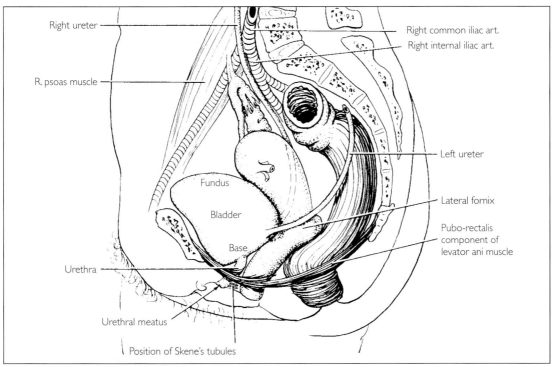

Fig 45.18 The relations of the urinary tract within the pelvis.

poorly supplied by autonomic nerves, and that forming the base (the detrusor muscle), which is richly supplied by autonomic nerves. The female urethra is a muscular tube, composed of two muscle layers. It is about 4cm long. The inner layer of muscle is longitudinal and is a direct continuation of the inner longitudinal layer of the detrusor muscle. It is embedded in dense collagen. The outer layer, which is a continuation of the outer layer of the detrusor muscle, is composed of semicircular fibres which never form a complete ring around the urethra. They loop around the urethra, at various degrees of obliquity, turning back to reach the bladder. Collectively they form a thick muscle layer, which encircles the urethra, to form a 'sphincter'.

Elastic tissue, collagen fibres and fascial attachments are intermingled with the involuntary semicircular fibres of the urethral muscle, and with the striated, voluntary fibres surrounding the mid-third of the urethra. This complex combination gives the urethra an 'inherent tone', or intra-urethral pressure, which is greatest at the mid-third of its length and which is important in maintaining urinary continence.

The voluntary muscle surrounding the mid-third of the urethra is part of the levator ani muscle (the puborectalis muscle), and its contraction cuts off micturition voluntarily. It also contracts to prevent urine leakage in response to the stress of coughing,

bearing down, sneezing or heavy lifting. It therefore acts as an external sphincter.

The external sphincter is under the control of the pudendal nerve; whilst the involuntary musculature is mainly under the autonomic control of the parasympathetic (cholinergic) nerves.

How does the urethra resist sudden increases in abdominal pressure? It is now known that as well as contraction of the voluntary external sphincter, the raised abdominal pressure is transmitted not only to the bladder but also to the proximal urethra, thus increasing the intra-urethral pressure as well as the intravesical pressure. This concept is important in understanding 'stress incontinence'.

The ureters pass from the renal pelves, behind the peritoneum, lying on the psoas muscle, to enter the true pelvis anterior to the sacro-iliac joint. They are separated from the joint by the ligaments of the joint, the psoas muscle and the common iliac vessels, and enter the pelvis in front of the common iliac artery at its bifurcation into the external and internal branches. Inside the true pelvis each ureter turns downward and runs on the medial side of the internal iliac artery. In the parametrium, as it courses forward to the bladder, it is crossed by the uterine artery, and lies 1cm lateral to the supravaginal cervix and 1cm above the lateral fornix. It passes obliquely through the bladder wall on the posterior aspect of its base, and the ureteric orifices mark the posterior

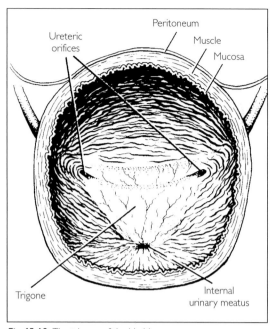

Fig 45.19 The trigone of the bladder.

points of thr trigone of the bladder *(Fig. 45.19)*. The ureter is lined with transitional epithelium, and the main coats of its wall consist of involuntary muscle which constantly moves as peristaltic waves pass along it. The obliquity with which the ureter enters the bladder acts as a valve preventing reflux of urine when the bladder is full.

INDEX

BIBLIOGRAPHY

Today with the availability of computer generated search programmes, I believe that students asked to explore a topic in greater depth are better served if they use these programmes, as references given in a textbook are often out of date. However, the list of books which follows, which are usually available in medical libraries may help students and interns access more information about a topic quickly.

GENERAL — Obstetrics

Chalmers, I., Enkin, M. & Keirse, M.J.N.C. *Effective Care in Pregnancy and Childbirth.* Oxford, Oxford University Press 1989 and subsequent data updated regularly and provided on disc, as the Oxford database of perinatal trials.

Cunningham, F.G. (Ed). Williams *Obstetrics.* 19th edn. New York. Appleton Lang 1993.

Enkin, M., Keirse, M.J.N.C. & Chalmers, I. A *Guide to Effective Care in Pregnancy and Childbirth.* Oxford, Oxford University Press 1989. This is a summarized version of the reference book.

De Swiet, M. & Chamberlain G. *Basic Science in Obstetrics and Gynaecology.* 2nd edn. Edinburgh: Churchill Livingstone. 1992.

GENERAL — Gynaecology.

Soutter, W.P., Shaw, R.W. & Stanton, S. (eds): *Gynaecology.* 1st edn. London: Longmans, 1992.

Woodruff, J.D. *Atlas of Gynaecological Pathology.* 1st edn. New York: Raven Press 1993.

Chapters 6 and 9

Hytten, H. & Chamberlain, G. *Clinical Physiology in Obstetrics.* 2nd edn. Oxford: Blackwell Scientific.

Chapter 10

Browning, P. *Pain Relief and Anaesthesia in Childbirth.* Melbourne, Ashwood Medical Library, 1994.

Chapter 16

Redman, C. & Walker, I. *Pre-eclampsia — the Facts.* 1st edn. Oxford: Oxford University Press, 1992.

Chapters 17, 18, 19

de Swiet, M. (ed). *Medical Disorders in Obstetric Practice.* 2nd edn. Oxford: Blackwell. 1989.

Chapter 28

Robertson, N.C.R. (ed). *Textbook of Neonatology.* 2nd edn. Edinburgh: Churchill Livingstone, 1992.

Chapter 30

Lewis, V.B. & Magos, A.L. *Endometrial Ablation.* 1st edn. Edinburgh: Churchill Livingstone, 1993.

Chapter 33

Drife, J.O. & Baird, D.T. (eds). *Contraception.* 1st edn. Edinburgh: Churchill Livingstone, 1993.

Filshie, M. & Guillebaud, J. (eds). *Contraception: Science and Practice.* 1st edn. London: Butterworths, 1989.

Chapter 34

Inster, V. & Lunenfeld, B. (eds). *Infertility: Male and Female.* 2nd edn. Edinburgh: Churchill Livingstone 1993.

Llewellyn–Jones, D. *Getting Pregnant.* 1st edn. New York. Bantam–Double Day. 1991.

Chapter 35

Berger, G.S. & Westrom, L.V. *Pelvic Inflammatory Disease.* 1st edn. New York: Raven Press 1992.

Chapter 39

Coppleston, M. (ed). *Gynaecology Oncology — Fundamental Principles and Practice.* 2nd edn. Edinburgh: Churchill Livingstone 1991

Chapter 41

Sutherst, J.R., Fraser, M.I., Richmond, R.S. & Haylen, B.R. *An Introduction to Gynaecological Urology.* 1st edn. London: Butterworths. 1991.

Chapter 42

Baum, M. *Breast Cancer — the Facts.* 2nd edn. Oxford: Oxford University Press, 1993.

Chapter 43

Carpenter, S.E. & Rock, J.A. *Pediatric and Adolescent Gynaecology.* 1st edn. New York: Raven, 1992.

Chapter 44

Burger, H.G. (ed). *Clinical Endocrinology and Metabolism.* London: Baillière Tindall, 1993.

Llewellyn–Jones, D. & Abraham, S. *Everywoman's Middle Years.* 1st edn. Melbourne: Ashwood Medical, 1992.

The use of misoprostol

Terminations after 16/40 for fetal anomalies

Induction. — DM and other indications.